Contrast Echocardiography in Clinical Practice

Springer-Verlag Berlin Heidelberg GmbH

José Luis Zamorano • Miguel Angel García Fernández

Contrast Echocardiography in Clinical Practice

Foreword by
Sanjiv Kaul

Springer

José Luis Zamorano
Director Echocardiographic Laboratory
Associate Professor of Medicine
University Clinic San Carlos
Plaza Cristo Rey
28040 Madrid, SPAIN

Miguel Angel García Fernández
Director Echocardiographic Laboratory
Associate Professor of Medicine
Department of Cardiology
Hospital General Universitario Gregorio Marañón
Calle Dr. Esquerdo 46
28007 Madrid, SPAIN

springeronline.com

Originally published by Springer-Verlag in 2004

ISBN 978-88-470-2174-7 ISBN 978-88-470-2125-9 (eBook)
DOI 10.1007/978-88-470-2125-9

Additional material to this book can be downloaded from http://extras.springer.com

 This textbook was funded in part by an educational grant from Bracco. Bracco, however, exercises no editorial comment, review, or any other type of control over the content of this textbook.

Editorial and production coordination: Springer Verlag, Milan
Typesetting: Graficando, Milan

SPIN: 10971079

Foreword

It gives me great pleasure to present the second publication by Springer-Verlag on contrast echocardiography in the last 3 years. The first one, *A Handbook of Contrast Echocardiography* by Peter Burns and Harald Becher, published in 2000, introduced many cardiologists and radiologists to the specialty of contrast echocardiography. This second publication, a multi-authored book entitled *Contrast Echocardiography in Clinical Practice*, will hopefully introduce more people to this exciting field.

José Luis Zamorano and Miguel Angel García Fernández have not only succeeded in bringing together coauthors from their own institutions but also in gathering contributions by specialists in the field from various centers worldwide. Because this field is changing so rapidly, a second book in just 3 years is both justified and welcome.

This book provides an update on the coronary circulation, types of microbubble contrast agents, the establishment of an echocardiography laboratory friendly to the use of contrast, and methods of quantification of contrast echo data, including simultaneous assessment of perfusion and function. It then discusses issues relating to left ventricular cavity opacification, assessment of coronary flow reserve, use in chronic coronary artery disease, assessment of myocardial viability, and stress perfusion imaging. Other topics include imaging of inflammation, acute myocardial infarction, and critically ill patients. The volume also covers the different approaches used in various laboratories and ends with a chapter on the therapeutic applications of microbubbles.

Being a multi-authored study, duplication of information is to be expected, as are different styles of presentation. Overall, the book provides an up-to-date review of important advances in contrast echocardiography, and newcomers to this field will find it very useful not only for understanding the basic concepts but also for finding relevant references. It will become apparent to most readers that this field requires an in-depth understanding of the interaction between ultrasound and microbubbles, acoustic physics and coronary physiology, which makes it both more complex and more exciting at the same time.

Because of the ongoing rapid technological advances in this field, coupled with an anticipation of the more widespread use of a contrast agent after it has been approved for myocardial opacification, another new volume or an addition to this book may yet be required in the next 3 years. In the meanwhile, the present volume serves an important purpose and I recommend it to all our colleagues interested in this field.

Charlottesville, October 2003 **Sanjiv Kaul, MD**

Acknowledgements

After nurturing the idea of doing a book on contrast echocardiography for a number of years, we are pleased to present *Contrast Echocardiography in Clinical Practice*. This textbook will be useful for individuals starting out in this new area of echocardiography and for those with previous experience who would like to explore this subject further. We believe that proper instruction is crucial before starting contrast echocardiography, and thus the present volume aims to serve as an educational tool in this field.

This book could not have become a reality without the efforts of its contributors on both sides of the Atlantic, all of them very well known in the contrast echo field. Their time, ideas and comments, as well as their enthusiasm during the preparation of the book are highly appreciated. In addition, we would like to acknowledge the valuable contribution of all the physicians and nurses in our echocardiography laboratories, who have worked hard in research and clinical studies in the contrast field. Their ideas and suggestions for this textbook are appreciated.

We would like to express our gratitude to Dr. Sanjiv Kaul, one of the pioneers in contrast echocardiography whose authoritative papers on contrast have been instructive for us all. Many of his first concepts and research work in contrast echocardiography are summarized here, and it is an honor to have his foreword in our book.

We gratefully acknowledge the staff of Springer-Verlag, especially Antonella Cerri who organized production of the book. It has been a real pleasure to work with her.

On a personal note, we would like to thank our wives, Charo and Margarita, and our children, Rocio and Miguel, Pepe, Jorge and Margarita, who always provided their support and understanding.

Finally, this book would not have been possible without the support of Bracco, in particular Fabio Pitzoi and Stefano Nervetti, who were involved in this project.

We hope that you will find this textbook of interest and that it will help you in your research and daily work.

José Luis Zamorano
Director Echocardiographic Laboratory
University Clinic San Carlos, Madrid

Miguel Angel García Fernández
Director Echocardiographic Laboratory
Hospital Gregorio Marañón, Madrid

Table of Contents

Contributors

LUCIANO AGATI
Echocardiography Laboratory
Department of Cardiology
"La Sapienza" University of Rome
Policlinico Umberto I
Via del Policlinico 155
00161 Roma, ITALY

JOSÉ AZEVEDO
Echocardiography Laboratory
S. Francisco Xavier Hospital
Estrada Forte do Alto do Duque
21449-005 Lisbon, PORTUGAL

HARALD BECHER
John Radcliff Hospital
Cardiac Investigation Annexe
Headington, Headley Way
Oxford OX3 9DU, UK

MANUEL DESCO
Laboratorio de Imagen Médica
Medicina y Cirugía Experimental
Hospital GU Gregorio Marañón
Calle Dr. Esquerdo 46
28007 Madrid, SPAIN

WILLIAM A.A. FOSTER
Cardiovascular Division
University of Virginia Health System
Charlottesville, Virginia 22908, USA

MARIO JORGE GARCÍA
Cleveland Clinic Foundation
9500 Euclid Avenue
Cleveland, OH 44195, USA

BIJOY K. KHANDHERIA
Mayo Clinic
200 First Street SW
Rochester, MN, USA

ROBERTO M. LANG
Noninvasive Cardiac Imaging Laboratories
Department of Medicine
University of Chicago
5841 S. Maryland Ave.
Chicago, IL 60637, USA

MARÍA J. LEDESMA-CARBAYO
ETSI Telecomunicación
Universidad Politécnica de Madrid
28040 Madrid, SPAIN

JONATHAN R. LINDNER
Cardiovascular Division
University of Virginia Health System
Charlottesville, Virginia 22908, USA

TERESA LÓPEZ FERNÁNDEZ
Laboratory of Echocardiography
Department of Cardiology
Hospital GU Gregorio Marañón
Calle Dr. Esquerdo 46
28007 Madrid, SPAIN

NORBERTO MALPICA
ETSI Telecomunicación
Universidad Politécnica de Madrid
28040 Madrid, SPAIN

PEDRO MARCOS-ALBERCA
Laboratorio de Ecocardiografia
Servicio de Cardiologia
Fundación Jimenéz Diaz
Avenida Reyes Católicos n°2
28040 Madrid, SPAIN

MARK J. MONAGHAN
Department of Cardiology
King's College Hospital
London, UK

VICTOR MOR-AVI
Noninvasive Cardiac Imaging Laboratories
Department of Medicine
University of Chicago
5841 S. Maryland Ave.
Chicago, IL 60637, USA

LUIS MOURA
Hospital Pedro Hispano
Rua Pedro Hispano 240
4100-393 Oporto, PORTUGAL

GIANNI PEDRIZZETTI
Dept. Civil Engineering
University of Trieste
P.le Europa 1
34127 Trieste, ITALY

ESTHER PÉREZ DAVID
Laboratory of Echocardiography
Department of Cardiology
Hospital GU Gregorio Marañón
Calle Dr. Esquerdo 46
28007 Madrid, SPAIN

LEOPOLDO PÉREZ DE ISLA
Laboratory of Echocardiography
University Clinic San Carlos
Plaza Cristo Rey
28040 Madrid, SPAIN

ROSA RÁBAGO
Laboratorio de Ecocardiografia
Servicio de Cardiologia
Fundación Jimenéz Diaz
Avenida Reyes Católicos n°2
28040 Madrid, SPAIN

MANUEL REY PÉREZ
Laboratorio de Ecocardiografia
Servicio de Cardiologia
Fundación Jimenéz Diaz
Avenida Reyes Católicos n°2
28040 Madrid, SPAIN

ANDRÉS SANTOS
ETSI Telecomunicación
Universidad Politécnica de Madrid
E-28040 Madrid, SPAIN

PARTHO SENGUPTA
Mayo Clinic
200 First Street SW
Rochester, MN, USA

ROXY SENIOR
Northwick Park Hospital
Watford Road
Harrow, HA1 3UJ, UK

VIVIANA SERRA
Laboratory of Echocardiography
University Clinic San Carlos
Plaza Cristo Rey
28040 Madrid, SPAIN

HELENE THIBAULT
John Radcliff Hospital
Cardiac Investigation Annexe
Headington, Headley Way
Oxford OX3 9DU, UK

JONATHAN TIMPERLEY
John Radcliff Hospital
Cardiac Investigation Annexe
Headington, Headley Way
Oxford OX3 9DU, UK

GIANNI TONTI
Echocardiography Laboratory
Division of Cardiology
S. Annunziata Hospital
Circonvallazione Occidentale 145
67039 Sulmona, ITALY

R. PARKER WARD
Noninvasive Cardiac Imaging Laboratories
Department of Medicine
University of Chicago
5841 S. Maryland Ave.
Chicago, IL 60637, USA

MAR MORENO YANGÜELA
Laboratory of Echocardiography
Department of Cardiology
Hospital GU Gregorio Marañón
Calle Dr. Esquerdo 46
28007 Madrid, SPAIN

Chapter 1
The Physiological Basis of Coronary Circulation

Pedro Marcos-Alberca • Manuel Rey Pérez • Rosa Rábago
José Luis Zamorano • Miguel Angel García Fernández

The high prevalence of cardiovascular diseases in developed countries, particularly coronary heart disease, has resulted in an increasing interest in the physiological basis of the circulatory system and coronary flow [1-4]. The study of the physiology helps us understand cardiovascular pathologic disorders and their clinical manifestations better. But it also allows us to learn about some aspects of the diagnostic tools applied in cardiovascular disease, since most of them aim to disclose abnormalities in coronary flow. These techniques use some type of tracer, a substance that travels through the coronary circulation and interacts with the cells of the vascular wall and the myocytes, reflecting the state, normal or abnormal, of the blood flow. This is the case of isotopic diagnostic techniques (SPECT, PET), the most recent technologies of cardiac magnetic resonance imaging or myocardial contrast-enhanced echocardiography – the topic of this book [5-7].

This chapter reviews the principal features involved in the regulation of coronary circulation. The anatomy of the coronary circulation, the regional nature of myocardial perfusion, the general basis of the regional regulation of the blood flow are important topics discussed. In addition, the specific landmarks involved in the control of regional myocardial blood flow, such as the metabolic demand, the role of the extravascular compressive forces, the characteristics of transmural myocardial perfusion, coronary autoregulation or the complex relationship between flow and contractile function, are described below.

Coronary Anatomy and the Regional Nature of Myocardial Perfusion

The coronary circulatory system includes the great epicardial vessels, the small vessels that are not imaged with angiography, the capillaries and the veins [8]. The epicardial vessels comprise the left and the right coronary arteries and their principal branches. Coronary arteries normally emerge from the ostia located at the corresponding left and right aortic sinus of Valsalva. In 50% of the population, there is a third ostia where the conus artery arises. In the rest, this vessel is the first branch of the right coronary artery (RCA).

The left coronary artery (LCA) runs a variable distance of some millimeters before subdividing into the left anterior descending (LAD) and left circumflex (LC) arteries. The size of the principal branches of the LCA decreases as they travel over the cardiac surface. The size of the RCA, loss of major bifurcation, remains constant until it arrives at the posterior area of the heart, the so-called *crux*, where the right posterior descendent artery (RPD) arises. The LCA and RCA run embedded in the epicardial fat and are located at the *A-V sulcus*.

The LAD arteries pass along the *interventricular sulcus*. From its origin, the most important branches are the anterior septal and diagonal arteries. The Anterior septal arteries, also called anterior perforator arteries, penetrate into the *interventricular septum*. Diagonal arteries runs over the anterolateral surface of the left ventricle.

The Circumflex artery goes into the *A-V sulcus* and along its way bifurcates into several marginal arteries, variable in number and of important size. These branches of the LC arteries perfuse the lateral and posterior region of the left ventricle. In 50% of the population, the LC is the origin of the sinus node artery and in 10%–15% the RPD arises from it, a condition called *left dominance.*

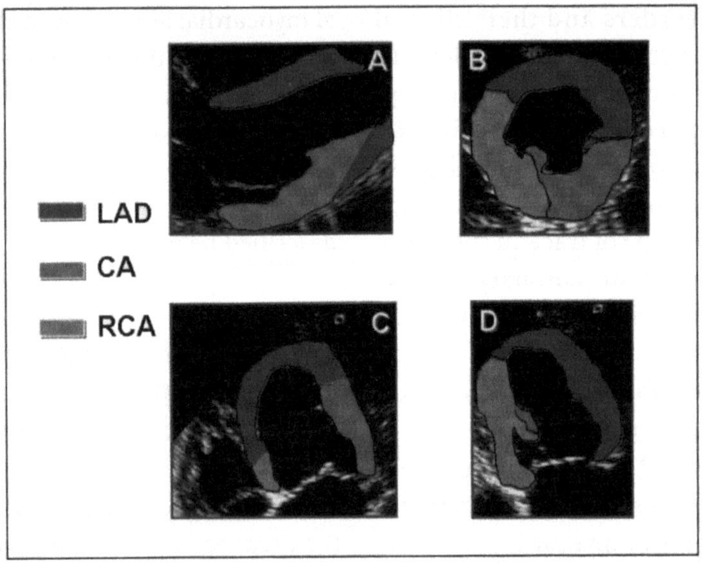

Fig. 1.1. Regional distribution of coronary flow. Echocardiographic views in parasternal long axis (**A**), parasternal short axis (**B**), apical four-chambers (**C**) and apical two-chambers (**D**). The areas of myocardium have been highlighted with the color corresponding to the major epicardial coronary artery responsible for their perfusion. *LAD*, left anterior descending coronary artery; *CA*, circumflex coronary artery; *RCA*, right coronary artery

The first branches of the RCA are, in 50% of the population, the conus artery and the sinus node artery. In the middle segment, the marginal artery emerges, irrigating the right ventricle. Nonetheless, the most important bifurcation appears at the *crux of the heart*. In this location, the RCA subdivides into the RPD and right posterolateral arteries toward the left ventricle. This is the most common anatomic distribution and is called *right dominance*.

The goal of treatment in acute coronary syndromes is to obtain a fast, complete and sustained opening of the totally or near occluded artery. Hence, terms such as "myocardial infarction-related artery" or "myocardial risk area" are very common. These terms point out the existence of a relationship between the implied coronary arteries and the myocardial area perfused by them. There is general agreement about the regional distribution of the coronary flow, that is, between the epicardial coronary arteries and the area of the myocardium irrigated [9-13]. The scheme in Fig. 1.1 is valid for the majority of the population, although with some variation with regard to several factors such as anatomic variations in a particular case or collateral vessels that could influence the final distribution of the regional flow.

Control of the Regional Flow: Physiological Basis

Blood flow is a term that expresses the relationship between volume and time. The hydraulic equivalent of Ohm's law links the flow with the pressure drop and the resistance as follows. Blood flow will be determined by the arterial pressure minus the venous pressure (normally depreciated, being near zero), called perfusion pressure, and the vascular resistance [1, 3, 14, 15]. Active resistance is secondary to the intrinsic properties of the vessel and opposite to passive resistance caused by other elements, e.g., the myocardium. This, the blood volume, adjusted to myocardial mass (ml/g) in a discrete time t depends on the perfusion pressure and the vascular resistance.

In hydrodynamics, resistance is the loss of energy of a volume V as it passes through the system. For continuous flow, resistance is expressed as the decrease in the perfusion pressure between two points adjusted to volume and time. In physiology, the flow is pulsatile, and the more appropriate term is *impedance,* which takes into account the rate of the driving force. Nonetheless, the relationship between flow, perfusion pressure and resistance are very complex. Pressure and flow relation is non linear and the resistance is also affected by the value of both the pressure and the flow. Pressure drops (loss of energy) across a stenosis are caused by viscous losses due to the friction and by the abrupt expansion and resulting separation and turbulence of the flow stream as it emerges from the stenosis. The magnitude of these losses will depend on the pressure, the length of the lesion or distance between the points of pressure drops, and the diameter of the vessel. Complex interactions within the stenosis and poststenotic vessel lumen occur as flow changes, introducing several other effects of variable magnitude. As a result, a simple estimation of the resistance is a great problem in hydrodynamics [16-18].

The association between all these factors has been profusely studied in fundamental physics and applied in physiology. This association, considering an ideal condition of a rigid tube and a constant and laminar flow, is defined by the equation of *Poiseuille*.

$$Flow=\frac{\pi(P_1-P_2)xR^4}{8xLxViscosity}$$

Flow is directly proportional to the pressure drop between points A and B and the fourth exponent of the radius of the tube, and inversely related with 8 times the distance between these points and the viscosity of the fluid. The relationship in this equation seems very simple and intuitive, but it cannot be strictly employed in the circulatory system. Why? Because the flow is not constant but pulsatile and it is not always laminar, and the vessels are neither rigid nor straight. Furthermore, the blood in the circulatory system adopts a distribution that makes it even more complex than a simple viscous substance. Nonetheless, the equation of *Poiseuille* provides an important fact: the weight of the vessel diameter, since the radius is elevated to the fourth power, influences to a large extent the final amount of flow [19].

There are other factors that differentiate physiology from fluid physics. The viscosity of the blood depends on the hematocrit, the body temperature, or the serum proteins. In addition, the vascular system is not a serial system but a parallel one, adding a new factor of complexity. Parallel disposition makes final resistance greater than the total individual resistance. In addition, recent studies using advanced techniques with stroboscopic illumination have suggested that resistance is controlled in different segments of the circulation, in different amounts in each of them. The consequence is that vascular resistance can be altered in a non uniform manner by a variety of physiological (autoregulation, oxygen consumption) and pharmacological stimuli (norepinephrine, adenosine, nitric oxide) [20, 21].

Perfusion pressure and flow are not related in a linear way, as is in the case of a rigid tube. The configuration of this relationship in experimental conditions is shown in Fig. 1.2. The curve discloses a complex interaction between these factors at the regional level.

Blood vessels are structures with elastic properties and distension capabilities. When pressure increases, it exerts a force against the wall of the vessel, resulting in an increase in the transmural pressure. Thus, the vessel, through stretch-mediated signals, distends and the diameter grows. The increase of the pressure results in an increase of the flow until the point of maximal dilation. At this point, the relationship reaches a steady state. Therefore, in a range of pressures from 50 mmHg to 200 mmHg, flow is constant. Mechanisms that maintain the constancy of blood flow for any previous increase or decrease (denoted in Fig. 1.2 by the dotted spikes) are termed autoregulation of regional flow. Autoregulation is an intrinsic property of some organs and systems and is par-

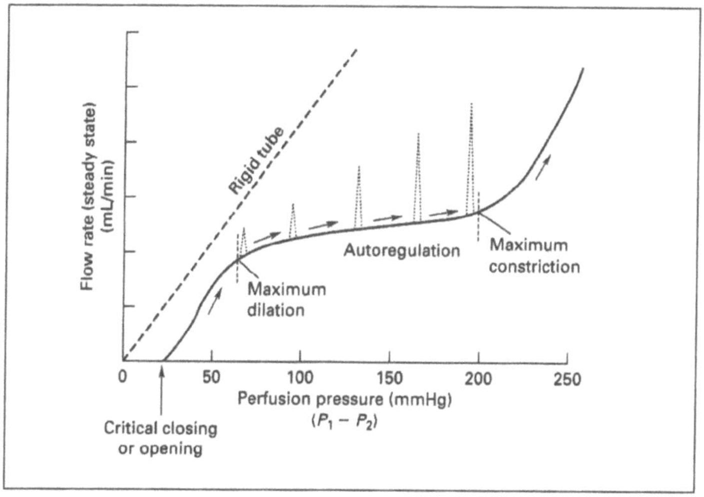

Fig. 1.2. Perfusion pressure and flow relationship in experimental conditions. *Dashed line* represents the ideal condition of a rigid tube and *continuous line* the relationship obtained in a vascular bed perfused with flow. *Dotted spikes* represent quick increases in blood flow with subsequent decline secondary to the vasomotor control returning the amount of flow to normal levels. Autoregulation can be maintained between limits of perfusion pressures corresponding to maximal constriction and dilation of the vessel (Reproduced from [14])

ticularly developed in coronary and cerebral vascular beds [3, 22, 23].

The inferior limit of pressure where coronary flow begins to decrease is 50 mmHg or less, which determines a hypoperfusion state. Below this value or *critical flow pressure*, coronary flow is close to zero, although it does not stop because the principal back force is sinus coronary pressure [20].

Autoregulation is a fundamental property of the cardiovascular system in general and the coronary vascular bed in particular. But, how can the vascular bed keep the flow constant against changes in perfusion pressure? Through the control and modification of the dilation of the vessels and the lumen size. There are several factors influencing the degree of distension and therefore the pressure/flow relationship.

1. The difference between intraluminal and extraluminal pressure or transmural distension pressure. Extraluminal pressure is partly the result of the intrinsic properties of the vascular wall, as cellular and interstitial composition, both determinants of their elastic properties; and partly the result of extrinsic factors, which in the case of the heart are the structure and properties of the myocytes and extracellular matrix as well as the sarcomeric contraction in systole.
2. The vascular compliance or vascular tone. Compliance is the result of the stiffness of the vascular wall and will determine the capability of the vessel to adapt its diameter to any increase in the intraluminal pressure. Vascular tone is a quality of the vascular bed supplied by the

contraction of the muscular layer of the vascular wall, with a fine molecular control; vascular tone is basic for the autoregulation of regional flow.

Transmural pressure and vascular tone are closely related. *Laplace's law* establishes the relationships between these factors. Wall tension, whose natural action is to distend the wall and increase the lumen size, is directly related to the transmural pressure and the vessel radius, but inversely related to the vessel thickness. Radius and thickness are determined by the composition of important elements, such as the cellular and interstitial content and vascular or myogenic tone [24-26].

The magnitude of autoregulation in a normal vessel is greater than in an atherosclerotic vessel, where there is a pronounced cellular proliferation and extracellular remodeling. Affected vessels show a decrease in radius and an increase in thickness, with a marked increase of the myogenic tone due to the loss of fine molecular control. All these factors make this vascular segment unable to modify its diameter in the presence of changes in intraluminal pressure, since the wall tension that can dilate it is minimal [27-33].

Control of Vascular Tone: Vasomotion

Vasomotion is regulated by a combination of physical and chemical properties of the endothelium and the smooth muscle fiber that control the stiffness and distensibility of the vessel.

Vascular tone promotes changes in the lumen size through several mechanisms:

1. Metabolites, hormones and chemical mediators carried in the blood or locally synthesized (Table 1.1), nitric oxide (NO), endothelin-1, adenosine being of

Table 1.1. Principal mediators implied in the control of vascular tone

Name	Action	Nature	Production or storage
Nitric oxide	Dilates	Gas	Endothelium
Hyperpolarizing factor	Dilates	Arachidonic acid metabolite	Endothelium
Prostacyclin	Dilates	Arachidonic acid metabolite	Endothelium
Endothelin-1	Constricts	Peptide (21 amino-acids)	Endothelium
Dopamine	Constricts (α1-receptors)	Catecholamine	Sympathetic nervous fibers
	Dilates (β1-β2 receptors)		
Acetylcholine	Dilates (NO pathway)	Choline derived	Parasympathetic nervous fibers
Angiotensin II	Constricts	Peptide (8 amino-acids)	Endothelium
Thromboxane A_2	Constricts	Arachidonic acid metabolite	Endothelium

major significance as well as others such as sprostaglandin, prostacyclin or thromboxane [35-38].
2. Wall strectch, through mechanisms of signaling in the smooth muscle cell [40].
3. Shear stress, at the endothelium, through flow-mediated vasodilation [41].
4. Nervous control, both sympathetic and parasympathetic fibers, releasing catecholamines and acetylcholine. Sympathetic control acts through the activation of specific α-receptors constricting arteries bigger than 150 mm but dilating vessels smaller than 100 mm. Cholinergic receptors produce modest but relatively uniform dilation of coronary microvessels, across all size classes. Evidence suggests that the action of acetylcholine is primarily endothelial dependent [42, 43].
5. Hypoxia and hypercapnia [44].

The endothelium plays a major role in the regional control of flow. The control of vascular tone by the endothelium depends on the equilibrium between vasodilators and vasoconstrictors.

The most important regulatory substance of vascular tone is a gas: nitric oxide (NO). NO is produced in the endothelium as a result of the metabolism of L-arginine to L-citruline, a reaction catalyzed by the enzyme NO-synthase. NO spreads quickly from the endothelium to the immediate inferior muscular layer. In the smooth muscle cell, NO stimulates the synthesis of GMPc, which removes calcium from the cytoplasm relaxing the cell and ultimately the vascular wall. Many substances exercise vasodilation using the NO-pathway: P-substance, bradykinin or serotonin. More importantly the endothelial cell has mechanisms able to sense the shear stress secondary to the increase of the blood flow, triggering NO synthesis and dilating the vessel. This mechanisms is called *endothelial flow-mediated vasodilation* and is primordial in the control of the coronary flow [35-37].

Vasoconstrictors act, in general, by promoting the entrance of calcium into the cytoplasm of the smooth muscle cell. The most powerful mediator is endothelin-1 [21, 38, 41].

Coronary Circulation

Coronary circulation is able to supply O_2 to the heart under a wide range of conditions and to increase the coronary flow by five to six times its value at rest. Coronary flow reserve or vascular reserve is the ability of the coronary vascular bed to provide additional O_2 to the myocardium when metabolic demand increases, increasing coronary flow through its own dilation. The provision of O_2 to the heart at rest has been calculated to range from 70 to 90 ml/100g/min. its consumption under the same conditions being from 8 to 10 ml/100g/min. The heart has an aerobic metabolism, thus the tissue extraction of O_2 is very high and the debt of O_2 very low, even at rest. In a steady state, the consumption of O_2 closely expresses its total metabolism. When metabolic demand increases, it is difficult for the myocardium to increase the tissue extraction. A higher supply of O_2 to the myocardium will only be possible through a parallel increase of coronary flow, that is, of the blood volume in the tissue per second. This strong relationship between metabolic demand and coronary flow is linked with several physicals and chemical mechanisms to control the amount of instantaneous coronary flow [3, 23, 34].

Determinants of MVO_2: Wall Tension, Contractility and Heart Rate

The consumption of O_2 in the non-beating heart is 1.5 ml/100g/min. This is the minimal amount that the heart needs to assess the maintenance of the physiologic process different to pure contraction–relaxation activity. Nonetheless, the consumption at rest ranges from 8 to 10 ml. That is, the major part of O_2 consumed is employed in contraction–relaxation activity. Determinants of O_2 consumption are listed in Table 1.2. The three most important factors are those at the top of the list (major determinants) [45].

The relationship between myocardial tension and MVO_2 is expressed, in a simple way, using *Laplace's law*; that is, tension increases proportionally to intraventricular pressure and the radius of the ventricular cavity. But this relationship is more complex. Indeed, the MVO_2 is closely related with myocardial tension, and this is the result of the pressure/volume interaction and the influence of other factors that affect pressure/volume relationship. Hence, the contractility (inotropism) changes this relationship switching the curve to the left (increase in contractility) or the right (decrease in contractility), and heart rate (chronotropism) increases or decreases the total generation of myocardial tension [46-48].

Table 1.2. Determinants of myocardial O_2 consumption

Major determinants
Wall tension (myocardium)
Contractility
Hear rate
Minor determinants
Afterload
Despolarization
Catecholamines
Fatty acid absorption

As a result, the heart consumes O_2 for the following reasons:

1. To generate a pressure work
2. To generate a volume work
3. To assure that pressure and volume works will be in a range that permits correctyl supply to organs and systems

This concept is well expressed by the close relationship between MVO_2 and the total area under the curve of pressure/volume or PVA (Fig. 1.3). Total area is equal to the sum of the O_2 consumption employed to generate pressure and volume works and the consumption to maintain the correct pressure/volume relationship and is represented by the maximal end-systolic pressure–volume line, called *end-systolic elastic potential energy of the ventricular wall*. The results indicate that PVA is a reliable and valuable predictor of myocardial oxygen consumption under different contractile states in human hearts [48, 49].

The alteration of the load conditions or the administration of positive inotropic agents, such as calcium, epinephrine or dobutamine, increase the consumption of

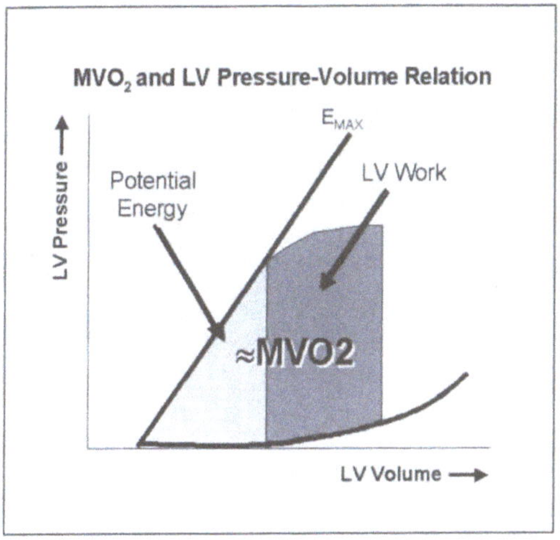

Fig. 1.3. Relationship between metabolic demand (*MVO*$_2$) and the total area under the pressure/volume curve of the left ventricle (*LV*). The total area is equal to the sum of the O_2 consumption employed to generate a work of pressure and volume and the consumption to maintain the correct pressure/volume relationship represented by the maximal end-systolic pressure–volume line, called end-systolic elastic potential energy of the ventricular wall (E_{MAX}) (Modified from [49, 50])

O_2 (Fig. 1.4). This is not the result of a direct action of these agents over the metabolism, but the action over exciting–contracting coupling mechanisms. The consumption of energy increases because contraction needs the mobilization of calcium toward the cytoplasm and the opposite for relaxation. Ionic interchangers coupled to enzymes that hydrolyze ATP perform this process generating an energetic debt. The changes in the inotropic state directly influence the pressure–volume relationship, switching to the left the regression line that reflects the end-systolic pressure–volume relationship [48].

As in any vascular bed, control of the coronary flow occurs on three levels:

1. Metabolic
2. Endothelial, whose importance has been mentioned above
3. Neuronal, through the sympathetic and parasympathetic neurotransmitters

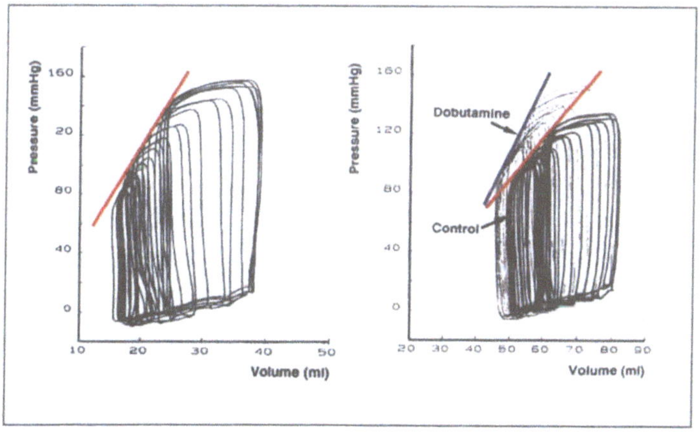

Fig. 1.4. Pressure–volume loops under different load conditions (*left*) and increasing contractility using dobutamine (*right*). Color lines represent the end-systolic pressure/volume relationship, reflecting the left ventricular performance. The total area under the pressure/volume relationship curve correlates closely with myocardial O_2 consumption, whose value modifies with the variations in the load conditions or in the contractile state (Reproduced from [57])

In the coronary vascular bed, metabolic control plays a major role. Coronary flow is closely related with O_2 consumption due to the aerobic condition of the heart, the low O_2 debt of the cardiac tissue, and its limited ability for energetic storage. Changes in O_2 consumption lead to changes in the coronary flow in a brief time interval. The most important mechanism that relates metabolism and flow is the adenosine-mediated pathway (Fig. 1.5). Adenosine is the final product of the metabolism of ATP used in all aerobic processes, in the heart mostly as a result of myocardial shortening. Adenosine acts directly on the smooth muscle cell through specific receptors dilating the vessel, without mediation of the endothelium. After the transitory total ligature of a coronary artery, the local production of adenosine is responsible for a 30% increase in the lumen

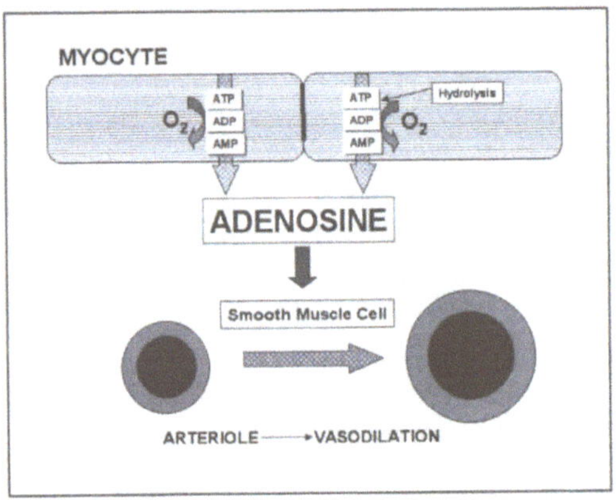

Fig. 1.5. Metabolic control of the coronary flow. Adenosine is locally produced by the myocyte as the final product result of the hydrolysis of ATP. ATP is necessary for all aerobic processes, but in the heart mostly for myocardial shortening through myosin-actin interactions. Adenosin exerts its action directly on the smooth muscle cell from the vascular wall, without mediation of the endothelium

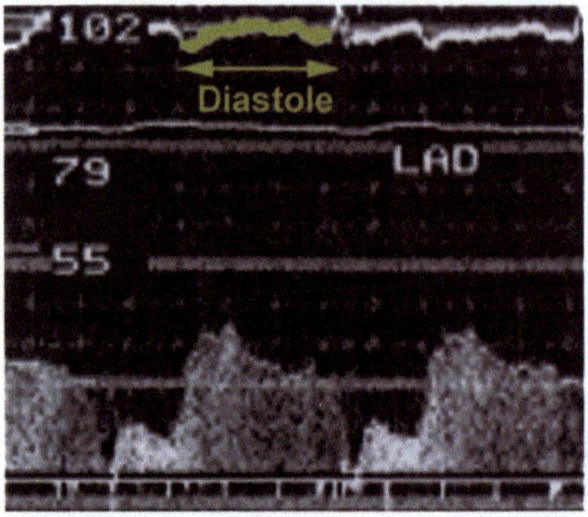

Fig. 1.6. Intracoronary Doppler registry obtained from the left anterior descending coronary artery (*LAD*) in a normal patient showing the predominant diastolic character of myocardial flow (Courtesy of Felipe Navarro, MD. Fundación Jiménez Díaz)

size, leading to reactive hyperemia [39, 50].

Coronary flow has a biphasic pattern (Fig. 1.6). The wall tension developed in systole compresses the intramyocardial vessels, there by closing them. Thus, most of the myocardial flow accounts for diastole. Extravascular compressive forces have two components:

1. Intraventricular pressure, which determines the establishment of a transmural pressure gradient from the endocardium, where it is maximal, to the epicardium, where it approaches atmospheric pressure level [3, 51].
2. Extrinsic myocardial compression due to myocardial shortening, which acts over the microvessels

The importance of the compressive forces is clear in conditions where intraventricular pressure is highest, such as ventricular pressure overload (aortic stenosis) or volume overload (aortic regurgitation), or when the total systolic time is increased (tachycardia) or the coronary flow reserve is decreased (exercise or vasodilator drugs) [3].

The effective perfusion accounts for diastole, since in this period, the drop in intraventricular pressure inverts the transmural gradient. Myocardial relaxation contributes to the increase in the capacitance of endocardial vessels, decreasing intraluminal pressure. Epicardial vessels will have a higher pressure. The inversion of the transmural gradient allows the principal amount of volume to be driven to the middle and inner layers of myocardium. Perfusion pressure must be above 50 mmHg to maintain an effective diastolic flow. In addition, end diastolic ventricular pressure (EDVP) is critical in maintaining a gradient that assures myocardial perfusion. An excessive increase of EDVP could compromise myocardial perfusion [3].

The extravascular compressive forces are greater in the endocardium than in the epicardium (greater degree of shortening and developed tension and greater transmission of the intraventricular pressure). Thus, the systolic flow is smaller in the endocardium than in the epicardium. In diastole, the amount of epicardial and endocardial flow increases, although proportionally more in the endocardium. It is secondary to a greater vasodilation of the vascular bed in diastole and secondary to a greater parietal stress and, therefore, a greater consumption of oxygen and local production of adenosine (Fig. 1.7) [3, 51, 52].

During exercise that causes tachycardia and shortens diastole, when there is steno-

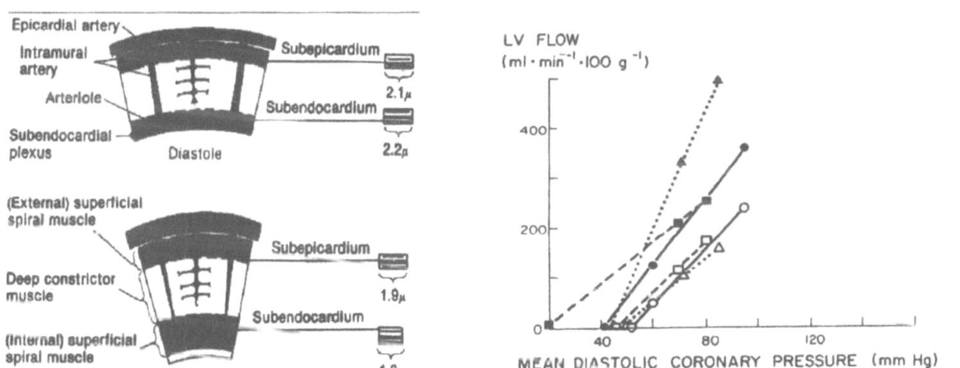

Fig. 1.7. Schematic representation of the action of the compressive extravascular forces over subepicardial and subendocardial vascular beds (*left*) and distribution of the coronary flow in such locations (*right*). In diastole (*left upper panel*), the mean diameter of subendocardial vessels is slightly bigger than subepicardial vessels (2.2 mm vs 2.1 mm) in concordance with the predominance of the metabolic control in this location secondary to the superior stress of subendocardial fibers during systole. In systole (*left lower panel*) there is a greater compression of the intramyocardial vessels and the subendocardial vascular bed (mean diameter 1.6 mm vs 1.9 mm in subepicardial bed). *Right panel* shows the flow–mean pressure in experimental conditions in the epicardial and endocardial vascular beds. For any value of mean diastolic pressure, flow is greater in the subepicardium than subendocardium (Reproduced from [54 and 3])

sis that causes a decrease in the perfusion pressure, or when the intraventricular pressure is too high, perfusion of the subendocardial layer is compromised. That is, the subendocardium is more susceptible to ischemia. Nevertheless, there are several control mechanisms to guarantee, up to a point, an adequate flow to the myocardium.

In the section describing the physiological properties of the vascular system, we depicted the mechanisms of autoregulation. Autoregulation is essential in the control of the coronary vascular bed, similar to the control of the blood flow in the brain. Autoregulation is the ability of the coronary circulation to keep the flow constant in response to variations in perfusion pressure [3, 20, 22, 23].

The interval of perfusion pressure in which the flow is constant in an experimental setting ranges between 60 and 130 mmHg. The mechanisms of autoregulation do not differ in the coronary circulation from other territories. They are rather complex, but the two most important are:

1. *Endothelial control,* mostly through the NO pathway and the flow-mediated control of vascular tone. Endothelium is sensitive to the changes in shear stress produced by the flow, modifying the production of NO acting on the content of calcium in the smooth muscle cell. In normal conditions, the inhibition of the mediators generated using the cyclooxygenase pathway (e.g. prostacyclin) does not seem to be very important, although if NO production is insufficient, their influence increases considerably. Endothelium balances the equilibrium between vasoconstrictor and vasodilator factors [35-38, 41].
2. *Myogenic control.* The smooth muscle cells can modify their degree of contraction in response to variations in the perfusion pressure through stretch signals. This is more important in vessels of greater diameter, since the thickness of the muscular layer is greater [41, 54, 55].

Coronary Flow and Myocardial Function

The close relationship between the metabolic demands of the myocardium, the requests of oxygen, and the coronary flow has been already mentioned. Modification of the three most important factors (wall tension, contractility, and heart rate) that determine the metabolic demand will increase the coronary flow. Under conditions of high wall tension, that is, as great as the area under the pressure/volume curve can be, the metabolic requests will be greater and also the volume by unit of time (flow). In normal physiology, they are adequately counteracted, but when the reserve of coronary flow is limited by different causes and the demand is high, they can lead to a situation of ischemia, of an insufficient volume blood supply to satisfy the needs of O_2 [56, 57]. In situations where there is an increase in the intraventricular pressure, such as in a ortic stenosis, or a rise in volume, such as in aortic regurgitation, the wall tension and O_2 consumption will be high. The stimulation of the contractile unit by catecholamines or the presence of calcium in the extracellular medium is translated into an energy debt that should be satisfied with an adequate blood supply. Finally, the heart rate is a determinant that also increases the consumption of O_2, since the main consequence of tachycardia is an increase in wall tension by unit of time.

One of the models that has contributed more to our understanding of the relationship between perfusion and contractile function has been the study of the hibernating myocardium [59, 60]. Hibernating myocardium is a condition characterized by a variable decrease in the contractile function in one or more areas of the myocardium, which impairs regional and, frequently, global ventricular function. It is produced by a metabolic adaptation of the myocyte in response to hypoxia secondary to a persistent decrease of the coronary flow. The study of the hibernating myocardium has led to a better characterization of the relationship between flow and contractility. Nevertheless, one of the principal problems in its study is the impossibility of employing animal models; thus, such adaptation is exclusive to the human species. In addition, we are short of tools that allow analysis of the regional dynamics of flow. One available tool is dynamic positron emission tomography (PET). PET has shown, not only that the nonviable and viable areas, areas with and without contractile reserve, are perfused, but also that the differences in the flow among viable and normal areas are quite subtle (relative difference 21–25%).

Under normal conditions there is a marked spatial heterogeneity in coronary flow (Fig. 1.8). This regional heterogeneous distribution of the flow has also been shown experimentally [60-62].

Spatial heterogeneity is critical in coronary heart disease, because of the inhomogeneous character of the myocardial damage

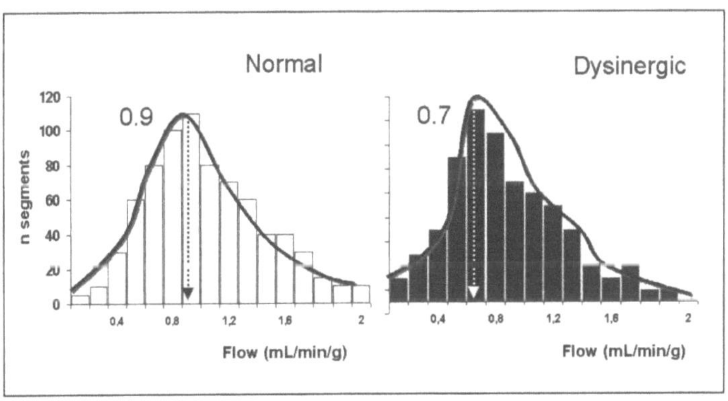

Fig. 1.8. Bar plot showing the distribution, in frequencies, of normokinetic segments of healthy patients for each one of the coronary flow values determined with water marked with O15 and employing PET (*left panel*). This heterogeneity is maintained when dysynergic segments were studied in patients with coronary heart disease and systolic left ventricular dysfunction (*right panel*). Note the tendency of the distribution to switch toward smaller coronary flow values in subjects with coronary heart disease. *n* is number of segments (Adapted from [61, 62, 63])

produced by the ischemia. One of the limitations of many techniques to assess the regional flow is that in the damaged areas there is a mixture of zones with lack of perfusion and zones that have survived the ischemic aggression and have preserved their microcirculation intact. This inhomogeneity of regional flow in a concrete area of myocardium, although not so marked, is also present in normal conditions [63].

On the other hand new innovative and refined techniques are emerging that focus on discerning not only the flow in a certain volume, but also whether this volume is really perfused (functionally viable) or not. With these techniques, ammonium-labeled tracers are replaced by water-labeled tracers (Fig. 1.9) [60, 64].

It is not easy to demonstrate if a dysynergic myocardial segment that shows a value of regional blood flow in normal limits is viable or not. In relation to this, there are some interesting data from the correspondence between the fact of a near-normal flow value in viable segments and the presence of redistribution with thallium or late capture of the isotope after reinjection. In 13 of 16 cases with late capture of thallium, the estimated regional flow using PET with the refined techniques mentioned employing marked H_2O was in the normal range (>0.7 ml/min/g) [65].

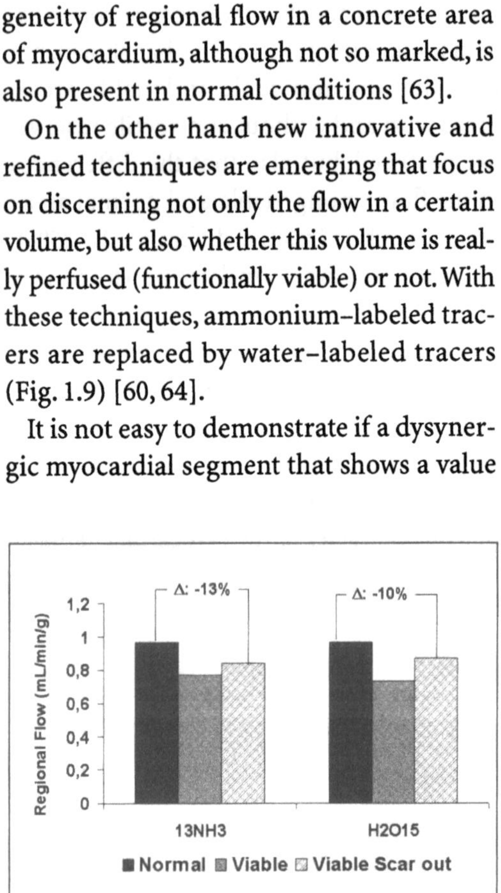

Fig. 1.9. Regional myocardial blood flow values obtained with PET. Excluding analysis of the portions of tissue corresponding to true scar, and that underestimate the quantification of the regional flow, differences between the values of flow in preserved distant areas and the damaged dysynergic segments that showed viability are near 10%, subtleties very difficult to appreciate at a glance with a qualitative approach (Adapted from [61, 65])

Although limited in spatial resolution, PET has provided valuable data on the flow–contractility relationship in normal conditions and under the effect of ischemia, not only in a region of interest or between regions, but also in the transmural dimension. These features are in concordance with previous experimental data (Fig. 1.10) [66, 67].

In both cases, a decrease in flow of at least 40% is necessary in order to observe a significant depression of the contractility. If the amount of flow decrease is around 20%, which has been calculated for the hibernating myocardium, a significant depression in contractility is not produced, *in experimental conditions*. Thus, we move to areas of the flow–function curve where the precision and validity of the instruments of measure are fundamental, since the differences are very subtle (relative reductions of 20–40%). This is one of the characteristics of the hibernating myocardium, the inability to create a consistent and reproducible experimental model. We should not forget that the hibernating myocardium has an autoregulation that is totally or nearly impaired. These increments in the meta-

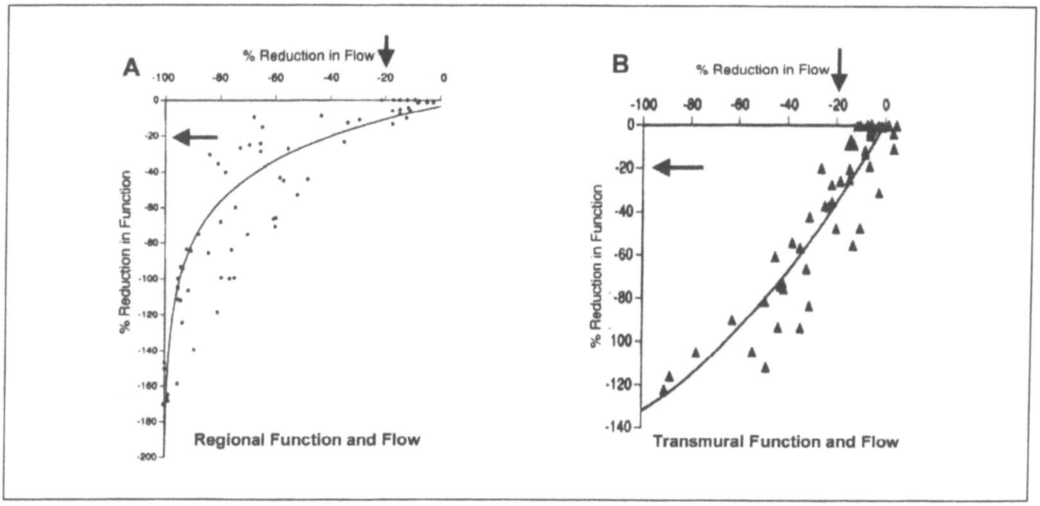

Fig. 1.10. Coronary flow and myocardial function (shortening and thickening). *Left panel* shows the close relationship between a decrease in the flow and a decrease in the myocardial shortening measured with microcrystals. *Right panel* discloses similar findings assessing the transmural decrease of the flow (subendocardial ischemia) and the decrease in the myocardial thickening (Reproduced from [67, 68])

bolic demand, sometimes of small magnitude, will produce ischemia and subsequent metabolic adaptative response, whose most emergent expression is the impairment of contractility. This can explain why, in the clinical setting, there is a depression in contractility with a decrease in coronary flow, which is difficult to carry out in an experimental setting.

Are SPECT and PET the best tools for assessing flow and contractile function? SPECT techniques lack the ability to quantify regional blood flow and could not detect subtle increases or decreases in coronary flow, showing parallel behavior in the flow of viable and normal segments. The lack of resolution for small increments in flow (10–20%) needed to detect endoepicardial differences limits its applicability. PET provides a quantitative approach to the study of regional flow and permits transmural analysis. However, it is expensive and not universally accessible [68].

Myocardial contrast-enhanced echocardiography emerges as a powerful technique that combines accessibility, low cost, and quantification, making it possible to discern normal and pathological conditions in both regional flow and contractile function.

References

1. Epstein SE, Cannon RO III, Talbot TL. Hemodynamic principles in the control of coronary blood flow. Am J Cardiol 1985 8;56:4E-10E.
2. Marcus ML, Chilian WM, Kanatsuka H, Dellsperger KC, Eastham CL, Lamping KG. Understanding the coronary circulation through studies at the microvascular level. Circulation 1990;82:1-7
3. Hoffman JI. Determinants and prediction of transmural myocardial perfusion. Circulation 1978;58:381-91
4. Chilian WM. Coronary microcirculation in health and disease. Circulation 1997;95:522-8
5. Schwaiger M, Muzik O. Assessment of myocardial perfusion by positron emission tomography. Am J Cardiol1991;67:35D-43D
6. Passariello R, De Santis M. Magnetic resonance imaging evaluation of myocardial perfusion. Am J Cardiol 1998;81:68G-73G
7. Kaul S. Myocardial contrast echocardiography: 15 years of research and development. Circulation 1997;96:3745-60
8. Waller BF, Schlant R. Anatomy of the heart. In: W Alexander, RC Schlant and V Fuster (eds.): Hurst's the heart, arteries and veins. 9th ed. McGraw-Hill, 1998:19-79
9. Waller BF. Anatomy, histology, and pathology of the major epicardial coronary arteries relevant to echocardiographic imaging techniques. J Am Soc Echocardiogr 1989;2:232-52
10. Waller BF, Orr CM, Slack JD, Pinkerton CA, Van Tassel J, Peters T. Anatomy, histology, and pathology of coronary arteries: a review relevant to new interventional and imaging techniques—Part I. Clin Cardiol 1992;15:451-7
11. Waller BF, Orr CM, Slack JD, Pinkerton CA, Van Tassel J, Peters T. Anatomy, histology, and pathology of coronary arteries: a review relevant to new interventional and imaging techniques—Part II. Clin Cardiol 1992;15:535-40
12. Waller BF, Orr CM, Slack JD, Pinkerton CA, Van Tassel JV, Peters T. Anatomy, histology, and pathology of coronary arteries: a review relevant to new interventional and imaging techniques—Part III. Clin Cardiol 1992;15:607-15
13. Waller BF, Orr CM, Slack JD, Pinkerton CA, Van Tassel J, Peters T. Anatomy, histology, and pathology of coronary arteries: a review relevant to new interventional and imaging techniques—Part IV. Clin Cardiol 1992;15:675-87
14. Schlant R, Sonnenblick EH, Katz AM. Normal physiology of the cardiovascular system. In: W Alexander, RC Schlant and V Fuster (eds.): Hurst's the heart, arteries and veins. 9th ed. McGraw-Hill, 1998:81-124
15. Young DF. Fluid mechanics of arterial stenosis. J Biomech Eng 1979;101:157
16. Gould KL. Pressure-flow characteristics of coronary stenoses in unsedated dogs at rest and during coronary vasodilation. Circ Res 1978;43:242-53
17. Gould KL. Dynamic coronary stenosis. Am J Cardiol 1980;45:286-92
18. Schwartz JS, Carlyle PF, Cohn JN. Effect of coronary arterial pressure on coronary stenosis resistance. Circulation 1980;61:70-6
19. Mates RE, Gupta RL, Bell AC, Klocke FJ. Fluid dynamics of coronary artery stenosis. Circ Res 1978;42:152-62
20. Chilian WM, Eastham CL, Marcus ML. Microvascular distribution of coronary vascular resistance in beating left ventricle. Am J Physiol 1986;251:H779-88
21. Lamping KG, Kanatsuka H, Eastham CL, Chilian WM, Marcus ML. Nonuniform vasomotor responses of the coronary microcirculation to serotonin and vasopressin. Circ Res 1989;65:343-51
22. Bellamy RF. Diastolic coronary artery pressure-flow relations in the dog. Circ Res 1978;43:92-101
23. Hoffman JI. Maximal coronary flow and the concept of coronary vascular reserve. Circulation 1984;70:153-9
24. Vatner SF. Regulation of coronary resistance vessels and large coronary arteries. Am J Cardiol 1985;56:16E-22E
25. Harrison DG, Marcus ML, Dellsperger KC, Lamping KG, Tomanek RJ. Pathophysiology of myocardial perfusion in hypertension. Circulation 1991;83(Suppl):III14-8
26. Wells R. Microcirculation and coronary blood flow. Am J Cardiol. 1972 Jun;29(6):847-50
27. Ludmer PL, Selwyn AP, Shook TL et al. Paradoxical vasoconstriction induced by acetylcholine in atherosclerotic coronary arteries. N Engl J Med. 1986;315:1046-51
28. Egashira K, Inou T, Hirooka Y et al. Impaired coronary blood flow response to acetylcholine in patients with coronary risk factors and proximal atherosclerotic lesions. J Clin Invest 1993;91:29-37
29. Cox DA, Vita JA, Treasure CB et al. Atherosclerosis impairs flow-mediated dilation of coronary arteries in humans. Circulation 1989;80:458-65
30. Nabel EG, Selwyn AP, Ganz P. Large coronary arteries in humans are responsive to changing blood flow: an endothelium-dependent mechanism that fails in patients with atherosclerosis. J Am Coll Cardiol 1990;16:349-56
31. Chilian WM, Dellsperger KC, Layne SM et al. Effects of atherosclerosis on the coronary microcirculation. Am J Physiol 1990;258:H529-39
32. Zeiher AM, Drexler H, Wollschlager H, Just H.

Endothelial dysfunction of the coronary microvasculature is associated with coronary blood flow regulation in patients with early atherosclerosis. Circulation 1991;84:1984-92.
33. Zeiher AM, Drexler H, Saurbier B, Just H. Endothelium-mediated coronary blood flow modulation in humans. Effects of age, atherosclerosis, hypercholesterolemia, and hypertension. J Clin Invest 1993;92:652-62
34. Hoffman JI, Buckberg GD. The myocardial supply:demand ratio. Am J Cardiol. 1978;41:327-32
35. Furchgott RF, Zawadzki JV. The obligatory role of endothelial cells in the relaxation of arterial smooth muscle by acetylcholine. Nature 1980;288:373-6
36. Palmer RM, Ferrige AG, Moncada S. Nitric oxide release accounts for the biological activity of endothelium-derived relaxing factor. Nature 1987;327:524-6
37. Ignarro LJ, Buga GM, Wood KS, Byrns RE, Chaudhuri G. Endothelium-derived relaxing factor produced and released from artery and vein is nitric oxide. Proc Natl Acad Sci U S A. 1987;84:9265-9
38. Yanagisawa M, Kurihara H, Kimura S et al.A novel potent vasoconstrictor peptide produced by vascular endothelial cells. Nature 1988;332:411-5
39. Berne RM. The role of adenosine in the regulation of coronary blood flow. Circ Res 1980;47:807-13
40. VanDijk AM, Wieringa PA, van der Meer M, Laird JD. Mechanics of resting isolated single vascular smooth muscle cells from bovine coronary artery. Am J Physiol 1984;246:C277-87
41. Kuo L, Davis MJ, Chilian WM. Endothelium-dependent, flow-induced dilation of isolated coronary arterioles. Am J Physiol 1990 Oct;259:H1063-70
42. Chilian WM, Layne SM, Eastham CL, Marcus ML. Heterogeneous microvascular coronary alpha-adrenergic vasoconstriction. Circ Res 1989;64:376-88
43. Myers PR, Banitt PF, Guerra R Jr, Harrison DG. Characteristics of canine coronary resistance arteries: importance of endothelium. Am J Physiol 1989;257:H603-10
44. Feigl EO. Coronary physiology. Physiol Rev 1983;63:1-2095
45. Braunwald E. Control of myocardial oxygen consumption: physiologic and clinical considerations. Am J Cardiol 1971;27:416-32
46. Sonnenblick EH, Ross J Jr, Covell JW, Kaiser GA, Braunwald E. Velocity of contraction as a determinant of myocardial oxygen consumption. Am J Physiol 1965;209:919-27
47. Boerth RC, Covell JW, Pool PE, Ross J. Increased myocardial oxygen consumption and contractile state associated with increased heart rate in dogs. Circ Res 1969;24:725-34
48. Takaoka H, Takeuchi M, Odake M et al. Comparison of hemodynamic determinants for myocardial oxygen consumption under different contractile states in human ventricle. Circulation 1993;87:59-69
49. Kameyama T, Asanoi H, Ishizaka S et al. Energy conversion efficiency in human left ventricle. Circulation 1992;85:988-96
50. Yada T, Richmond KN, Van Bibber R, Kroll K, Feigl EO. Role of adenosine in local metabolic coronary vasodilation. Am J Physiol 1999;276:H1425-33
51. Hess DS, Bache RJ. Transmural distribution of myocardial blood flow during systole in the awake dog. Circ Res 1976;38:5-15
52. Bache RJ, Cobb FR. Effect of maximal coronary vasodilation on transmural myocardial perfusion during tachycardia in the awake dog. Circ Res 1977;41:648-53
53. Bell JR, Fox AC. Pathogenesis of subendocardial ischemia. Am J Med Sci 1974;268:3-13
54. Jones CJ, Kuo L, Davis MJ, Chilian WM. Myogenic and flow-dependent control mechanisms in the coronary microcirculation. Basic Res Cardiol 1993; 88:2-10
55. Rajagopalan S, Dube S, Canty JM. Regulation of coronary diameter by myogenic mechanisms in arterial microvessels greater than 100 microns in diameter. Am J Physiol 1995;268:H788-H793
56. Little WC, Cheng CP, Mumma M, Igarashi Y, Vinten-Johansen J, Johnston WE. Comparison of measures of left ventricular contractile performance derived from pressure-volume loops in conscious dogs. Circulation 1989;80:1378-87
57. Kass DA, Maughan WL, Guo ZM, Kono A, Sunagawa K, Sagawa K. Comparative influence of load versus inotropic states on indexes of ventricular contractility: experimental and theoretical analysis based on pressure-volume relationships. Circulation 1987;76:1422-3
58. Grandin C, Wijns W, Melin JA, Bol A, Robert AR, Heyndrickx GR et al. Delineation of myocardial viability with PET. J Nucl Med 1995;36(9):1543-52
59. Yamamoto Y, de Silva R, Rhodes CG, Araujo LI, Iida H, Rechavia E et al. A new strategy for the assessment of viable myocardium and regional myocardial blood flow using 15O-water and dynamic positron emission tomography. Circulation 1992;86:167-78
60. Marinho NV, Keogh BE, Costa DC, Lammerstma AA, Ell PJ, Camici PG. Pathophysiology of chronic left ventricular dysfunction. New insights from the measurement of absolute myocardial blood flow and glucose utilization. Circulation 1996;93(4):737-44
61. Ghaleh B, Shen YT, Vatner SF. Spatial heterogeneity of myocardial blood flow presages salvage versus necrosis with coronary artery reperfusion in con-

scious baboons. Circulation 1996;94:2210-5

62. Bassingthwaighte JB, Li Z. Heterogeneities in myocardial flow and metabolism: exacerbation with abnormal excitation. Am J Cardiol 1999;83:7H-12H
63. Camici PG, Wijns W, Borgers M, De Silva R, Ferrari R, Knuuti J et al. Pathophysiological mechanisms of chronic reversible left ventricular dysfunction due to coronary artery disease (hibernating myocardium). Circulation 1997;96:3205-14
64. Gerber BL, Vanoverschelde JL, Bol A, Michel C, Labar D, Wijns W et al. Myocardial blood flow, glucose uptake, and recruitment of inotropic reserve in chronic left ventricular ischemic dysfunction. Implications for the pathophysiology of chronic myocardial hibernation. Circulation 1996;94:651-9
65. Marin-Neto JA, Dilsizian V, Arrighi JA, Freedman NM, Perrone-Filardi P, Bacharach SL et al. Thallium reinjection demonstrates viable myocardium in regions with reverse redistribution. Circulation 1993;88:1736-45
66. Vatner SF. Correlation between acute reductions in myocardial blood flow and function in conscious dogs. Circ Res 1980;47:201-7
67. Gallagher KP, Matsuzaki M, Koziol JA, Kemper WS, Ross J. Regional myocardial perfusion and wall thickening during ischemia in conscious dogs. Am J Physiol 1984;247:H727-38
68. Bonow RO. Contractile reserve and coronary blood flow reserve in collateral-dependent myocardium. J Am Coll Cardiol 1999;33:705-7

Chapter 2
Microbubbles: Basic Principles

Viviana Serra • Miguel Angel García Fernández • José Luis Zamorano

Introduction

Echocardiography represents a basic tool for diagnosis of cardiac pathology. During the last few years technological advances have led to new imaging methods with more applications. The availability of wide-band transducers has been fundamental for the utilization of ultrasound contrast agents.

In this chapter, we analyse the basic principles of microbubbles so as to understand their behaviour in an ultrasound field, as well as the origin, evolution and development of contrast agents and the technological advances that have led to their clinical application.

Basic Principles

Backscatter Signal

When an even wave is transmitted through a medium and crosses an interface with a different acoustic impedance, a reflection wave is produced in the first medium and a transmitted wave is produced in the second medium. Depending on the interface extent and the signal wave length, the ultrasound reflection may be specular or non-specular [1]. Specular reflection means the interface is longer than the wave length and the reflection angle is similar to the angle of incidence. On the other hand, non-specular reflection or scattering is produced when the interface is smaller than the wave length and the ultrasound is reflected in all directions.

The signal reflected back to the transducer is called backscatter.

Fundamental Imaging

The ultrasound transmitted through the medium produces reflection and transmission phenomena. The echographic image is produced by the reflection echo. "Fundamental image" is the image that is produced by the specular ultrasounds, which means that the specular interfaces are longer than the wave length and have the same frequency as the transmitted ultrasound. As we have already mentioned, the specular reflection is angle dependent, thus the reflection will be longer when the reflecting interface is more perpendicular to the sound beam.

With fundamental imaging, the anterior and lateral wall of the left ventricle are more difficult to visualize due to the parallel direction of the wall and sound beam. Limited visualization of the apical segment is often a result of clutter and near-field artefact [2].

Harmonic Imaging

Harmonic imaging is an echocardiographic skill different from fundamental imaging, because it transmits the ultrasound at a certain frequency and receives it at twice the transmitted frequency. To generate a pure harmonic image, it is necessary to suppress the returning fundamental signal, which is often stronger than the harmonic signal. This can be achieved with different techniques: filtering the signal at the fundamental frequency, power modulation, pulse inversion imaging, coherent contrast imaging and contrast pulse sequencing (CPS).

Harmonic imaging was first intended to be used with utrasonographic contrast agents. However, it has been shown that harmonic imaging improves tissue visualization even before the contrast injection stage [2-3]. In human tissue, the sound transmission is not linear, which results in a change of the ultrasound waves transmitted. During the pressure period, the tissues become thick and the ultrasound waves cross the tissue faster than during the rarefaction period; thus the sound wave distortion during transmission results in a progressive energy change from fundamental to high harmonics [4].

The amount of harmonic signal produced depends on the incident acoustic pressure, the transmitted frequency, the distance the wave has been transmitted and the tissue non-linearity [5].

Acoustic Pressure

There is a strong dependence of the tissue behaviour on the acoustic pressure. Thus, at a low mechanical index, the tissue signal is mainly linear, and at a high mechanical index, a significant non-linear signal is produced through the tissue.

Fundamental Frequency

The generation of non-linear signals in the tissue is greater at lower frequencies.

Also, when imaging for tissue harmonics, the attenuation, which is dependent on the frequency, is minimized by transmitting at relatively low frequency.

Wave Transmission Distance

The second harmonic intensity signal depends its distance from the transducer: the signal is stronger from the basal than from the apical part of the left ventricle. This is because the ultrasound pulse is distorted more and more as it continues travelling along the tissue, which implies a higher nonlinear frequency content.

However, it is important to take into account that the attenuation of the returning harmonic signal also increases with the distance from the transducer; therefore, if a structure is too far away, the returning harmonic signal will not be strong.

In summary, we receive less harmonic signal from the near and far field than from the mid field.

It has been shown that tissue harmonic imaging improves image quality and may be used to enhance the left ventricular endocardial border definition. Because the harmonic beams are narrower and have lower side lobes than the fundamental ones, there is also an enhancement of lateral resolution, which allows a better definition of lateral and anterior walls. The basal segments are better defined because the amount of harmonic signal increases with the transducer distance propagation. The reverberations are almost entirely made up of ultrasound energy at the fundamental frequency, therefore noise and artefacts are reduced allowing a better definition of apical view.

The development of this imaging technique has been of great clinical relevance, being a useful tool for assessing both global and regional left ventricular function [6, 8].

Ultrasound Contrast Agents

Definition

Contrast agents are encapsulated microbubbles filled with either air or high-molecular- weight gas. They range in diameter from 1 to 10 μm, are innocuous, biologically inert and when administered intravascularly, the sound backscatter from the blood pool is enhanced.

Echocardiographic Contrast Agents: Historical Development

In 1968, Gramiak and Shah [9] reported an effect they called "contrast effect", which is the aortic and cardiac chamber opacification after injection of saline solution in the aortic root during angiography. Early contrast agents included hand-agitated saline solutions, hydrogen peroxide, 5% dextrose, indocyanine green, iodinated contrast and blood. However, these microbubbles were not small and stable enough to survive transpulmonary crossing and to reach the left cardiac chamber.

In 1983, Feinstein et al. [10] developed the use of sonification to produce more microbubbles with higher stability; the microbubbles are produced when the air in the liquid medium is exposed to high-energy ultrasound. In 1984, Feinstein took part in the commercial development of sonicated human albumin marketed under the name Albunex®. Albunex® and Levovist® were the first agents able to reach the left cardiac chambers after intravenous administration (first-generation contrast agents).

The main limitation of the first-generation contrast agents is that the air in the microbubbles is highly diffusible from the microbubbles when mixed with blood. Thus, the loss of air with consequent decrease in bubble size results in the decrease of its backscattering properties [11]. The bubbles' dissolution time decreases with a higher surface tension, which is in part determined by the surfactant molecule concentration on the bubble–liquid interface.

Attempts to maximize the persistence of microbubbles included high-density gases with low diffusion and solubility. These contrast agents are called second-generation contrast agents [12], and have proved to be useful in myocardial opacification after intravenous administration [13, 14].

De Maria et al. [15] reported the first experiments encouraging the potential use of microbubbles for myocardial opacification. Over the years, technical progress and the development of enhanced contrast agents have led to several advances in myocardial perfusion evaluation.

Some new applications of microbubbles include drug delivery, endothelial function evaluation, tissue-targeted gene therapy, angiogenesis and vascular remodelling, tumour destruction, inflammation assessment and thrombus targeting [16].

Physical Properties in the Determination of the Reflecting Capability of Microbubbles

The ultrasonic contrast agents are microbubbles that resonate when excited by diagnostic ultrasound frequencies (non-linear acoustic behaviour) producing an increasing ultrasound backscatter from the blood [17, 18]. The enormous reflective ability of microbubbles is due to a large acoustic impedance mismatch between the bubble gas content and the surrounding blood. The non-linear potency of the microbubbles depends on several factors: the microbubble diameter, frequency and ultrasound power applied, as well as compressibility and gas density and shell composition.

Microbubble Diameter

The scattering cross section is extremely dependent on the bubble size and is directly proportional to the sixth power of its radius [19]. Thus, larger microbubbles produce higher ultrasound signal and any reduction in microbubble size results in a marked decrease of its reflection ability. However, bubbles larger than 8 μm become entrapped in the pulmonary microcirculation. On the other hand, very small microbubbles have less reflective ability and less stability. The microbubble size may also change with the milieu (higher pressure levels add to microbubble shrinkage). Based on these principles, the ideal diameter of microbubbles is approximately 4 μm.

Ultrasound Frequency

Microbubbles undergo changes because under ultrasound interaction (radial oscillation) they are compressed during pressure peaks and expand during pressure nadirs. This microbubble behaviour is called resonance phenomenon [20]. Oscillation of the microbubbles may produce a wide range of harmonic frequencies: subharmonic [21, 22], second harmonic [23], ultraharmonic [24] and super harmonic (third, fourth, fifth). The resonance frequency, which is related to the microbubbles radius, is achieved with frequencies commonly used in echocardiography.

Compressibility
The ability of microbubbles to produce strong backscattered acoustic signal is based on their compressibility, which depends on the viscoelastic and pressure properties of the shell and gas.

Stability
Microbubbles in the blood pool are rather unstable due to gas diffusion which causes microbubble collapse. Changes in microbubble shell content (thicker and less flexible), gas content (less diffusibility) or both have improved bubble stability [25].

Shell
Microbubble encapsulation is required to increase stability and persistence. The persistence depends on rigidity, which is the ease with which a microbubble dissolves or is disrupted when exposed to ultrasound energy [26]. There is no agreement about the nature of the shell surrounding microbubbles for achieving the best result. One approach involves the use of polymeric shells where thickness and flexibility may be controlled with more accuracy (Sonovist, Cardiosphere). Rigidity is an important characteristic that provides persistence and good resistance to blood pressure changes and ultrasound pressure waves. However, since microbubble crack is required for perfusion studies, a degree of fragility is needed to allow the destruction and posterior myocardial refilling. It has been shown that the optimal power for achieving maximal signal intensity with minimal microbubble destruction is influenced by the shell's elastic properties [27]. Soft-shell agents such as SonoVue (Bracco Italy) have high echogenicity at low mechanical index (0.2), and tend to be destroyed at high mechanical index [28]. Effective agents at low mechanical index have the advantage of the absence of harmonic signal proceeding from the tissue.

On the other hand, the microbubbles' surface characteristics influence their ability to cross the pulmonary microvasculature (endothelial adhesion, leucocyte phagocytosis, and glycocalyx interaction) [29, 30].

Gas
One of the approaches to extend microbubble survival is the use of gas with low solubility and diffusibility. Because gas diffusion is inversely proportional to the square root of its molecular weight [31], the microbubbles with higher molecular weight gas will have more survival. The gases most commonly used for this purpose include sulphur hexafluoride (SonoVue) and perfluorocabons such as perfluoropropanate (Definity), perfluorohexane gas and nitrogen gas (Imagent), octafluoropropane (Optison).

Mechanical Index
Mechanical index (MI) is defined as the peak of negative pressure divided by the square root of the ultrasound frequency. The negative pressure measurement is expressed in Kilopascals. In an acoustic field, bubbles have different responses depending on MI. For low ultrasound acoustic pressure (<100 kPa; MI<0.1), the microbubble behaviour is linear oscillation (contraction and slackness are similar in amplitude). When peak pressure is between 100 kPa–1 MPa (MI 0.1-1),

expansion is higher than contraction (non-linear oscillation) and produces signals whose frequencies are a multiple of the emitted frequency and are called harmonics. When the pressure peak is higher than 1 MPa (MI>1), bubbles are destroyed producing a brief non-linear response and the harmonic signal has high amplitude [32, 33].

In summary, depending on acoustic pressure, these particles may remain with stable resonance during ultrasound exposure period (resonance frequency) or be destroyed producing a brief non-linear response.

Microbubble Concentration

The signal intensity depends on the microbubble concentration. At low concentration the signal intensity increases linearly. As the concentration increases, the relationship between microbubbles and signal intensity becomes curvilinear until it reaches a plateau, where the contrast effect may actually decrease. This phenomenon suggests that microbubbles attenuate ultrasound signal at higher concentration [12].

Types of Contrast Agents

According to the behaviour of microbubbles when crossing the microcirculation, we may classify them as free flow or deposit tracers.

Free-Flow Microbubbles

Free-flow microbubbles are considered true red blood tracers because their rheological properties and size are similar to the red cell, they cross the microcirculation freely and are not caught by myocytes. These properties are particularly useful to enhance Doppler signal [34], the left heart chamber definition [35, 37] and the myocardial perfusion issue [38, 39].

Deposit Tracers

It has been demonstrated that several new agents persist in the microcirculation and are selectively collected by the tissue cells or adhere to the endothelium. The combination of the attaching properties of some microbubbles with the ultrasound which destroys them, would be useful in future applications such as specific site delivery of therapeutic agents, genetic material and growth factors. Moreover, the cell's assimilation of bubbles would have great diagnostic utility.

Artefacts

Artefact is an image feature which does not correspond to reality. We will describe the most common artefacts that should be taken into account when working with contrast agents.

Attenuation (Shadowing)

Attenuation can be defined as a reduction in backscatter signal produced by bubbles reflecting in the near field. This event may occur due to high concentration of strongly scattering microbubbles, which could produce far-field shadowing. In addition, in vitro studies suggest differences in the degree of attenuation among different microbubble agents [26]. Porter et al. have shown that attenuation of the posterior wall is reduced by high-molecular-weight perfluorocarbons [40].

Attenuation is particularly evident in the basal segments (apical views) and posterior wall (parasternal view) producing "pseudo" defects in subjects with normal perfusion.

An enormous variability in the degree of attenuation in different patients was observed, thus it is very important to individualize the doses in order to obtain less attenuation.

There are two approaches to contrast agent administration: bolus injection and continuous infusion. Out of the two, continuous infusion would be the best option to adjust the individual dose to a level at which adequate myocardial opacification could be reached with minimal attenuation.

Swirling

Swirling is an apical attenuation caused by bubble destruction in the near field. There are several factors that may produce this artefact such as: mechanical index, frame rate, line intensity, insufficient contrast agent or very low flow at the apex. Changing the focal zone and adjustment of the rate of contrast infusion could change these factors [41].

Blooming

The cavity blooming artefact is due to the high difference of reflectivity in the interface between the myocardial and ventricular cavities [42]. Thus the high signal from the cavity exceeds the endocardial border showing a false myocardial opacification. This is mainly due to the quick infusion of contrast, whereas with an adequate infusion rate, cavity blooming is less frequently seen.

Wall Artefact

Motion artefact is observed mainly with the Power Doppler Harmonic (PDH) mode [42]. This technique, contrary to traditional Doppler that detects velocity and flow direction, detects only the presence of flow. Thereby, the Doppler signal is displayed in one colour and its presence indicates flow. However, once Doppler detects movement, it may display, in colour, the movement produced by the heart wall, breath, patient and operator's hand.

To reduce the possibility of movement artefact it is important to note the following procedures:

1. The colour may be adjusted before injection of contrast, showing the myocardium without colour.
2. It is important to ask the patient to breath shallowly to avoid artefact caused by breath movement.
3. Delay of triggering may be gated during the cardiac cycle with less movement (end- systole or end- diastole).
4. The filter threshold may be optimized before contrast injection.
5. Due to the fact that PDH uses packet of pulses, the image creation may be delayed depending on the number of pulses. During this time lag, tissue motion may occur which may lead to the artefact generation. To avoid this problem, we can reduce the sector size and examine different myocardial regions at different times. Another option is the use of a small pulse packet thereby reducing the time of

image acquisition; however, there is a decrease in sensitivity.

Rib Artefact

The rib artefact is caused by the blocking of the scan line by the ribs and it appears as a dark region that does not enhance with contrast. This is easily recognized and solved by changing the transducer position.

Clinical Aspects of Contrast Agents

The ideal contrast agents should be non-toxic, intravenously injectable, able to cross the pulmonary capillary after a peripheral injection, and stable enough to achieve enhancement during the examination. There are some products on the market and several agents under development. The potential utility of these agents depends on the pharmacokinetic and pharmacodynamic properties of the products.

They are currently made up of encapsulated microbubbles filled with air (first-generation contrast agents) or an inert gas (second-generation contrast agents).

We will describe the characteristics of SonoVue®, one of the most commonly used second-generation agent in Europe.

Characteristics of SonoVue®

SonoVue® is a new second-generation contrast agent with elevated resistance to pressure [42]. This agent is made up of microbubbles stabilized by a thin phospholipids monolayer and containing sulphur hexafluoride (SF6), a poorly soluble and totally innocuous gas. SF6 was selected because of its good resistance to pressure changes (left ventricle, pulmonary microvasculature bed and coronary circulation) and its good tolerability in clinical practice.

With a mean diameter of 2.5 µm and more than 90% of bubbles smaller than 8 µm, these bubbles are small enough to prevent trapping in the capillary vasculature. The high bubble concentration ($2x10^8$ / ml) combined with a favourable size distribution results in highly echogenic suspensions with a very low relative bubble volume.

The suspension of gas microbubbles is reconstituted before use by introducing 5 ml of 0.9% sodium chloride followed by hand agitation. The white milk suspension is stable for hours at room temperature and only a minimal decrease (10%) in echogenicity is noted after 8 h.

However, because the product does not contain a sterilizing agent, the maximum time of use for reconstituted SonoVue® should be limited to 6 h.

SonoVue® does not diffuse into the extravascular compartment but remains within the blood vessels until the gas dissolves and is eliminated in expired air. More than 80% of the administered gas is exhaled through the lungs after 11 min.

SonoVue® shows essentially constant echogenic properties over the entire medical frequency range. The maximum attenuation and backscatter was found to extend over a wide range of frequency of 4–9 MHz and is around 4–4.5 MHz, thus indicating that the majority of microbubbles resonate in this frequency range.

Extensive studies in animals and humans

have confirmed the outstanding safety profile of SonoVue® and its capability of providing a clinically useful signal at 0.03 and 0.3 ml, which are the expected clinical dose and 10 times the clinical dose, respectively [43, 44].

SonoVue® can provide ventricular opacification and improve endocardial border definition [45] and Doppler signal. Moreover its utility was shown in myocardial perfusion studies [46, 47].

Contrast Administration Methods

The discussion of the ideal administration method is relevant in myocardial perfusion studies.

The bolus administration is an injection of a small amount of contrast material during a short time period (20–30 seconds), followed by a flush of 10–20 ml of normal saline solution. However, the duration of the injection of contrast and saline solution can also be extended. In this way it is possible to avoid attenuation and blooming artefacts. Moreover, for bolus injection, a reduction in microbubble destruction has been shown, with the use of a three-way stopcock to inject the saline flush solution at a 90° angle [41].

During continuous infusion, the dose of microbubbles may be customized to individual patients.

Continuous infusion could be the best option for contrast administration because it reduces artefacts (shadowing, blooming) and it has an important implication for quantification of myocardial blood flow [48, 49].

Available Methods to Detect Myocardial Bubbles

There are two main categories of methods for the detection of myocardial contrast: the so-called high-MI contrast imaging (intermittent triggered imaging and pseudo real time with monitoring mode and auto beat sequence), and the low-MI contrast imaging (real-time imaging and triggered low-MI imaging) (Table 2.1).

Table 2.1. Methods for detecting myocardial bubbles

High MI contrast imaging
Intermittent triggered imaging
• Harmonic power Doppler
• Ultraharmonic
Pseudo real-time (with monitoring mode and Autobeat sequence)
• Harmonic power Doppler
• Ultraharmonic
Low MI contrast imaging
Real-time imaging
• Power modulation
• Pulse inversion
• Coherent contrast imaging
• Contrast pulse sequencing
Triggered low-MI imaging or triggered replenishment imaging (TRI)

High-MI Contrast Imaging

Intermittent Triggered Imaging

Microbubble destruction is directly related to acoustic power (mechanical index) and inversely related to transducer frequency [32]. Thus microbubble destruction is more evident at lower frequencies and higher acoustic power.

A large number of microbubbles are destroyed when using a high-MI technique. With this method, the bubbles are destroyed when the image is being formed. Therefore, in order to allow a replenishment of the myocardium by microbubbles, it is necessary to use a triggering mode that creates an image with a pulsing interval previously determined [50]. Thus, two images are obtained (on the left and on the right of the screen, before and after the bubble destruction, respectively). It is also possible to obtain only one image or more than two.

In order to allow the quantification of the microbubble refilling curve, the pulsing interval should be increased (51), for instance, from every 1 heart beat (1:1) to every 2(1:2), 4(1:3), 7(1:7), and 10(1:10).

The major inconvenience of this method is the loss of the original image plane as a consequence of breathing, heart movement, patient movement or even the movements of the physician's hand.

Pseudo Real-Time Imaging (with Monitoring Mode and AutoBeat Sequence)

The new technique applied to some triggering modes is the "monitoring mode", which allows a continuous low-MI monitoring of the image during the examination. With this method, we may visualize a real-time 2D image that can be used as reference and is visualized between the triggered perfusion frames (previously the blinded period). The monitoring mode image is obtained with very low-MI, so the bubbles are not being destroyed and therefore the replenishment of the myocardium is not affected.

The two high-MI techniques more commonly used are harmonic power Doppler (Angio) and ultraharmonic mode.

Harmonic Power Doppler

As mentioned above, when using high-MI, the tissue has a strong non-linear behaviour and therefore the signal-to-noise ratio between the tissue and the contrast agent in B-mode harmonic imaging is not as high as desired. However, there is a new Doppler technique for detecting microbubbles called harmonic power Doppler [52] that appears to be promising for the assessment of myocardial perfusion [42]. This Doppler method detects Doppler shift (using *decorrelation* techniques), therefore the display is proportional to the number of scatters that have moved or that have been destroyed (microbbubles). For this to be achieved, the equipment sends several pulses along the scan line. If a scatter detected by the first pulse has moved or has been destroyed, the second pulse detects the change after comparing both pulses. The colour depicted on the myocardium is influenced by the number of such events (more bubbles will result in greater signal amplitude). On the contrary, if there are no bubbles due to the lack of blood flow, that region is depicted without colour (Fig. 2.1).

This technique has the advantage of being highly sensitive but movement artefacts are often higher than in ultraharmonics and

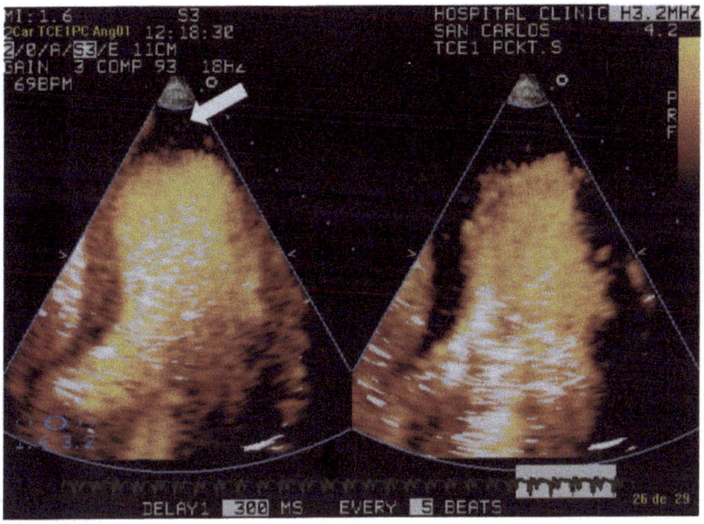

Fig. 2.1. An example of intermittent harmonic power Doppler imaging in a patient with a prior infarction. On the *left*, an apical perfusion defect is seen (*arrow*), with homogeneous contrast enhancement in the other segments in this view. On the *right*, segments are depicted without colour due to microbubble destruction in the first one

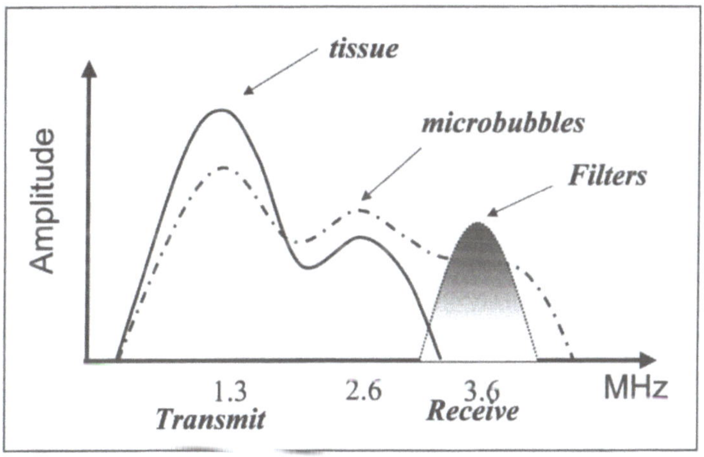

Fig. 2.2. The graphic shows that ultraharmonic signal mainly proceeds from microbubbles. The tissue harmonic signals do not include ultraharmonic frequency

more care may be required so as to minimize these potential artefacts.

Ultraharmonics

This technique also uses a high-MI, and therefore the bubbles are destroyed. When the transmission power (MI) is increased beyond the point of oscillation, the microbubbles respond directly with a transient, high-amplitude signal before they collapse. These transient signals have a broadband signal that include ultraharmonic fre-

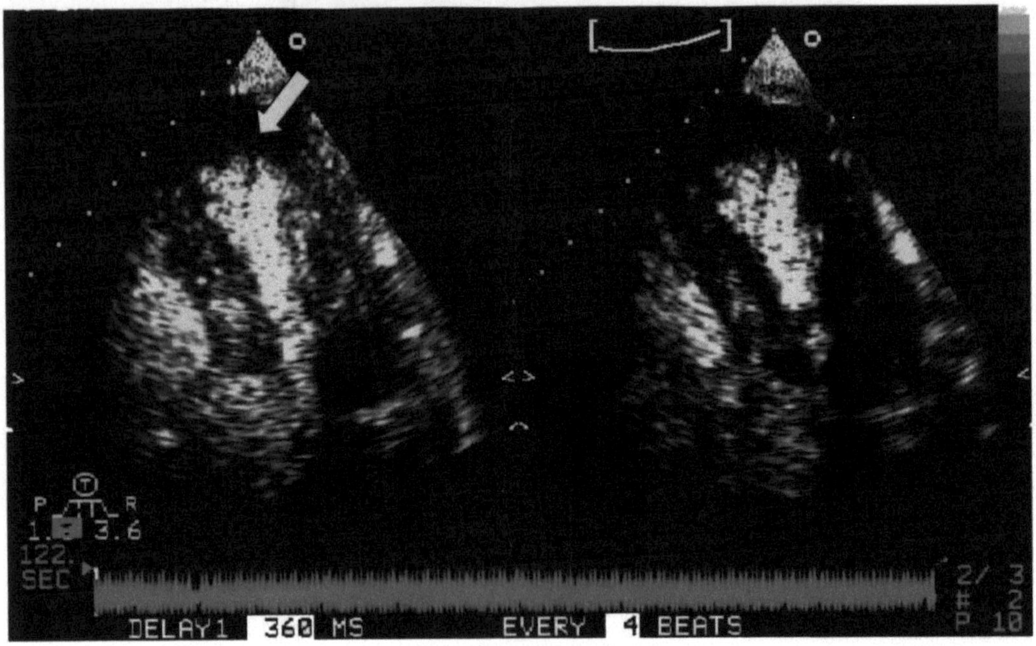

Fig. 2.3. Apical perfusion defect in a patient with anterior myocardial infarction evaluated by ultraharmonic imaging (*left*). The lack of signal in the apical wall indicates the existence of a perfusion defect (*arrow*). The other segments displayed in this view show a normal myocardial opacification. The *right image* shows an absence of microbubbles in all the segments displayed as it has been taken immediately after the microbubble destruction. When compared with the *right image*, there is no myocardial opacification because the microbubbles have been destroyed in the first one

quency (the probe emits and receives at 1.3 and 3.6 MHz respectively); therefore, the returning signal has a frequency beyond the second harmonic but below the third harmonic frequency of the incident ultrasound waves [24, 53] (Fig. 2.2).

As the tissue returns to a very low signal at the ultraharmonic frequency, the microbubbles may be detected with high sensitivity and precontrast while the myocardium appears darker (Fig. 2.3).

With this technique, images with a high frame rate and no movement artefact (since we are not using Doppler), may be obtained. However it has a lower sensitivity than harmonic angio due to the fact that fewer pulses are used per scan line. Resolution is higher than harmonic angio because of the higher receiving frequency.

Multiple Frame Triggering Image

Acquisition Protocol

After opacification of the left heart chamber by the contrast agent, two images are obtained (on the left and on the right of the screen). On the left image the myocardial display is on a grey scale (ultraharmonic) or colour (harmonic power angio) representing the presence of microbubbles. The second image, which is created shortly after the first image, displays a darker myocardium (without colour) because the microbubbles have been destroyed during the creation of the first image. Thus the second image is useful as a control. The absence of myocardial opacification confirms that the signal detected in the first image was in fact generated by microbubbles being destroyed. In contrast, the persistence of myocardial opacification suggests artefact by either high gain or tissue signals.

Low-MI Contrast Imaging

Because the microbubble behaviour depends on ultrasound acoustic power, lower-MI minimizes microbubble destruction and allows detection of backscatter signal from oscillating microbubbles at frame rates of 10–30 Hz. The techniques that use low-MI include Real-Time Imaging (power modulation, pulse inversion, coherent imaging and contrast pulse sequencing (CPC)) and Triggered Replenishment Imaging (TRI).

Real-Time Imaging

Real time imaging is a multipulse technique which uses a MI low enough to suppress tissue signal while allowing the detection of microbubble signal. However, unlike the strong signal produced by microbubble destruction, the signal at low-MI is less robust and it is often necessary to use higher doses of microbbubles which may produce attenuation in the far field. In order to allow the assessment of the regional reperfusion rate, this technique uses a flash of high-energy ultrasound pulses that destroys the microbubbles. The replenishment rate can then be qualitatively assessed or measured. Real-time imaging can be used to accurately quantify relative myocardial blood flow velocity (MFV) and myocardial blood volume (MBV) [54].

Power Modulation

Power modulation is a new technique which selectively detects backscatter signal generated by microbubbles, while suppressing reflections from cardiac structures and tissue. To accomplish this aim, the transducer sends two or more successive pulses of identical shape along each scan line, the second pulses being half of the amplitude of the first. The smaller reflection (second pulses) is multiplied by 2 and subtracted from the large one (first presses reflection). Assuming the tissue lineal behaviour at lower MI, the subtraction of the smaller pulses from the larger one results in zero signal (Fig. 2.4). On the contrary, because of the non-linear signal generated by microbubbles, the reflecting pulses would differ from each other not only in amplitude but also in their shape. As a consequence, the subtraction results would be non-zero and the contrast agent signal would be detected (Fig. 2.5). The great sensitivity of power modulation at lower MI (0.1–0.2) provides selective real time detection of microbubble signal (Fig. 2.6). This novel technique appears to be promising for the clinical assessment of myocardial perfusion. Studies with

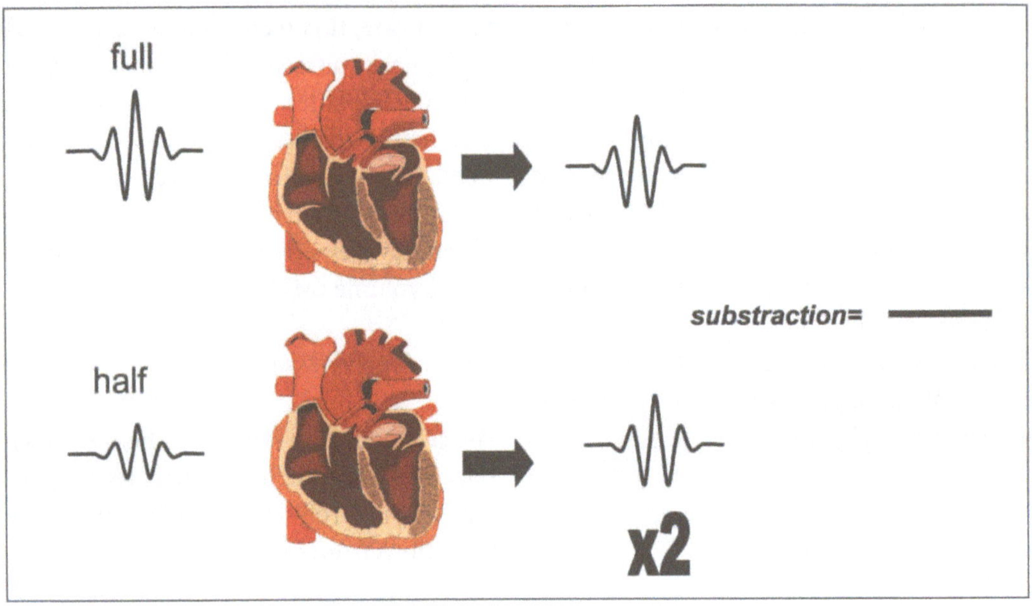

Fig. 2.4. Tissue suppression when power modulation is used. Due to the linear behaviour of cardiac tissue at low mechanical index, the subtraction of the larger pulse minus twice the smaller one results in a near complete signal elimination

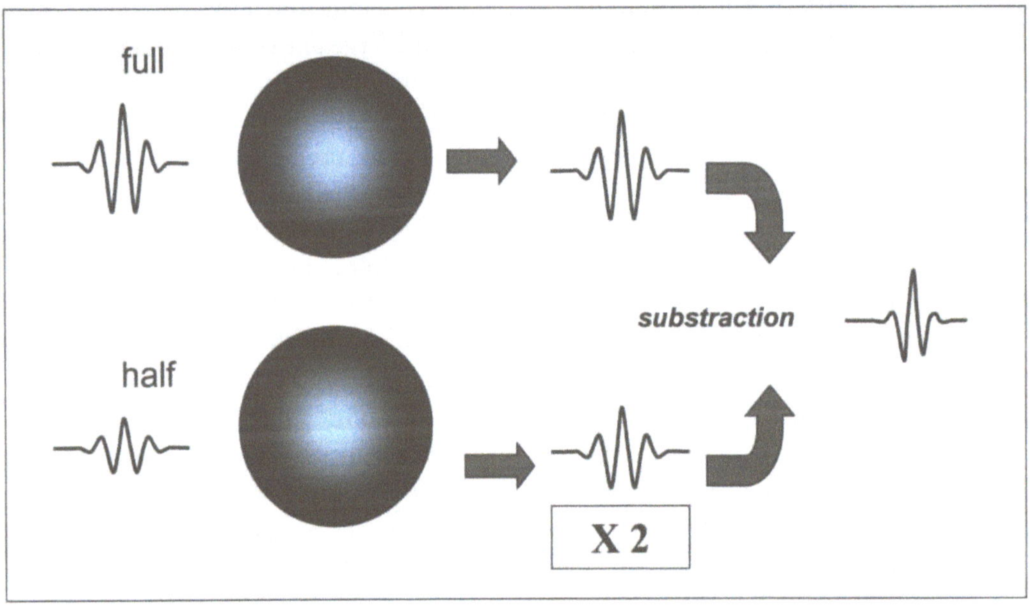

Fig. 2.5. Power modulation technique allows detection of non-linear signal from microbubbles. Two pulses are emitted, one of them being half the amplitude of the other. The reflected pulses are a compound of a fundamental signal plus a harmonic signal. Fundamental signals from both pulses are eliminated (subtraction) and only the harmonic signal remains

animals and humans have shown the feasibility of this mode in the assessment of myocardial perfusion [39, 56, 57].

Recent improvements in power modulation imaging technology in grey-scale provide advantages such as higher frame rate, better spatial and temporal resolution and more sensitivity (signal-to-noise ratio) (Fig. 2.7).

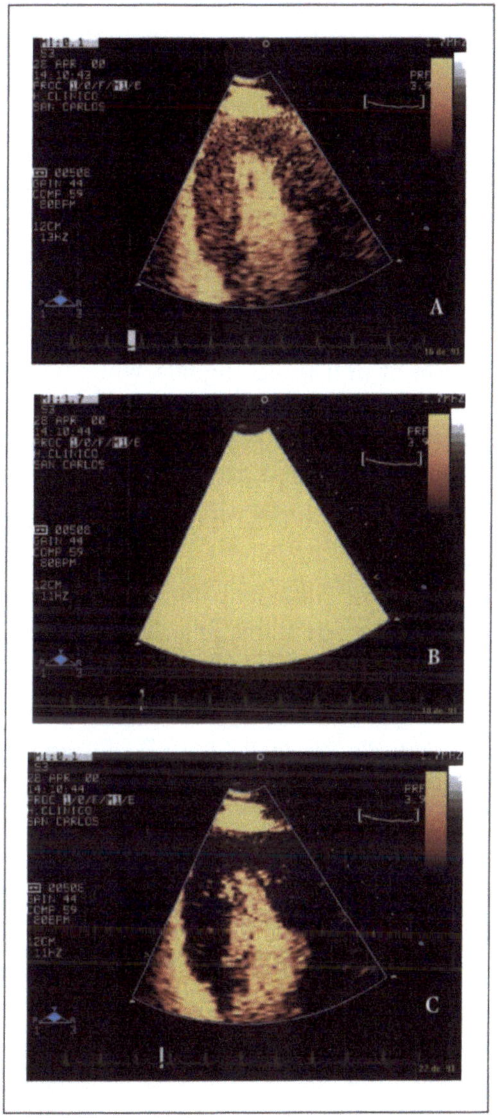

Fig. 2.6. An example of power modulation imaging (angio). **A.** Contrast enhancement is seen at low mechanical index. **B.** Impulse at high mechanical index. **C.** Myocardium depicted without color view to the microbubbles destructions with high mechanical index impulse

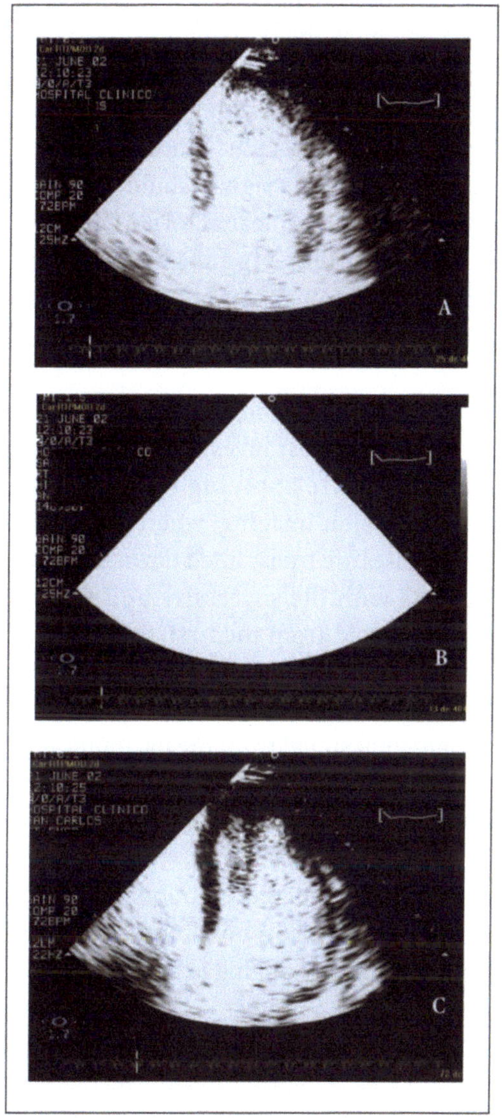

Fig. 2.7. An example of power modulation imaging using gray-scale. **A.** The segments are depicted in gray color except the apical region, where perfusion defect is seen in a patients with myocardial infarction. **B.** Impulse at high mechanical index. **C.** Myocardium without color due to the absence of microbubbles in all the segments

Pulse Inversion or Phase Inversion

Pulse inversion is another pulse cancellation technique that transmits alternatively two identical pulses per image line, each being of opposite polarity to the preceding pulses. Because the returning tissue signal at low MI (0.1) is the fundamental frequency (lineal behaviour), adding the pulses after they return from the tissue cancels the signal; therefore, the tissue signal would be eliminated because it is linear at low MI. However, the nonlinear signal generated by microbubble resonance is not cancelled, and is thereby displayed on the screen [58].

Coherent Contrast Imaging (CCI)

Until recently, most investigations on contrast agent were applying some form of phase inversion imaging; whereby two (or more) pulses are transmitted down the same scan line with the successive pulse being phase inverted from the first. By means of comparison of the datasets received along that same scan line, one could separate the fundamental signal from the harmonic signal. Although effective, there were issues related to the fact that each scan line needed to be pulsed multiple times, which reduced frame rate and increased bubble destruction. There was also a possibility for "flash" artifacts if the area being examined moved quickly between pulses.

Cadence Coherent Contrast Imaging (CCI) is a proprietary non-linear imaging technology, that provides cancellation of the fundamental signal with only a single transmit pulse. This technique provides high-resolution images in grey scale, instead of Doppler processing, eliminating many of the limitations of Doppler cancellation methods. CCI offers less bubble destruction and higher imaging frame rates due to this "single pulse cancellation" technology.

There are two specific technologies that make Coherent Contrast Imaging possible:

- *Transmit Pulse Shaping*, that enables precise control of the pulse phase and amplitude as well as the spectral shape of the pulse.
- *Single Pulse Cancellation*, a coherent imaging technology that achieves the cancellation of linear signals and detection of non-linear signals, while using only a single transmit pulse.

Coherent image processing is then applied to achieve cancellation of the linear tissue echoes similar to the Doppler cancellation methods.

Since *Single Pulse Cancellation* is only possible with coherent imaging technology, it's important to review coherent image formation, which is at the core of *Single Pulse Cancellation*. We can begin by reviewing the conventional form of image formation. As we can see in figure 2.8-A, a beam former is used to acquire phase and amplitude information by transmitting and receiving sound along a specific scan line. This information along the line is used to form a scan line, which only preserves the amplitude information of the image. The phase information is not preserved for scan conversion, so each scan line in the image is essentially phase independent of the next. To be more specific in conventional image formation, the system transmits and receives ultrasound along a discrete scan line. Processing of the phase and amplitude information received is restricted to that scan line. This is because the limited phase information acquired for each line is specific to that line and has no relationship to neighboring lines.

In Coherent Image Formation (Fig. 2.8-B) multiple beam formers are used to sample the phase and amplitude information in the image plane. There are no discrete and independent scan lines used. The phase and amplitude samples are used to define a coherent image plane of phase and amplitude information fully characterizing the image plane under study. This means that after acquiring the image data, one can arbitrarily choose any point in the coherent image plane and sufficient information is available to know exactly what the image phase and amplitude is at that point. After acquiring the phase and amplitude image samples, the next step is to coherently form the image. The revolutionary concept of a coherent image plane where all the acquired data has a definite relationship to it and is tied together (i.e. is coherent) enables coherent processing to form a coherent image. Since both phase and amplitude information is available, coherent processing uses the phase information, along with the amplitude information, to form the diagnostic image.

As in the case of conventional image formation, one still transmits and receives ultrasound, but the purpose is now to sample the image phase and amplitude in a par-

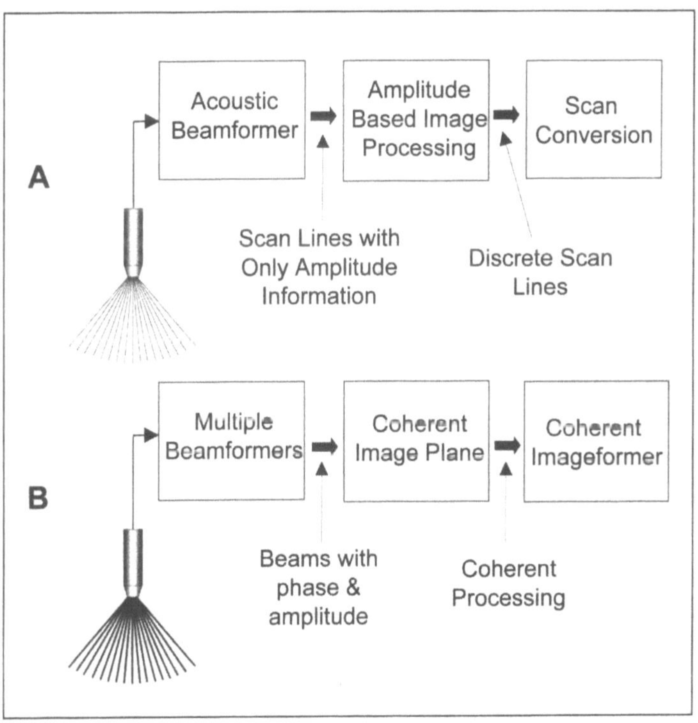

Fig. 2.8. A Conventional image formation. **B** Coherent image formation

ticular "pie" section of the image as opposed to forming a discrete scan line. Coherent processing is not limited to specific lines, but can operate across the image.

Coherent Imaging Technology achieves excellent performance and sensitivity in 2D, NTHI (Native Tissue Harmonic Imaging), Color and Contrast Imaging. When Single Pulse Cancellation is used in combination with transmit pulse shaping, these two coherent imaging technologies provide very high sensitivity to weak non-linear signals like those found in NTHI and Contrast agent imaging applications.

Single Pulse Cancellation is a paradoxical concept when viewed from a more conventional image formation standpoint, but with coherent image processing, it makes perfect sense. Let's step through a very simple example of how Single Pulse Cancellation can cancel linear tissue echoes using only a single transmit pulse in any one direction.

We start with a wideband imaging pulse and spectrum overlapping the resultant harmonic signal spectrum (Fig. 2.9). Using precise transmit pulse shaping, CCI is able to separate the fundamental and harmonic signal spectrums by shaping the transmit spectrum. In addition to removing high frequency components, other portions of the spectrum can be sharpened to effectively widen the harmonic signal spectrum making it wider band and also increase the harmonic response of contrast agents. In NTHI applications, this removal of high frequencies does not have any affect on the imaging harmonic signal spectrum, because these high frequencies are highly attenuated and fail to generate native tissue harmonics during propagation. Once the two spectra are separated, Single Pulse Cancellation is used to remove the fundamental signal.

To better understand the nature of transmit pulse shaping, we can look at actual transmit pulses and the corresponding frequency spectrum (Fig. 2.10). The pulse in the upper left is a normal imaging pulse with a fundamental and harmonic signal spectrum. By precisely adjusting the phase and amplitude of the transmit pulse, one can separate the fundamental and harmonic spectra while also increasing the overall bandwidth of the harmonic spectrum. In this manner, transmit pulse shaping enables very wide bandwidth harmonic imaging. Once the fun-

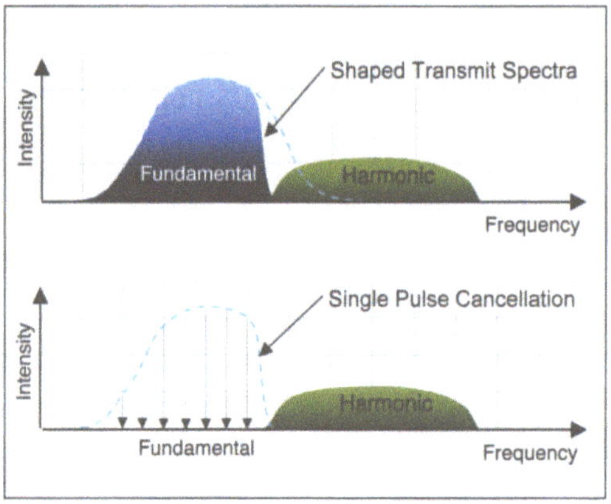

Fig. 2.9. Single Pulse Cancellation. This picture shows how Single Pulse Cancellation can cancel linear tissue echoes using only a single transmit pulse in any one direction. We start with a wideband imaging pulse and spectrum overlapping the resultant harmonic signal spectrum. Using precise transmit pulse shaping, Acuson is able to separate the fundamental and harmonic signal spectrums. In addition to removing high frequency components, other portions of the spectrum can be sharpened to widen the harmonic signal spectrum. Once the two spectra are separated, Single Pulse Cancellation is used to remove the fundamental signal

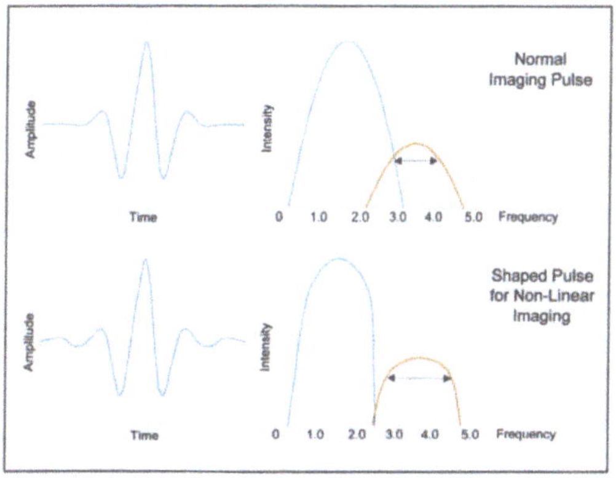

Fig. 2.10. Transmit pulse shaping. To better understand the nature of transmit pulse shaping, we can look at actual transmit pulses and the corresponding frequency spectrum. The pulse in the upper left is a normal imaging pulse with a fundamental and harmonic signal spectrum. By adjusting the phase and amplitude of the transmit pulse, one can separate the fundamental and harmonic spectra while also increasing the overall bandwidth of the harmonic spectrum. In this manner, transmit pulse shaping enables very wide bandwidth harmonic imaging

damental and harmonic spectra are separated, Single Pulse Cancellation is used.

Single Pulse Cancellation (Fig. 2.11) begins with a broadened transmit pulse (with a positive phase) that insonifies a pie section of the image plane. Next, a negative phase pulse is transmitted in a direction adjacent to the previous transmit pulse. Once this is completed, we have image samples, in the coherent image plane, corresponding to a positive phase pulse and also corresponding to a negative phase pulse.

Using coherent processing, we can achieve single pulse cancellation of the linear response over the entire region between the two transmit pulses.

We are also able to detect the non-linear response to coherently form the harmonic image. Single Pulse Cancellation is continued across the image with successive pulses using alternating phase. For each transmit pulse, there is another region over which we complete single pulse cancellation.

As with other cancellation techniques, motion in the image can cause incomplete cancellation of the fundamental signal spectrum (Fig. 2.12). However, since transmit pulse shaping was used previously to separate the signal spectra, there is no overlap, no flash artifact and no need to use a complex Doppler wall filter. A simple (frequency domain) filter can be used to remove the

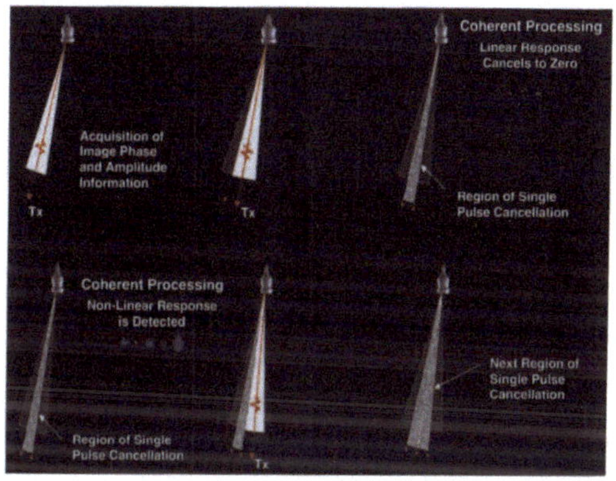

Fig. 2.11. Single Pulse Cancellation begins with a broadened transmit pulse (with a positive phase) that insonifies a pie section of the image plane. Next a negative phase pulse is transmitted in a direction adjacent to the previous transmit pulse. Once this is completed, we have image samples, corresponding to a positive phase pulse and also corresponding to a negative phase pulse. Using coherent processing, we can achieve single pulse cancellation of the linear response over the entire region between the two transmit pulses. We are also able to detect the non-linear response to coherently form the harmonic image. Single Pulse Cancellation is continued across the image with successive pulses using alternating phases. For each transmit pulse, there is another region over which we complete single pulse cancellation

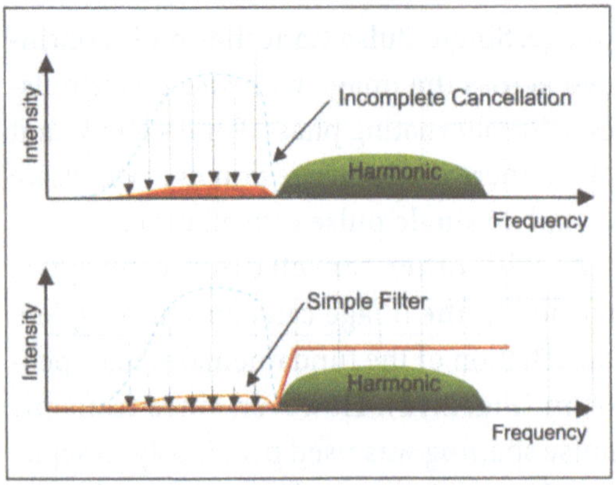

Fig. 2.12. Coherent contrast imaging. Motion in the image can cause incomplete cancellation in the fundamental signal spectrum. However, since transmit pulse shaping was used to separate the signal spectra, there is no overlap, no flash artifact and no need to use a complex Doppler wall filter. A simple (frequency domain) filter can be used to remove the motion noise without requiring any additional transmit pulses

motion noise without requiring any additional transmit pulses as often required in Doppler pulse cancellation methods.

Contrast Pulse Sequencing (CPS)

Contrast pulse sequencing (CPS) is a new, real time, non-linear imaging technique for contrast agent studies. It provides an easy maintenance of the 2D image plane mixing simultaneously myocardial contrast echocardiography with the wall motion evaluation based on a strong detection of non-linear fundamental and harmonic energy. The image, optimised for low mechanical index, shows and echo-free non-contrast myocardium that increases in intensity and textural appearance as contrast is detected, with real-time perfusion frame rates.

CPS technology is based on receiving multiple pulses per image line while precisely controlling, simultaneously, the phase and amplitude of the transmitted and received signals. The unique pulse sequences allow detection of non-linear fundamental energy and higher order harmonic energy. It detects all non-linear responses and rejects linear responses.

Because the non-linear fundamental response from the contrast agent is much stronger than their harmonic responses (Fig. 2.13), CPS processing utilizes all non-linear responses; fundamental and higher orders harmonics to produce high sensitivity contrast agent images with excellent agent-to-tissue specificity at very low mechanical index (0.16-0.23). With this approach, it can enhance agent detection while preserving bubble life.

Non-linear fundamental energy provides advantages over inversion techniques, for example it improves sensitivity and penetration, which are based on detecting only 2nd harmonic energy.

With the CPS technology we can work at two frequency options, P1.5 and P 2MHz (improved detail resolution), and we can choose three different display options: contrast only (CA), contrast and fundamental tissue imaging (Mix) and only fundamental 2D tissue image (2D).

Compare with CCI technology, Cadence CPS has more sensitivity, specificity and penetration (Fig. 2.14). CPS allows easy transition of wall motion analysis and MCE. This new technology increases agent preservation and thus contrast agent MCE dosing requirements are less, especially with SonoVue, (currently available in Europe). The benefit of CPS over standard pulse cancellation studies (CCI) is important in patients with poor acoustic

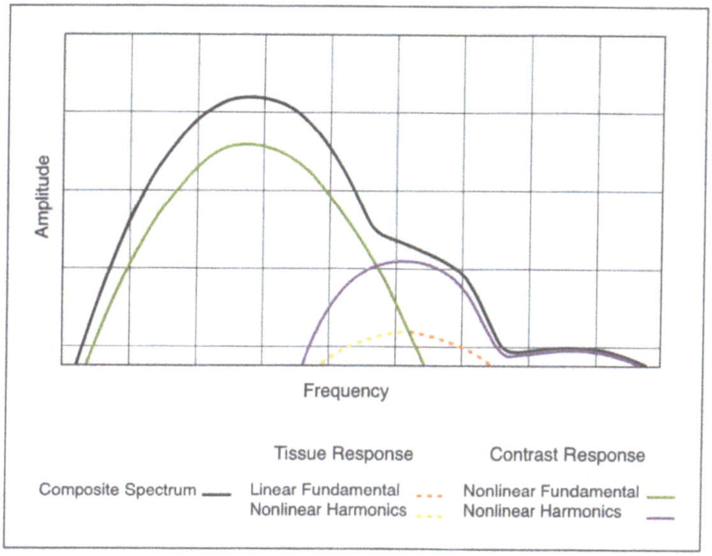

Fig. 2.13. Cadence Contrast Pulse Sequencing (CPS) is a real time, non-linear imaging technique based on receiving multiple pulses per image line while precisely controlling, simultaneously, the phase and amplitude of the transmitted and received signals. Because the non-linear fundamental response from contrast agent is much stronger than its harmonic responses, CPS processing utilizes all non-linear responses; fundamental and higher orders harmonics, to produce high sensitivity contrast agent images with excellent agent-to-tissue specificity at very low mechanical index

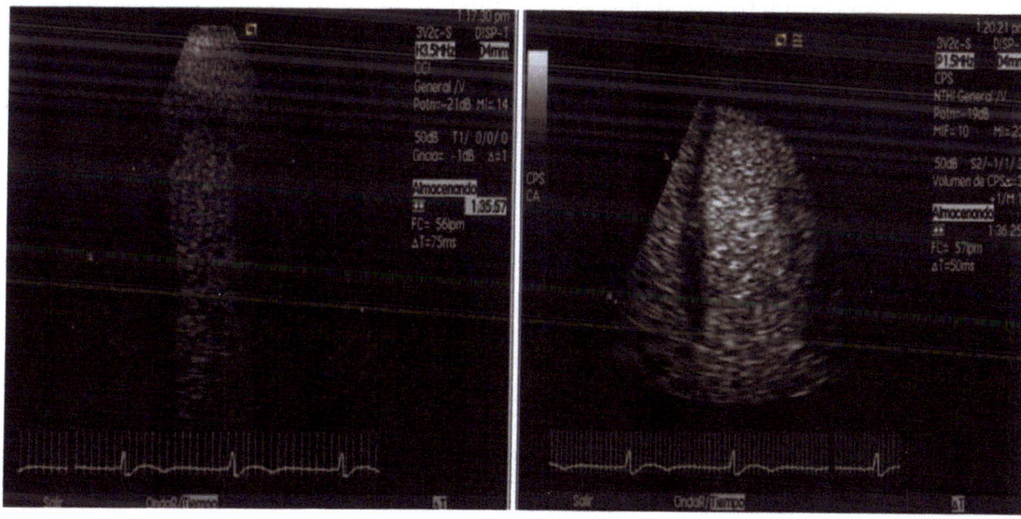

Fig. 2.14. This picture shows MCE images in the same patient performed with CCI technology in the left and CPS technology in the right. Compare with CCI, Cadence CPS has more sensitivity, specificity and penetration, which is more evident, like in this case, when the patient has a poor acoustic window. CPS allows also a better delineation of endocardial border

windows, especially in apex and inferior wall.

CPS overcomes the limitations of current "singular" methodologies, reducing motion artefacts and increasing sensitivity to contrast agents (Fig. 2.15), while maintaining a higher frame rate.

The B mode imaging is performed using fundamental imaging, with a transmit frequency of 1.5 or 2 MHz. The dynamic range is 50dB, Space/ Time, of S1, 0 Edge, O persistence and a post processing of 0. The Delta setting used is 3. The mechanical index is decreased to 0.22. Before commencing the infusion of SonoVue, the B-mode overall gain is decreased until only no information is visible on the screen in the CA mode and the equalize gain is activated. The DGC is adjusted to obtain a diagonal curve from left to right.

The micro bubble destruction phase is carried out by entering in Colour Doppler microbubble destruction (MBD) mode. Time triggers are employed to allow specific control of frame rates and minimise micro bubble destruction. Time triggers are set at 50 milliseconds. Regional Expansion Selection (RES) is also used to increase resolution and overall quality of the B-mode image.

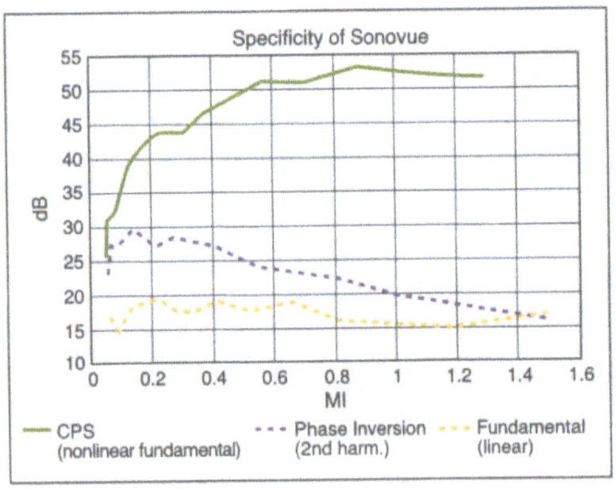

Fig. 2.15. CPS overcomes the limitations of current "singular" methodologies, increasing sensitivity to contrast agents

Triggered Replenishment Imaging

Until recently, the protocols of intermittent imaging required gate acquisition up to one frame for multiple cardiac cycles because the use of high MI involves bubble destruction. Triggered replenishment imaging (TRI) is an acquisition mode with the pulsing interval at every heart beat (1:1) during telesystole and does not involve bubbles destruction because it uses a lower MI (0.3).

Conclusions

Understanding the behaviour of the microbubbles when they interact with the ultrasound as well as knowledge of the differences in the properties of the various contrast agents provide the basis for the correct selection of applications.

There are several methods for evaluating myocardial perfusion by echo contrast imaging. When deciding which method to use, one must take into account the aim of the study, the patient's characteristics, as well as the type of contrast agent and its method of administration. In the next few years we expect to see a practical development in all these techniques so that we may incorporate them into our daily clinical practice. The continuous search for new alternative tools for clinical applications is very promising.

References

1. Villarraga H, Foley D, Chung S, et al. Harmonic imaging during contrast echocardiography: basic principles and potential clinical value. In Kluwer Academic Publishers(ed). Advances In echo imaging using contrast enhancement 2nd ed. Nanda N, Schlief R, and Goldberg B.1997:433-450
2. Spencer K, Berdnarz J, Rafter P, et al. Use of harmonic imaging without echocardiographic contrast to improve two-dimensional image quality. Am J Cardiol 1998;82(6):794-799
3. Caidahl K, Kazzam E, Lidberg J, et al. New concept in echocardiography: harmonic imaging of tissue without use of contrast agent. The Lancet 1998;352(9136):1264-70
4. Carerj S, Trono A, Zito C, et al. The second tissue harmonic signal: from physics principles to clinical aplication. Ital Heart J 2001;2(10 suppl):1078-86
5. Karsprzak J, Paelinck B, Folkert J, et al. Comparison of native and contrast-enhanced harmonic echocardiography for visualization of lef ventricular border. Am J Cardiol 1998;83(2):211-217
6. Kornbluth M, Liang D, Paloma A, Schnittger I. Native tissue harmonic imaging improves endocardial border definition and visualization of cardiac structures. J Am Soc Echocardiogr 1998;11:693-701
7. Senior R, Soman P, Khattar RS, and Lahiri A. Improved endocardial visualization with second harmonic imaging compared with fundamental two dimensional echocardiographic imaging. Am Heart J 1999;138(1Pt1):163-8
8. Skolnick D, Sawada S, Feingenbaum H, and Segar S. Enhanced endocardial visualization with noncontrast harmonic imaging during stress echocardiography. J Am Soc Echocardiogr 1999;12(7):559-63
9. Gramiak R, Shah PM. Echocardiography of the aortic root. Invest Radiol 1968;3:356-366
10. Feinstein SB, Ten Cate FJ, Zwehl W et al. Two dimensional contrast echocardiography. In vitro development and quantitative analysis of eho contrast agent. J Am Coll Cardiol 1984;3:14
11. Porter T, Xiei F, Kilzer K: intravenous perfluoropropane-exposed sonicated dextrose albumin produces myocardial ultrasound contrast that correlates with coronary blood flow. J Am Soc Echocardiogr 1995;8(5Pt1):710-718
12. Cheng S, Dy T, and Feintein S. Contrast echocardiography: Review and future directions. Am J Cardiol 1998;81(12A):41G-48G
13. Firschke C, Lindner J, Wei K, et al: Myocardial perfusion imaging in the setting of coronary artery stenosis and acute myocardial infarction using venous injection of a second generation echocardiographic contrast agent. Circulation 1997;96(3):959-67
14. Skyba DM, Camarano G, Goodman NC, et al: Hemodynamic characteristics, myocardial kinetics and microvascular rheology of FS-069, a second generation echocardiographic contrast agent capable of producing myocardial opacification from a venous injection. J Am Coll Cardiol 1996;28:1292-300
15. DeMaria AN, Bommer WJ, Riggs K et al. Echocardiography visualization of myocardial perfusion by left heart and intracoronary injections of echo contrast agents (abstr). Circulation 1980 ;62(suppl II):143
16. Lindner J. Evolving applications for contrast ultrasound. Am J Cardiol 2002;90(suppl):72J-80J
17. Burns PN, Powers JE, Simpson DH , et al. Harmonic imaging: principles and preliminary results. Clin Radiol 1996;51(suppl):50-5
18. Porter TR, Xie F, Kricsfeld D et al. Improved myocardial contrast with second harmonic transient ultrasound response imaging in humans using intravenous perflorocarbon-exposed sonicated dextrose albumin. J Am Coll Cardiol 1996;27:1497-501
19. Kaul S: myocardial contrast echocardiography. Curr Probl Cardiol 1997; 22:549-640
20. De Jong N, Frinking PJ, Bouakaz A, et al. Optical imaging of contrast agent microbubbles in an ultrasound field with a 100-MHz camera. Ultrasound Med Biol 2000;26(3):487-92
21. Forsberg F, Shi W and Goldberg B. Subharmonic imaging of contrast agents. Ultrasonics 2000;38(1-8):93-8
22. Chomas J, Dayton P, May D, and Ferrara K, Nondestructive subharmonic imaging. IEEE Trans Ultrason Ferroelectr Freq Control 2002;49(7):883-92
23. Calliada F, Campani R, Bottinelli O, and Sommaruga MG Ultrasound contrast agents: basic principles. Eur J Radiol 1998;27 suppl 2:S157-60
24. Kuersten B, Murthy T, Li P, et al. Ultraharmonic myocardial contrast imaging. In vivo experimental and clinical data from a novel technique.J Am Soc Echocardiogr 2001;14:910-6
25. Lindner J Contrast echocardiography. Curr Probl Cardiol 2002;27:449-520
26. Raisinghani A and DeMaria A. Physical principles of microbubbles ultrasound contrast agents. Am J Cardiol 2002;90(suppl 10 A):3J-7J
27. Leong Poi H, Song J, Rim SJ, et al. Influence of microbubble properties on ultrasound signal: implications for low-power perfusion imaging. J Am Soc Echocardiogr 2002;15(10 Pt 2):1269-76.
28. Michel Schneider. Design of an ultrasound contrast agent for myocardial perfusion. Echocardiography 2000;17(6 pt2):S11-S16
29. Villanueva FS, Jankowski RJ, Manaugh C, Wagner WR. Albumin microbubble adherence to human

coronary endothelium: implications for assessment of endothelial function using myocardial contrast echocardiography. J Am Coll Cardiol 1997;30:689-93
30. Fisher NG, Christiansen JP, Klibanov A, et al. Influence of microbubbles surface charge on capillary transit and myocardial contrast enhancement. J Am Coll Cardiol 2002;40(4):811-9
31. Porter TR, Xie F: Visually discernible myocardial echocardiographyc contrast after intravenous injection of sonicated dextrose albumin microbubbles containing high molecular weight, less soluble gases. J Am Coll Cardiol 1995;25(2):509-515
32. Wei K, Skyba D, Firschke C, et al. Interaction between microbubbles and ultrasound: in vitro and in vivo observations. J Am Coll Cardiol 1997;29(5):1081-1088
33. De Jong N, Bouakaz A, Ten Cate FJ. Contrast harmonic imaging. Ultrasonics 2002;40(1-8):567-73
34. Von Bibra H, Sutherland G, Becher H , et al. Clinical evaluation of left heart Doppler contrast enhancement by a saccharide-based transpulmonary contrast agent. The Levovist Cardiac Working Group. J Am Coll Cardioll 1995;25(2):500-508
35. Porter TR, Xie F, Kricsfeld et al: improved endocardial border resolution during dobutamine stress echocardiography with intravenous sonicated dextrose albumin. J Am Coll Cardiol 1994;23 (6):1440-1443
36. Moreno R, Zamorano J, Almería C et al. Usefulness of contrast agents in the diagnosis of left venticular pseudoaneurysm after acute myocardial infarction. Eur J Echocardiogr 2002;3(2):111-6
37. Zamorano J, Sanchez V, Moreno R, et al. Contrast agents provide a faster learning curve in dipyridamole stress echocardiography. Int J cardiovasc imaging 2002;18(6):415-9
38. Heinle S, Noblin J, Goree-Best P, et al. Assessment of Myocardial Perfusion by Harmonic Power Doppler Imaging at Rest and During Adenosine Stress. Comparison with ^{99m} Tc Sestamibi SPECT Imaging. Circulation 2000;102:55-60
39. Moreno R, Zamorano J, Serra V, et al. Weak concordance between wall motion and microvasculature status after acute myocardial infarction. Study with myocardial contrast echocardiography in real time with power modulation. Eur J Echocardiogr 2002;3:89-94
40. Porter TR, Xie F, Kricsfeld A, et al. Reduction in left ventricular attenuation and improvement in posterior myocardial contrast with high molecular weight intravenous perfluorocarbon-exposed sonicated dextrose albumin microbubbles. J Am Soc Echocardiogr 1996;9:437-441
41. Witt S. Implementing microbubble contrast in the echocardiography laboratory: a sonographer's perpective. Am J Cardiol 2002;90(supp);15j-16j
42. Senior R, Kaul S, Soman P and Lahiri A. Power Doppler harmonic imaging: a feasibility study of a new technique for the assessment of myocardial perfusion. Am Heart J 2000;139:245-51
43. Schneider M, Arditi M, Barrau M-B, et al. BR1: A new ultrasonographic contrast agent based on sulfur hexafluoride-filled microbubbles. Invest Radiol 1995;30(8):451-457
44. Morel D, Schwieger I, Hohn L, et al. Human Pharmacokinetics and safety evaluation of SonoVue™, a new contrast agent for ultrasound imaging. Invest Radiol 2000;35(1):80-85
45. Senior R, Andersson O, Caidahl K, et al. Enhanced left ventricular endocardial border delineation with an intravenous injection of SonoVue, a new echocardigraphic contrast agent: a European multicenter study. Echocardiogr 2000;17(8):705-11
46. Broillet A, Puginier J, Ventrone R, and Schneider M. Assessment of myocardial perfusion by intermittent harmonic power Doppler using SonoVue, a new ultrasound contrast agent. Invest Radiol 1998;33(4):209-215
47. Bokor D. Diagnostic efficacy of SonoVue. Am J Cardiol 2000;86(suppl):19G-24G
48. Kuersten B, Nahar T, and Vannan m. Methods of contrast administration for myocardial perfusion imaging: continuous infusion versus bolus injection. Am J Cardiol 2002;90(suppl):35j-37j
49. Wei K, Jayaweera A, Firoozan S, et al. Basis for detection of stenosis using venous administration of microbubbles during myocardial contrast echocardiography: bolus or continuous infusion? J Am Coll Cardiol 1998;32(1):252-260
50. Mayer s and Grayburn P. Myocardial contrast agents: recent advances and future directions. Progress in cardiovascular diseases 2001;44(1):33-44
51. Wei K, Ragosta M, Thorpe J et al. Noninvasive quantification of coronary blood flow reserve in humans using myocardial contrast echocardiography. Circularion 2001;103:2560
52. Rubin J, Bude R, Carson P et al. Power Doppler US: a potentially useful alternative to mean frequency-based colour Doppler US. Radiology 1994;190(3):853-6
53. Moreno R, -Zamorano JL, Serra V, et al. Evaluation of myocardial perfusion with grey-scale Ultra-harmonic and multiple-frame triggering. Is there a need for quantification. Int J Cardiol 2003. In press
54. Poi H, Le E, Rim S-J, et al. Quantification of myocardial perfusion and determination of coronary stenosis severity during hyperemia using real-time myocardial contrast echocardiography. J Am Soc Echocardiogr 2001;14:1173-82

55. Kaul S. Myocardial contrast echocardiography: basic principles. Progress in Cardiovascular Diseases 2001;44(1):1-11
56. Mor-Avi V, Caiani E, Collins K, et al. Combined assessment of myocardial perfusion and regional left ventricular function by analysis of contrast-enhanced power modulation images. Circulation 2001;104:352
57. Moreno R, Zamorano JL, Serra V, et al. Myocardial perfusion in real-time using Power Modulation. Evidence for a microvasculature damage after acute myocardial infarction. Int J Cardiol 2003. In press
58. Masugata H, Peters B, Lafitte S, et al. Quantitative assessment of myocardial perfusion during graded coronary stenosis by real-time myocardial contrast echo refilling curves. J Am Coll cardiol 2001;37:262-9
59. Desco M, Ledesma-Carbrugo MJ, Santos A, García-Fernández MA, Marcos-Alberca P, Malpica N, Antoranz C, García-Barreno P. Coherent contrast imaging quantification for myocardial perfusion assessment. J Am Cold Cardiol 2001;37(suppl):495A

Chapter 3

Organization of the Contrast Echocardiography Laboratory: Tips and Tricks

Teresa López Fernández • Esther Pérez David • Mar Moreno Yangüela
José Luis Zamorano • Miguel Angel García Fernández

Introduction

Recently, developments and advances have been made in echocardiography so as to improve the diagnostic evaluation of cardiac structures and function. Among these new innovations during the last decade, the use of contrast echocardiography (CE) has gained great interest because it can provide, non-invasively, new information about coronary microcirculation and myocardial perfusion. Started in 1968, with the use of hand-agitated saline as a source of ultrasonic contrast, CE was based on the concept of creating a gas–blood interface for enhancement of blood within the heart [1]. By injecting small amounts of physiologically safe microbubbles for visualization of tissues and chambers, a new level of physiological imaging has been developed.

The delay in the application of this technique was caused by complications concerning stability, inherent in the volatile nature of the bubbles. Fortunately, the stability of the bubbles has improved recently with the use of gases with a low level of diffusion instead of air. On the other hand, improvement of contrast agents that are able to pass the pulmonary microcirculation and reach the left ventricle and the coronary arteries after intravenous administration has been essential in the spreading of this technique.

Moreover, it is important to emphasize that, with the introduction of second harmonic imaging, it has become possible to obtain good-quality images of myocardial perfusion. Because these images are acquired and displayed in the same format as conventional echocardiography, myocardial contrast echocardiography (MCE) offers the possibility to assess functionality and perfusion simultaneously.

Specific requirements are necessary in an echocardiography-laboratory interested in clinical application of contrast echo. Different methodologies and techniques have been developed, which are essential for standardization in contrast administration and image acquisition, for a correct interpretation of contrast echo studies. Among the determining factors for obtaining greater imaging quality we can include an adequate system set-up. As much for the cardiologist as for the nurse, some previous training is required before getting accustomed to this technique. In this chapter, the echo laboratory organization will be discussed, with special emphasis on contrast agent administration and protocols for acquisition imaging.

Echocardiographic Equipment Settings

Contrast echocardiography is the only clinical imaging technique in which the imaging modality can cause a change in the contrast agent [2]. A gas bubble is highly compliant and therefore it contracts when the pressure rises and expands when the pressure is lowered [3-5]. Thus, unlike tissue, a bubble does not scatter in the same way if it is exposed to weak sound than to high amplitude. The signal from the bubbles depends on the degree of change the bubble undergoes and on its durability. Thus, contrast imaging cannot be performed effectively without a basic understanding of this interaction and how it is exploited by the new imaging modes.

Echocardiographic equipment settings are patient, agent and system dependent. Figure 3.1 shows the most important settings that we need to adjust before initiating

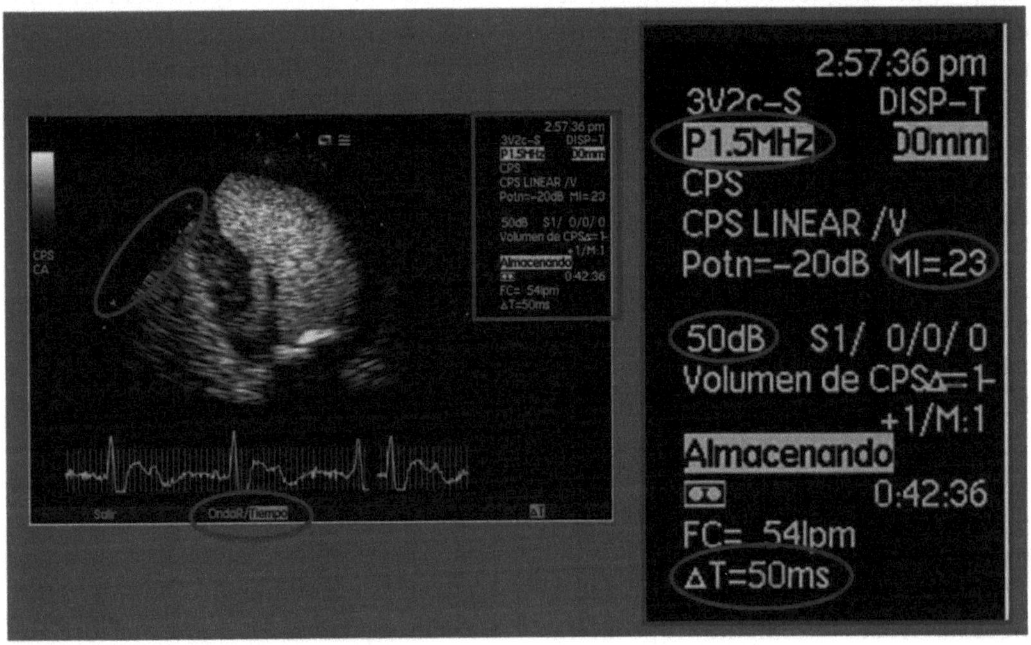

Fig. 3.1. The most important settings that we need to control before initiating a contrast echocardiography study. ▸: Focus position; P1.5MHz: ultrasound transmit frequency; MI = 0.23: mechanical index; 50 dB: dynamic range; ΔT = 50ms: triggering mode; Δ = 1: degree of contrast resolution (Delta); receive gain; S1: space/time; 0/0/0: edge/persistence/postprocessing

a contrast echocardiographic study. Ultrasound scanners carry an on-screen label of the estimated pressure to which tissue is exposed, termed *mechanical index* (MI). In absence of attenuation, the mechanical index is maximum in the focus of the beam, and decreases with increasing depth and towards the sector edges. In a clinical ultrasound system, this index usually lies somewhere between 0.1 and 2.0. Because imaging quality is proportional to mechanical index, conventional echocardiography usually operates with the maximum output power. However, when we use a contrast agent it is necessary to achieve an equilibrium between imaging quality and contrast agent durability and we need to work at a lower mechanical index.

Adjusting the *image depth* and the *RES® function* (regional expansion selection) we can increase or decrease the field of view, and in most cases ameliorate the resolution of the region that we need to study. The *focus* position determines the line in which the system concentrates the ultrasound beam. New technologies incorporate a double focus position, which allows a more homogeneous distribution of bubble destruction, avoiding some attenuation artefacts.

The *emission frequency* determines the behaviour of bubbles, and only with certain transmit intensities does bubble backscatter begin to show non-linear characteristics, such as the emission of harmonics. Overall echocardiographic equipment with contrast software works in the 1.5–2–MHz range. During the study it is indispensable to regulate the overall 2-D *gain* so as to receive the image with a suitable bright intensity. It is also important to maintain a uniform and high-level *dynamic range*, because if we reduce it, the echo intensity signal turns towards black and it is very difficult to distinguish structures or quantify perfusion.

Other important settings are: *space/time* that controls the balance between spatial resolution and temporal resolution; *edge* function varies the degree of sharpness of borders and thus lower edge levels produce a less detailed image; *persistence* smoothens the image changes over time, and the *post-processing* curves are used to define the relationship between the echo amplitude and the displayed grey level. With the CPS technology, we usually perform the myocardial contrast studies with a higher temporal resolution (S1), edge 0 (sharper image), persistence 0 and post-processing 0.

Finally, myocardial contrast echocardiographic images can be acquired in real-time or with different *triggering modes*, performed with R-wave ECG-triggering or time-triggering settings (mseg). Both methods are equal in their ability to identify coronary stenosis and quantify altered myocardial blood flow [6, 7]. Triggered imaging increases the prevalence of bubbles and results in more effective detection of ultrasound contrast [8, 9], but with this method the dynamic character of the echocardiographic examination cannot be used. If the mechanical index is set low enough, the image acquisition can be continuously performed, and real-time data on both wall motion and perfusion can be obtained [10]. Independently of the chosen method, myocardial contrast echocardiography is based on the comparison between the baseline images without contrast and the images heightened with contrast. Differents studies confirm that the duration of the *destructive pulse* is essential for obtaining a good imaging quality. The longer the destructive pulse, the closer the post-destructive pulse is to the true baseline, and thus we can improve the quantification methods [11].

Contrast echocardiography quality is dependent on the quantity and rate of the injected/infused contrast agent and proper adjustment of the ultrasound system settings. In reality, the manufacturer's recommended settings for contrast echocardiograms are only guidelines; the image itself dictates the appropriateness of the settings.

Contrast Agent Administration

Most contrast agents consist of free gas or encapsulated gas microbubbles, but their composition is quite heterogeneous. This implies that pharmacokinetic and acoustic properties can also be quite dissimilar, and different contrast agents injected at different pressures or volumes, in a certain contrast software, may require different doses, dilutions or infusion rates. The signal amplitude of contrast echocardiography is related to the microbubble properties and stability [12].

Regarding the use of echocardiographic contrast for left ventricular opacification, both bolus and infusion administrations are effective, although in specific clinical circumstances, one may be preferred over the other [13].

Bolus Infusion

A bolus administration of contrast entails an intravenous injection of a small amount of contrast over a period of 20–30s, followed by a flush using normal saline solution. An infusion of contrast may involve administration of contrast diluted in normal saline solution at a prescribed rate.

When a bolus injection of microbubbles is performed, via the intra-aortic or intracoronary route, it produces a rapid increase in signal intensity in the myocardium until a plateau is reached, followed by a decay function, defined as the time intensity curve (Fig. 3.2) [14]. Different parameters extracted from this curve are able to estimate the mean myocardial transit time and myocardial blood volume. Mean myocardial transit time correlates with myocardial blood flow, when coronary blood volume is held constant. In the same way, if myocardial blood flow is held constant, the changes in mean myocardial transit time reflect changes in coronary blood volume. It is on this basis that non-critical stenosis (where coronary blood volume increases) can be detected at rest. However, mean myocardial transit times cannot be obtained from time intensity curves derived from an intravenous injection, since the bolus injection is dispersed by intrapulmonary filtering. Therefore, with intravenous injections, myocardial blood volume (peak intensity) can be estimated but it is not possible to quantify myocardial blood flow [15].

Regardless of the route of injection, an accurate definition of bubble concentration

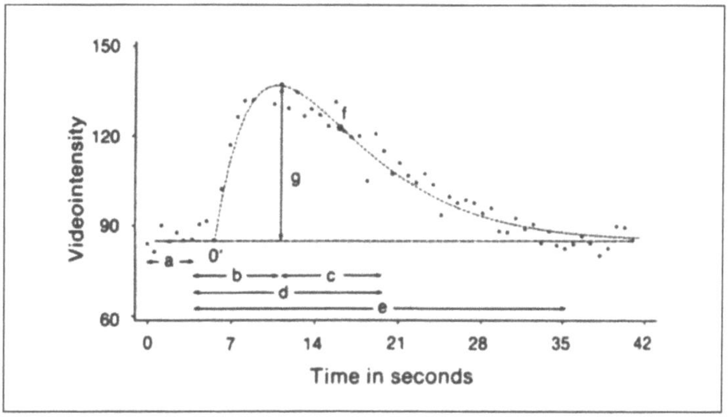

Fig. 3.2. This curve shows the different parameters that we can measure after intra-aortic or intracoronary injection of echocardiographic contrast:
a: time for injection to appearance of contrast agent in the myocardium; *b:* time from appearance of contrast agent in the myocardium to peak contrast agent effect; *c:* half-life of contrast agent in the myocardium; *d:* time from appearance of contrast agent in the myocardium to half of maximal contrast agent effect; *e:* time from appearance to disappearance of contrast agent from the myocardium; *f:* 2/a, which are derived from the curve fit shown by the dotted line; *g:* peak amplitude of contrast agent (Reproduced from [14])

in the myocardium requires that the relationship between the concentration and the signal intensity be linear. This precondition is fulfilled at low intramyocardial bubble concentration. With bolus injection, transient high concentrations can be reached even in regions with reduced myocardial blood flow because echocardiographic systems reach a saturation point, where video intensity is no longer proportional to the microbubble concentration. It is not until the microbubble concentration falls, during the washout period, that differences in microbubble concentration are visually evident. This is the point where there is a linear relationship between concentration and signal intensity and that analysis of perfusion should be performed with bolus injections [16]. However, optimal bolus injection cannot be predicted because myocardial video intensity is influenced by a whole host of factors, including cardiac output and the inhomogeneity of the ultrasound field. In addition, bolus injection does not allow the measurement of myocardial volume because a steady state is required to calculate this measurement.

Continuous Peripheral Venous Infusion

The difficulties arising from the thresholding effect and saturation point of echocardiographic systems can be partially avoided by using a continuous peripheral venous infusion of microbubbles instead of a bolus injection [17, 18]. This method assumes a constant input of microbubbles into the myocardium, thus reducing attenuation artefacts. During continuous infusion, the rate can be adjusted to prevent shadowing from excessive left ventricular microbubble concentration and also to maintain the myocardial video intensity within the detection and attenuation thresholds for a prolonged period [19] (Fig. 3.3). Moreover, the contrast dosage administered can easily be adjusted to the individual imaging conditions of different patients [20].

With a continuous venous infusion we can achieve a semi-quantitative assessment of myocardial blood flow. After contrast administration, a high mechanical index is used, which results in almost complete bubble destruction with every pulse. Triggering at a sequence of incrementally longer cardiac cycles allows a replenishment of contrast agent corresponding to a flow to the given region during that time sequence. The longer the triggering intervals are set, the more bubbles fill up the capillaries and the higher the signal intensity until finally a plateau phase is reached. To this point, the signal intensity of a given myocardial region is related to the cross-sectional capillary area. The rate at which this plateau is achieved (slope) is proportional to the blood flow velocity in that region [21] (Fig. 3.4). Since the peak background-subtracted myocardial video intensity is directly related to the capillary cross-sectional area, the slope time's peak or plateau myocardial video intensity represents a measure of myocardial blood flow. The most important problem is incomplete destruction of the bubbles which leads to a significant underestimation of myocardial blood flow abnormalities [22].

In addition, there are practical reasons

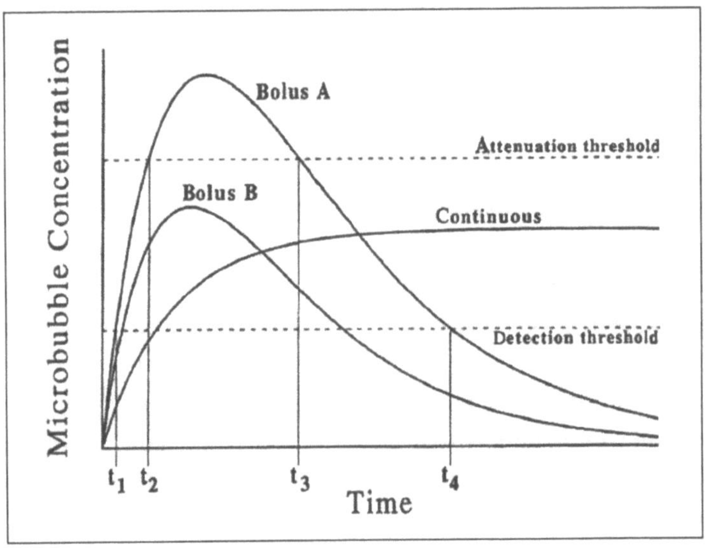

Fig. 3.3. Differences between continuous infusion and bolus injections in optimal myocardial opacification. T_2-T_1 and T_4-T_3 represent intervals during which optimal myocardial opacification can be achieved with bolus (Reproduced from [20])

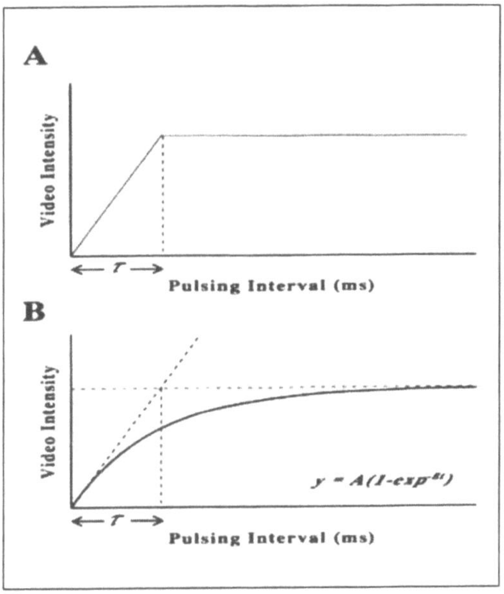

Fig. 3.4. *Curve A:* Theoretical relation between pulsing interval and myocardial video-intensity.
Curve B: relation in vivo between pulsing interval and myocardial video-intensity.
(**A**, plateau; **B**, slope) (Reproduced from [21])

why continuous infusion of contrast agent is preferred to bolus injection. Once the system is set up, it is possible for a single operator to both image and control the infusion rate of contrast. Frequently, the infusion rate that produces the best myocardial opacification, with minimal attenuation over the myocardium in the apical views, is different from the infusion rates required in the parasternal short-axis view. Whereas the infusion rate can be adjusted during a continuous infusion, the regulation is impossible after a bolus injection. On the other hand, due to the time that is needed to optimize the image, continuous infusion is the only method that allows enough time for satisfactory results to be obtained. Although bolus injection is attractive and easy there are many disadvantages with regards to myocardial perfusion imaging [23] that deny its clinical utility. The continuous infusion of contrast has important implications for quantification of myocardial blood flow and also it assures efficient and optimal data acquisition during clinical studies.

In our echocardiographic laboratory, most of the experience was gained with SonoVue (Bracco). This contrast agent consists of stabilized sulphur hexafluorure (SF6) microbubbles. The blood kinetics of SF6 was not dose dependent, and the gas was rapidly removed from the blood by the pulmonary route, with 40% to 50% of the injected dose eliminated within the first minute after administration and 80% to 90% eliminated by 11 minutes after administration. SF6 is a poorly diffusible gas, resistant to very high pressures. This feature makes SonoVue ideal to work with in the high-pressure left ventricle. When working with low mechanical index, such as 0.1, the best images have been acquired with continuous infusion.

Bolus injection may still be used for a rest study in acute transmural myocardial infarction providing qualitative information as to whether there is a perfusion defect or reperfusion (Fig. 3.5). In conclusion, bolus is enough for a qualitative analysis of MCE and for left ventricular opacification studies, thrombus detection or for Doppler enhancement signal. For all other indications, such as in myocardial perfusion studies and analysis of coronary flow reserve, the contrast agent, administered as an infusion, is mandatory.

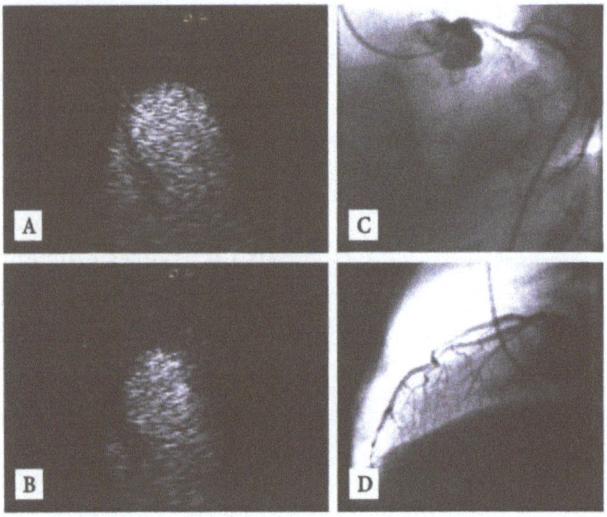

Fig. 3.5. A. A myocardial perfusion image with an apical defect, due to an occlusion of the proximal segment of the anterior descending coronary artery (**C**). After primary PTCA (**D**) the perfusion defect resolves (**B**). In the setting of an acute myocardial infarction, MCE performed with bolus injections allows quick identification of perfusion defects, even though the image quality is not optimal for quantification of myocardial perfusion

In Table 3.1 we summarize the reasons for using bolus or infusion [18].

Tips and Tricks: Pitfalls in Myocardial Contrast Echocardiography

There is no question that the majority of difficulties that occur when a contrast agent is first used in the clinical echocardiography laboratory can be attributed to problems with the preparation and administration of the injected material itself. Weak or absent contrast does not always mean impaired myocardial perfusion, but may be caused by technical problems. When we have this effect in the entire myocardium or after an initial adequate display, it is necessary to re-check the instrument controls and scan-plane in harmonic B-mode. Only after ensuring that the venous line and infusion pump are correct, should inadequate contrast dose be considered.

SonoVue® is prepared by simply mixing 25 mg of lyophilized powder (which contains a mixture of phospholipids and polyethylene glycol with sulphur hexafluoride, a low molecular-weight gas) with 5 ml of normal saline, achieving a concentration of 8 ml of SF6 microbubbles per millilitre. The bubbles are buoyant and the preparation of quite low viscosity, thus the bubbles float rapidly. It can be infused effectively using an infusion pump but care should be taken to ensure that the direction of the infused output is vertical so that bubbles do not become trapped. For continuous infusion we use a syringe pump from Bracco with a continuous oscillatory movement that keeps the contrast agent agitated. Table 3.2 shows

Table 3.1. Pros and cons of using bolus or infusion administration

Bolus administration	**Pros**	**Cons**
	Easy to perform	Contrast effect short life
	Highest peak enhancement	Contrast effects changing during study
	Wash-in and wash-out visible	Timing of bolus difficult
	Agent is used quickly with no stability problems	Comparative contrast studies difficult
Infusion administration	**Pros**	**Cons**
	Extends time of enhancement	More complex to perform; may require pump
	Provides consistent effect Losing the scan plane does not result in loss of the study Recording can be repeated under comparable conditions	Titration of infusion takes time and effort
	Blooming and contrast shadowing can be reduced	
	Continuous oscillatory movement of the syringe pump allows contrast agent stability throughout the study	Stability of agent over infusion period can be a problem if infusion pump is not well adjusted
	It is relatively easy to adjust the dose of contrast agent to the patient imaging conditions and agent is used more efficiently	
	A quantification of myocardial contrast effect can only be achieved by using a stable contrast infusion	

Table 3.2. Dosage for SonoVue® administration

	Contrast agent administration	**Dosage (ml of SonoVue® solution)**	**Comments**
Enhancement of Doppler signals	Bolus	0.1-0.3ml	V_{max} 1ml/sec
Enhancement of endocardial border	Bolus	1ml	V_{max} 1ml/sec
Perfusion during stress test	Continuous infusion	0.9 ml/min	
Acute myocardial perfusion study	Bolus/continuous infusion	1ml/1.1ml/min	
Myocardial contrast echocardiography perfusion	Continuous infusion	1.1ml/min	In some cases it is preferable to administer a slight bolus (0.5ml) first

V_{max} maximal velocity of bolus administration

differents dosages of SonoVue®, depending on the type of contrast study needed.

The decision to perform a contrast echocardiographic study may be reached in consultation with the patients and the physicians. The quality of the non-enhanced endocardial visualization image and the specific clinical issues at hand determine whether or not administration of contrast is justified [24]. The entire contrast procedure must be explained to the patient. It is necessary that they understand its rationale, possible side effects and adverse reactions to the contrast agent [25]. A registered nurse performs the intravenous insertion and also obtains the patient's consent to the procedure. Documentation on a procedural worksheet that the patient has no known contraindications to the ultrasound contrast agent is an alternative to a signed formal consent form.

There are not many definitive contraindications for SonoVue® administration except documented previous allergic reactions. Among relative contraindications we can include severe pulmonary hypertension or distress syndrome and advanced renal or hepatic failure. There are no studies of SonoVue® in pregnant women.

In the case of SonoVue®, side effects are unusual and generally consist of headache, dizziness, weakness or blush at the site of injection. Some patients experience thoracic or abdominal pain, restlessness or sleeplessness. There is only one case documented of a possible anaphylactic shock after its administration.

The sonographer and the nurse must be thoroughly acquainted with the package insert of the contrast agent. Best results are achieved if the contrast syringe and saline flush solution set-up are located as close as possible to the vein, because this shortens the length of intravenous tubing. With all agents, the use of smaller diameter needles should be avoided, to prevent bubbles damage because of the large pressure drop due to the Bernoulli effect. A 22-gauge or large needle is most suitable. It should be borne in mind that the smaller the needle lumen, the slower the injection should be so as to avoid inadvertent bubble destruction. Because the total injection volume for some studies can be less than 1ml, a flush of normal saline is needed to push the agent into the central venous stream. Five to ten millilitres of saline administered through a three way stopcock at the end of a short line is often best.

A number of common artefacts frequently appear in the initials studies, until the sonographer is fully trained (Table 3.3). Usually, artefacts can be resolved by adjusting equipment settings and contrast concentration. The most frequent error is leaving the transmit power on the same level as in tissue harmonic mode and not changing the focus position. If this measure does not produce better left ventricular opacification, administration of a higher dose of contrast should be considered. The receive gain should be reduced to a level where myocardial tissue only produces weak signals. On the other hand, nearfield defects, inhomogeneous opacification or systolic reduction or disappearance of contrast are all artefacts due to inadequate bubble disruption [26]. Because of the higher local acoustic pressures close to the transducer, more bubbles are destroyed in the near field and during systole. In apical views, inho-

Table 3.3. Frequent artefacts in contrast echocardiography

Artefact	Causes	Solution
Setting artefacts	• Inadequate focus position	
	• Inadequate ultrasound transmit frequency	
	• Excessive receive gain	
Attenuation (shadowing)	• Overabundance of contrast agent in left ventricular cavity	• Slower contrast agent administration • Decrease contrast dosage • Wait for washout of contrast agent • Continuous infusion instead of bolus
	• Focus position in the near field	• Move the focus position towards the base
Blooming	• Cavity signals of neighbouring compartments exceed endocardial borders	• Slower contrast agent administration • Continuous infusion instead of bolus • Break off the ultrasound emission 4-5 s when contrast appears in the right ventricle
	• Overabundance of contrast when we use contrast agent to enhance Doppler signal	• Wait for contrast agent washout • Adjust Doppler gain
Swirling	• High mechanical index (MI)	• Decrease mechanical index
	• Focus position in the near field	• Move the focus position towards the base
		• Increase contrast dosage
	• Insufficient contrast agent	
	• Left ventricular dysfunction	
Chest wall artefacts	• Ribs or pulmonary tissue artefact	• Adjust the transducer position in the chest wall
Wall motion artefacts	• Respiratory or thoracic movement	• Adequate breathing regimen or hold respiration during image acquisition

mogeneous opacification may be seen, reflecting mixing of apical blood containing low amounts of bubbles with blood from deeper regions with more bubbles.

Attenuation and Shadowing

Attenuation is an artefact caused by the high echogenicity of an elevated concentration of bubbles. It is often observed after a bolus injection. For a short time the overabundance of contrast agent in the cavity reflects most of the ultrasound. Thus, ultrasound is completely scattered and absorbed by the bubbles in the near field, with no ultrasound penetrating into the deeper regions of the image. Strong signals are found in the near field, whereas the deeper parts are weakly contrasted or even not visualized. Thus, when cavity bubbles *shadow* distal regions, the basal septum and basal inferior and antero-lateral walls can have "pseudo" perfusion defects [27]. The problem is more serious for parasternal views because the ultrasound must penetrate both the right ventricle and the left ventricular cavities to reach the infero-posterior wall.

Shadowing is difficult to compensate. Perhaps with the use of the lowest effective dose of contrast agent we can, almost partially, obviate masking. Implementing a slow bolus or infusion technique to minimize left heart chamber attenuation enables a slow increase of the contrast concentration until the entire cavity is opacified without swirling. Waiting for washout is the best way to resolve this problem. As the contrast agent dilutes with blood, this attenuation typically resolves itself.

In some instances, focus position in the near field can result in similar contrast imaging; thus it is necessary to move the focus towards the base of the scan plane.

Swirling

The bubble destruction in the near field causes an artefact known as *swirling*, generally caused by a combination of factors: high mechanical index, frame rate, insufficient contrast agent or left ventricular dysfunction with low flow at the apex. Changing the machine settings, such as the focal zone, may alter these factors and resolve the problem.

On the other hand, enough agent should be injected to opacify the entire cavity without apical swirling. Best results are obtained when we administer contrast agent with a slow bolus. When contrast appears in the right ventricle, it is advisable to stop bolus administration as well as ultrasound emission for a few seconds. This allows bubbles to fill up the left ventricular cavity, minimizing their destruction in right-side cavities.

Blooming

Blooming [28] describes the appearance of contrast signals which originate from the myocardial tissue, but spread into neighbouring compartments. With blooming, the cavity signals exceed the endocardial borders to a certain extent and resemble myocardial opacification. Cavity blooming is caused by strong echoes, which lie above or below the scan plane. These echoes can be formed particularly in the septum from blooming of the right ventricle cavity. Such septal blooming then occurs simultaneously with the maximum contrast effect in the right ventricle, clearly before the time at which myocardial perfusion is displayed. This phenomenon is more common with bolus injection and accounts for false-positive results [29].

In spectral Doppler, the overabundance of contrast also produces a blooming artefact. It is caused by a returning Doppler signal that is too strong. A relatively low contrast concentration and careful adjustment of the Doppler gain settings may eliminate this artefact.

Chest Wall and Wall Motion Artefacts

Apparent defects in the lateral wall often do not represent a real perfusion deficit but inadequate myocardial contrast due to attenuation by cavity contrast or extra-cardiac structures such as the ribs and pulmonary tissue. Adjusting the scan plane before contrast agent administration has a substantial impact on the success of a myocardial contrast study. Sometimes a slight change in the scan-head position and moving the antero-lateral wall further in the middle of the imaging sector, are necessary so as to minimize ribs artefacts, seen as a dark and non-enhanced region in the lateral wall, and to achieve an optimal grey scale in all segments. This grey level is a good indicator of how well these segments can be filled with contrast.

It has recently been suggested that post-processing of myocardial contrast echocardiography images could reduce the occurrence of theses artefacts and enhance our ability to identify true perfusion abnormalities. One such approach uses a parametric display of microbubble kinetics after their initial destruction by ultrasound [30]. Parametric images of β (an index of myocardial blood velocity, represented by the rate of rise of myocardial contrast intensity) and A (a measure of myocardial blood volume, represented by the plateau of myocardial contrast intensity reached) allow a reduction of the heterogeneity of the contrast effect seen, even in the healthy subject, thus improving image quality [31].

During assessment of myocardial perfusion, *wall motion artefacts*, caused by respiratory or thoracic movements, can alter the contrast display. They can mimic tissue perfusion signals if they are not eliminated before myocardial contrast quantification. The movement of the myocardial tissue may produce Doppler signals, which are different from cavity blooming and from the signals originating from contrast in myocardial vessels. However, fast movements of the heart during deep respirations and coughing, or exaggerated cardiac motion during physical or dobutamine stress, result in wall motion velocities which exceed the threshold of the wall filter of the ultrasound system. Wall motion artefacts can easily be recognized, because they produce dark areas, which often overlay epicardial or pericardial layers in the lateral wall (four-chamber view), but they may also be found in other regions such as near the mitral valve and the septum. Wall motion artefacts can be seen before contrast administration. Proper adjustment of the settings before the injection suppresses most of the signals caused by wall motion. Performing studies with shallow breathing is usually sufficient. If not, patients should hold their breath for 5–10s to achieve an adequate image.

If these measures are not effective, a different scan plane may bring the echo-dense structures into a position where their movement is more perpendicular to the beam.

It is more difficult to suppress wall motion artefacts during stress. It may be possible to control the breathing regimen but the wall motion artefacts caused by increased inotropy may still hinder wall motion analysis.

Indications and Protocols for Myocardial Contrast Echocardiography

With or without contrast, the echocardiographic interpretation depends on experience. Widespread use of contrast echocardiography could even be hazardous in some clinical situations, because bubble artefacts can obscure the diagnostic capabilities of contrast agents if we are not accustomed to this technique. Thus, when an echocardiographic laboratory wants to introduce contrast techniques in its daily clinical practice, it is necessary to bear in mind several indications and protocols.

Enhancement of Doppler Signals

Doppler forms an essential part of all echocardiography examinations, but in some cases the Doppler signal cannot be detected adequately. For successful Doppler detection of blood flow, the velocity of blood must be sufficient to give a detectable Doppler shift, the strength of the blood echo must be sufficient for detection, and tissue motion must be quite slow so that its Doppler shift can be distinguished from that of blood flow.

The injection of a contrast agent into the blood results in a substantial enhancement of the blood echo. With the advent of second-generation contrast agents, the enhancement of Doppler signals has been a reality even in left cardiac chambers. In a Doppler examination this is seen as an intensifying dose dependent on the grey scale of the spectrum or of the colour signal. Since the development of contrast echocardiography, several studies have demonstrated the capacity of contrast agents to increase the technical success of Doppler assessment [32, 33].

Usually, pulsed-wave Doppler study at the mitral valve provides adequate signals without contrast enhancement even in patients with poor acoustic windows. However, contrast administration improves Doppler accuracy in the evaluation of other valvular heart diseases such as aortic stenosis [34] or mitral or pulmonary regurgitation [35] in patients for whom native Doppler curves are not problem solving. Administration of contrast should be considered so as to enhance pulmonary venous Doppler in patients presenting with heart failure and normal left ventricular ejection fraction or in those with significant mitral regurgitation [36]. Suspected tamponade and restrictive or constrictive cardiomyopathies are rare but important indications for contrast echocardiography when Doppler parameters are not diagnostic. Moreover, microbubbles constitute a useful tool for the non-invasive assessment of pulmonary pressure in patients with poor acoustic window or in those without baseline tricuspid regurgitation [37].

Enhancement of Doppler signals is the contrast method that requires the fewest instrument controls. Only the receive gain should be adjusted. A reduction is necessary so as to avoid spectral blooming and saturation of the spectrum, which cause an unreliable spectral envelope. The study can be performed during washout to improve diagnostic confidence.

Protocol for Enhancement of the Doppler Signal: Limitations

Indications

- Administration in patients with technically difficult studies, to improve recordings and diagnostic confidence of both colour Doppler and spectral Doppler signals.

Dosage and Administration

- In general the administration of a contrast bolus of 0.1–0.3 ml of SonoVue® is enough to improve Doppler signals in difficult studies.
- Because the total injection volume can be less than 1ml (usually 0.5 ml), a flush of normal saline is needed to push the agent into the central venous stream. Five to ten millilitres of saline administered through a three-way stopcock at the end of a short line is often best.
- The receive gain should be reduced so as to optimize the brightness of the spectral display.

Limitations

- Spectral Blooming: gain too high
- Signals too weak: inadequate effect
- Contrast dosage too high: attenuation (use the minimum dose needed)
- Irredeemably inadequate native recordings

Enhancement of Endocardial Border

Accurate measurement of left ventricular volumes and systolic function provides valuable diagnostic and prognostic information in patients with cardiovascular diseases. Poor acoustic windows produce inadequate visualization of the endocardial border in roughly 20% of cases, caused by obesity, chronic lung disease or chest wall deformities [38]. Despite the use of second harmonic imaging, optimal delineation of the endocardial border is not achieved in several patients [39]. Even if the development of automated endocardial border detection has contributed towards overcoming the subjective nature of traditional left ventricular function assessment, it has not been fully integrated into routine clinical practice, mainly because endocardial visualization is not consistent throughout the cardiac cycle in a significant proportion of cardiac patients.

Adequate endocardial visualization is essential for accurate interpretation of regional wall motion abnormalities and for reproducible assessment of left ventricular ejection fraction. In these patients, echocardiographic contrast agents capable of producing left ventricular cavity opacification from venous injection can be helpful in delineating endocardial border [40]. Different studies confirm that contrast enhancement resulted in significantly higher segmental evaluation scores compared with harmonic imaging alone [41, 42]. At present, the ability to achieve left ventricular opacification has improved to the point that a technically difficult study is nearly a thing of the past.

Hundley et al. [43] measured, after intravenous contrast injection, the cardiac volumes and left ventricular ejection fraction in 40 patients, referred for echocardiography. Immediately after echocardiography, each patient underwent a gated cardiac cine resonance imaging (MRI) to determine whether enhanced endocardial border definition by contrast echocardiography resulted in more accurate measurement of left ventricular function. The correlation coefficients between echocardiography and MRI were more than 0.92. Before contrast administration, left ventricular ejection fraction by echocardiography and MRI differed by more than 0.10 in 31% of patients and after contrast administration differed by more than 0.10 only in one patient (3%).

The ability to enhance the endocardial border can also improve the accuracy for regional wall motion analysis. Hundley et al. [44] evaluated the wall motion score in a total of 420 segments and they compared basal echocardiography with contrast echocardiography and MRI. They concluded that contrast echocardiography has greater utility in lateral and anterior walls. In these regions, the ability to distinguish normal from abnormal systolic thickening increased from 78% to 98% and 65% to 88%, respectively.

Recently, two multicentre studies evaluated the safety and efficacy of SonoVue® for left ventricular opacification. In Nanda's study of 264 patients [45], complete left ventricular opacification was seen in 34%–87% of patients receiving SonoVue® (they assessed four different dosages: 0.5, 1, 2 and 4 ml), compared with 0%–16% of patients receiving Albunex, a first-generation contrast agent. Senior et al. [46] concluded that SonoVue® is safe and effective for endocardial border enhancement in patients (218 patients) with sub-optimal images.

Contrast echocardiography is practical for evaluating left ventricular function or regional wall motion. Moreover, in difficult patients, the ability to achieve a better delineation of the endocardial border allows for a more precise definition of cardiac anatomy, identifying conditions such as hypertrophic cardiomyopathy or arrhythmogenic right ventricular dysplasia [47]. Administration of contrast may be helpful in the diagnosis of an intra-cavitary thrombus by showing a filling defect. Alternatively, contrast administration is useful to rule out a diagnosis of thrombus made because of a near-field clutter artefact or false tendon imaging [48]. When imaging left ventricular thrombus, it is necessary to avoid apical destruction of bubbles by reducing the mechanical index. In some cases it is helpful to use modified scan planes to improve visualization of the region with suspected thrombus.

In critically ill patients, transthoracic echocardiography frequently provides sub-optimal information for many reasons: mechanical ventilation, bandages, emphysema, chest tubes or inadequate positioning in the left lateral decubitus. In intensive care unit settings, the use of contrast echocardiography improves the feasibility of transthoracic exams and provides an alternative to transoesophageal echocardiography, which often requires sedation and carries a small risk of complications [49-50].

Protocol for Enhancement of the Endocardial Border: Limitations

Indications

- Assessment of left ventricular function in patients with sub-optimal recordings in two to six segments.
- Delineation of left ventricular thrombi.
- Delineation of left or right ventricular morphology.

Dosage and Administration

- Slow contrast bolus of 1 ml of SonoVue®. In cases of severe left ventricular dysfunction with left ventricular enlargement higher doses are usually needed (1.5–2ml).
- Reduce mechanical index to 0.2–0.3 and the receive gain (image nearly black before contrast administration). The DGC is adjusted to obtain a diagonal curve from left to right. When bubbles reach the right ventricle it is advisable to stop the ultrasound emission for 4-5s, so as to allow the contrast agent to fill up the left ventricle, and thus minimize bubble destruction.

Limitations

- Contrast study is not indicated if it is anticipated that image improvement will not alter patient management or when native images are totally inadequate.
- Contrast artefacts: attenuation (which is a great problem in parasternal views because contrast in the right ventricle renders the left ventricular posterior wall difficult to visualize); blooming; inhomogeneous opacification; motion artefacts.
- Systolic reduction or disappearance of contrast. Left ventricular outflow tract defect in aortic regurgitation.

Contrast Stress Echocardiography

Confirming or excluding coronary artery disease in patients with chest pain remains a challenge, because this disease is still the leading cause of death in the Western world [51]. Large numbers of patients referred for evaluation of chest pain are unable to perform adequate exercise testing, mainly because of deconditioning or neurologic, respiratory, peripheral vascular or orthopaedic limitations. In these patients, echocardiographic pharmacological stress represents a non-invasive alternative test, perhaps the best alternative if we complement the study performing an evaluation of the myocardial perfusion status at rest and during peak stress.

The ability to improve regional wall motion scoring and inter-observer variability has important implications for stress echocardiography [52]. During stress, the interpretation of regional wall motion becomes more difficult, because of chest wall motion during hyperventilation and tachycardia. Rainbird et al. [53] evaluated the use of contrast during dobutamine stress testing in 300 unselected patients. They demonstrate that, in this setting, bubbles significantly improve wall segment visualization and image quality at rest and at peak stress, resulting in a more confident interpretation. Importantly, the use of contrast agents during stress echocardiography is cost effective. The cost of the contrast agent itself is more than counterbalanced by savings made by reducing repetitive testing [54].

During myocardial contrast echocardiography (MCE), stress can be performed with any of the available methods; however, the special imaging conditions, make pharmacological stress more suitable.

Even if exercise provides the greatest myocardial oxygen consumption compared to other methods, scanning is difficult during and after exercise because of increased respiratory and cardiac motion. Dobutamine infusion only slightly reduces these difficulties. Thus vasodilators stress, usually dipyridamole or adenosine, is our method of choice for performing a perfusion study during stress. However, for patients with relative contraindications to these direct vasodilators, dobutamine stress myocardial perfusion echocardiography represents an excellent alternative.

During dipyridamole or adenosine administration, the changes in heart rate are moderate and the inotropic state is not altered significantly. Because of their superiority in creating blood flow heterogeneity, a perfusion defect can be displayed with high sensitivity. Blood flow in the perfusion bed supplied by a significantly stenosed artery increases only marginally or even decreases when steal phenomenon develops, compared to the three-to four-fold increase in areas supplied by non-stenotic arteries. The reduction of contrast in a region of interest and the reduced velocity of the bubbles can be used to detect significant stenosis of the epicardial vessel [55].

At present, MCE should be used in combination with a regular pharmacological stress echo protocol when detection of inducible ischaemia is indicated. With real-time perfusion imaging, we can achieve simultaneous assessment of perfusion and wall motion during a constant infusion of contrast [56].

Protocol for Contrast Administration During Echo Stress: Limitations

Indications

- Improves diagnostic accuracy in the assessment of regional left ventricular wall motion.
- Detection or exclusion of myocardial ischaemia with a perfusion study during stress (to exclude myocardial ischaemia, optimal display of the entire myocardium is necessary, a prerequisite not usually fulfilled).

(We use the same protocol as for conventional pharmacologic stress echocardiography).

Dosage and Administration

- The preferred method for contrast administration is a continuous infusion of 0.9 ml/min of SonoVue® for endocardial border delineation and increased dosage of 1.1 ml/min to perform MCE.
- *Recommended image files to document changes in regional wall motion* are baseline, middle stress and peak stress: parasternal long and short axis, and four- and two-chamber apical views. If echocardiographic windows are inadequate in the parasternal region, it is advisable to attempt the subcostal plane. *Machine settings are similar to those described for enhancement of the endocardial border.*
- *Recommended image files to document a*

MCE study are baseline and peak stress: four-chamber view, two-chamber view and if imaging quality is adequate long-axis view. *We will describe machine settings for MCE using CPS technology.*

Limitations

- For perfusion stress echocardiography, patient limitations are identical to those of a non-contrast study.
- See limitations of endocardial border delineation.
- A particular aspect of contrast stress echocardiography is that following contrast administration at basal stage (to improve endocardial border delineation and to perform a perfusion study) the washout produces a swirling artefact lasting several minutes.

Myocardial Perfusion Imaging

Myocardial perfusion imaging has two major objectives: the assessment of ischaemia and the estimation of myocardial viability. In clinical cardiology there are different methods to achieve these objectives: stress ECG, stress echo, nuclear scintigraphy, contrast echo or cardiac magnetic resonance.

Stress ECG has limited sensitivity [57]. Stress echo allows evaluation of wall motion as an indirect marker of perfusion. But even under optimal imaging conditions, analysis of left ventricular wall motion is inferior to the display of a perfusion mismatch, because flow must be reduced to 50% in at least 5% of the myocardium so as to detect new wall motion abnormalities, and because a reduced perfusion precedes, in the ischaemic cascade, the wall motion abnormalities. Thus, an echocardiographic perfusion method should enable us to detect myocardial ischaemia earlier and with higher sensitivity. Moreover, there are some important situations in which wall motion cannot be used as an indicator of perfusion. One is the evaluation of patients following thrombolysis of an acute myocardial infarction. Stunned myocardium has the same pathologic movement as necrotic myocardium.

The potential of myocardial contrast echocardiography (MCE) has been demonstrated in numerous animal and human studies. Myocardial perfusion with contrast echocardiography offers a pure intravascular tracer, better spatial resolution (transmural distribution of perfusion is shown), and the potential for quantification and real-time imaging during rest, stress and interventional studies. It is more widely available, portable and less costly than other methods, and remains in the hands of the cardiologist.

Perfusion imaging in the setting of acute myocardial infarction provides incremental physiologic and clinical information for conventional assessment of the angiographic patency of the infarct-related artery and left ventricular systolic function. The accuracy of MCE in defining the functional area at risk for necrosis during coronary occlusion is now established. The identification of a perfusion defect in a patient presenting with chest pain and ECG changes can be helpful in the triage of patients. Furthermore, resolution of the defect after thrombolysis would confirm non-invasively the recanalization of the infarct-related artery and the integrity of the microvasculature in the ischaemic region. Because bubbles will not enter a region in which the microvasculature is destroyed, a persistent perfusion defect after reperfusion therapy means necrotic myocardium. Presently, MCE is gaining importance in the evaluation of microvasculature derangements after acute myocardial infarction [58], which is related to the extent of viable myocardium as well as to the long-term prognosis of post-infarction patients [59].

Protocol for Myocardial Perfusion Studies: Limitations

Indications in the Setting of Acute Myocardial Infarction

- MCE can be used to determine *infarct size* and to *assess reperfusion* [60] or non-reflow phenomenon. Several studies have shown that the area of risk correlates well with that demonstrated using thallium imaging [61].
- MCE is useful following reperfusion for assessing myocardial salvage. The presence of contrast indicates *myocardial viability* in patients presenting with an acute myocardial infarction [62, 63].
- Potential uses of MCE include the evaluation of clinical conditions associated with impaired coronary flow reserve, such as hypertrophy, infiltrative cardiomyopathies, acute cardiac rejection or syndrome X.

Dosage and Administration

- Contrast administration with continuous infusion is recommended. Optimization of infusion rate is performed by visual evaluation of contrast intensities in the apical and basal segments. An optimal infusion results in homogeneous contrast enhancement in the apical and basal segments.
- Normally, SonoVue® dose consist of 1.1 ml/min.
- At least two apical views are necessary and it is important to bear in mind that modified scan planes can improve display of lateral and anterior walls.

Machine Settings for CPS Perfusion Studies

With the CPS technology, *B-mode imaging* is performed using fundamental imaging. We can work at two *transmit frequency options*, P1.5 and P 2 MHz (improved detail resolution). With the exception of an excellent echocardiographic window, we use P1.5 MHz. The *dynamic range* is 50 dB, *space/time*, of S1, 0 *edge*, 0 *persistence* and a *post-processing* of 0. The *Delta setting* used is 3. The *mechanical index* is decreased to 0.22. Before commencing the infusion of SonoVue, the B-mode overall *gain* is decreased until no information is visible on the screen in the CA mode and the equalize gain is activated. The DGC is adjusted to obtain a diagonal curve from left to right. The double focus is adjusted to the level of the mitral valve.

The microbubble destruction phase is carried out by entering in the *colour Doppler microbubble destruction (MBD) mode*. The colour box must embrace the entire myocardium of interest. *Time triggers* are employed to allow specific control of frame rates and to minimize microbubble destruction. Time triggers are set at 50 ms. *Regional expansion selection* (RES) is also used to increase the resolution and overall quality of the B-mode image.

With CPS we can choose three different display options: contrast only (CA), contrast and fundamental tissue imaging (Mix) and only fundamental 2-D tissue image (2-D). With this option we can confirm during the study that the scan plane is correct.

Limitations

- If the acoustic window is poor, MCE usually is sub-optimal, mainly at the basal and lateral segments.
- Several artefacts (previously explained) can obscure the diagnostic accuracy of MCE.

Conclusions

Over the past quarter of a century, echocardiography has become a major tool in the armamentarium of clinical cardiology. With the advent of new technological developments, MCE will become a powerful clinical application. It is used in the diagnosis of coronary disease through the enhancement of endocardial borders during rest and stress echocardiograms, making regional wall motion abnormalities and wall thickening easier to evaluate. In fact, contrast echocardiography should soon virtually eliminate the technically difficult echocardiogram.

Analysis of images obtained during MCE studies allow us to measure quantitative indices of perfusion and also to quantify changes in regional left ventricular function. Even if further work is essential, the simultaneous availability of objective information of myocardial perfusion and function should improve the accuracy of echocardiographic diagnosis of coronary artery disease. In the acute setting, the development of new technologies allows us to evaluate more reliably the efficacy of myocardial reperfusion treatments and thus the long-term prognosis of ischaemic patients.

References

1. Feigenbaum H, Stone J, Lee D, Nasse W, Chang S: Identification of ultrasound echoes from the left ventricle by use of intracardiac injections of indocyanine green. Circulation 1970; 41: 615-621
2. Kaul S. Instrumentation for contrast echocardiography: technology and techniques. Am J Cardiol 2002; 90(suppl): 8J-14J
3. Wei K, Skyba DM, Firschke C, Lindner JR, Jayaweera AR, Kaul S. Interaction between microbubbles and ultrasound: in vitro and in vivo observations. J Am Coll Cardiol 1997; 29: 1081-1088
4. Skyba DM, Price RJ, Linka AZ, Skalak TC, Kaul S. Direct in vivo visualization of intravascular destruction of microbubbles by ultrasound and its local effects on tissue. Circulation 1998; 98: 290-293
5. Tamyel A, Havaux X, Van Camp G, Campanelle B, Gisellu G, Pasquet A, Denf JF, Melen JA, Vanoverschelde JL. Destruction of contrast microbubbles by ultrasound. Effects on myocardial function, coronary perfusion pressure and microvascular integrity. Circulation 2001; 104: 461-466
6. Masugata H, Lafitte S, Peters B, Strachan GM, DeMaria AN. Comparison of real-time and intermittent triggered myocardial contrast echocardiography for quantification of coronary stenosis severity and transmural perfusion gradient. Circulation 2001; 104: 1550-1556
7. Aggeli CJ, Shimon S, Nagueh SF, Zoghbi WA. Quan-

titative parameters of myocardial perfusion with contrast echocardiography in human beings: influence of triggering mode. J Am Soc Echocardiogr 2002; 15: 1432-1439
8. Porter TR, Xie F, Li S, D'Sa A, Rafter P. Increased ultrasound contrast and decreased micro bubble destruction rates with triggered ultrasound imaging. J Am Soc Echocardiogr 1996; 9: 599-605
9. De Jong N. Imaging methods for MCE: what to expect in near future. Eur J Echocardiography 2002; 3: 245-306
10. Porter TR, Li S, Jiang L, Grayburn P, Deligonul U. Real-time visualization of myocardial perfusion and wall thickening in human beings with intravenous ultrasonographic contrast and accelerated intermittent harmonic imaging. J Am Soc Echocardiogr 1999; 12: 266-271
11. Bahlmann EB, Mc Quillan BM, Handschumacher MD, Chow CM, Guerrero JL, Picard MH, Weyman AE, Scherrer-Crosbie M. Effect of destructive pulse duration on the detection of myocardial perfusion in myocardial contrast echocardiography: in vitro and in vivo observations. J Am Soc Echocardiogr 2002; 15: 1440-1447
12. Kaul S. Myocardial contrast echocardiography: 15 years of research and development. Circulation 1997; 96: 3745- 3760
13. Kuersten B, Nahar T, Vannan MA. Methods of contrast administration for myocardial perfusion imaging: continuous infusion versus bolus injection. Am J Cardiol 2002; 90 (suppl): 35J-37J
14. Kaul S, Kelly P, Oliner JD, Glasheen WP, Keller MW, Watson DD. Assessment of regional myocardial blood flow with myocardial contrast two-dimensional echocardiography. J Am Coll Cardiol 1989; 13:468-482
15. Wiencek JG, Feinstein SB, Walker R, Aroson S. Pitfalls in quantitative contrast echocardiography: the steps to quantification of perfusion. J Am Soc Echocardiogr 1993; 6(4): 395-416
16. Skyba DM, Jayaweera AR, Goodman NC, Ismail S, Caramaro GP, KaulS. Quantification of myocardial perfusion with myocardial contrast echocardiography from left atrial injection of contrast: implications for venous injection. Circulation 1994; 90:1513-1521
17. Weissman NJ, Mylan CC, Hack TC, Gillam LD, Cohen JL, Kitzman DW. Infusion versus bolus contrast echocardiography: a multicenter, open-label, crossover trial. Am Heart J 2000; 139: 399-404
18. Wei K, Jayaweera AR, Firoozan S, Linka A, Skyba DM, Kaul S. Basis for detection of stenosis using venous administration of microbubbles during myocardial contrast echocardiography: Bolus or continuous infusion? J Am Coll Cardiol 1998; 32: 252-260
19. Murthy TH, Li P, Locvicchio E, Baisch C, Dairywala I, Armstrong WF, Vannan M. Real time myocardial blood flow imaging in normal human beings with the use of myocardial contrast echocardiography. J Am Soc Echocardiogr 2001; 14: 698-705
20. Lindner JR, Villanueva FS, Dent JM, Wei K Sklenar J, Kaul S. Assessment of resting perfusion with myocardial contrast echocardiography: theoretical and practical considerations. Am Heart J 2000; 139: 231-240
21. Wei K, Jayaweera AR, Firoozan S, Linka A, Skyba DM, Kaul S. Quantification of myocardial blood flow with ultrasound-induced destruction of microbubbles administered as a contrast venous infusion. Circulation 1998; 97: 473- 483
22. Porter TR, Xie F, Li S, Kricsfeld D, Deligonul U. Effect of transducer standoff on the detection, spatial extent and quantification of myocardial contrast defects caused by coronary stenosis. J Am Soc Echocardiogr 1999; 12: 951-956
23. Coggins MP, Sklenar JD, Le E, Wei K, Lindner JR, Kaul S. Non-invasive prediction of ultimate infarct size at the time of acute coronary occlusion based on the extent and magnitude of collateral-derived myocardial blood flow. Circulation 2001; 104: 2471-2477
24. Witt S. Implementing microbubble contrast in the echocardiography laboratory. A sonographer's perspective. Am J Cardiol 2002; 90 (suppl): 155-165
25. Burgess P, Moore V, Bednarz J, Carney D, Floer S, Gresser C, Jasper S, Moos S, Odabastian J, Sisk E, Trough M, Waggoner A, Witt S, Adams D. Performing an echocardiographic examination with a contrast agent: a series on contrast echocardiography II. J Am Soc Echocardiogr 2000; 13: 629-634
26. Beker H, Burns PN. Assessment of myocardial perfusion by contrast echocardiography. Left ventricular function and myocardial perfusion. Beker H, Burns PN editors. Handbook of contrast echocardiography. 2000; 128-133
27. Lindner JR, Villanueva FS, Dent JM, Sklenar J, Kaul S. Assessment of resting perfusion with myocardial contrast echo: theoretical and practical considerations. Am Heart J 2000; 139: 231-240
28. Paré JC, Saquete N, Sirges M, Velamazán M. Organización del laboratorio de ecocardiografía de contraste. García-Fernández MA, Zamorano JL. Editors. Práctica de la ecocardiografía de contraste. Madrid: ENE, 1999:107-113
29. Lutz C, Tie Mann K, Kosher J, Schlosser T, Grenache J, Belcher H. Does colour blooming limitate the assessment of myocardial perfusion using harmonic power Doppler? Euro Heart J 1999; 20(abstract supplement): 359

30. Sklenar J, Jayaweera AR, Linka Az, Kaul S. Parametric imaging for myocardial contrast echocardiography: pixel-to-pixel incorporation of information from both spatial and temporal domains: method for the myocardial perfusion evaluation during myocardial contrast two-dimensional echocardiography. J Am Soc Echocardiogr 1998; 25: 461-464
31. Ay T, D'Hondt AM, Pasquet A, Melin JA, Vanoverss-chelde JL. Heterogeneity of contrast effect during intermittent second harmonic myocardial contrast echocardiography in healthy patients. J Am Soc Echocardiogr 2002; 15:1448-1452
32. Kerber R, Kioschos J, Lauer R. Use of an ultrasound contrast method in the diagnosis of valvular regurgitation and intra-cardiac shunts. Am J Cardiol 1974; 34:722
33. Hagler DJ, Currie PJ, Seward JB, Tajik AJ, Mair DD, Ritter DG. Echocardiographic contrast enhancement of poor or weak continuous-wave Doppler signals. Echocardiography 1987; 4:63
34. Nakatani S, Imanishi T, Terasawa A, Beppu S, Nagata S, Miyatake K. Clinical application of trans-pulmonary contrast enhanced Doppler technique in the assessment of severity of aortic stenosis. J Am Coll Cardiol 1992; 20:973
35. Tanabe K, Asanuma T Yoshitomi H. Doppler estimation of pulmonary artery end-diastolic pressure using contrast enhancement of pulmonary regurgitation signals. Am J Cardiol 1996; 78:1145
36. Lambertz H, Schumacher U, Tries H, Stein T. Improvement of pulmonary venous flow Doppler signal after intravenous injection of Levovist. J Am Soc Echocardiogr 1997; 10:891
37 Rey JR, García-Fernández MA, Pérez E. Utilidad de la inyección de ecopotenciadores de la señal Doppler en la estimación de la presión sistólica pulmonar en pacientes sin insuficiencia tricúspide. Rev Esp Cardiol 1998; 51 (supl5):31
38. Schiller N, Shah P, Crawford M, DeMaria A, Devereux R, Feigenbaum H for the American Society of Echocardiography Committee on Standards, Subcommittee on Quantification of Two-dimensional Echocardiograms. Recommendations for quantitation of the left ventricle by two-dimensional echocardiography. J Am Soc Echocardiogr 1989; 2:358-367
39. Lang RM, Mor-Avi V, Zoghbi WA, Senior R, Klein AL, Pearlman AS. The role of contrast enhancement of left ventricular function. Am J Cardiol 2002; 90 (suppl): 28J-34J
40. Lindner JR, Dent JM, Moos SP, Jayaweera AR, Kaul S. Enhancement of left ventricular cavity opacification by harmonic imaging after venous injection of Albunex. Am J Cardiol 1997; 79:1657-1662
41. Spencer KT, Bednarz J, Mor-avi V, Weinert L, Tan J, Godoy I, Lang RM. The role of echocardiographic harmonic imaging and contrast enhancement for the improvement of endocardial border delineation. J Am Soc Echocardiogr 2000; 13: 131-135
42. Fernández Portales J, García Fernández MA, Moreno M, González Alujas MT, Placer JL, Allue C, Bermejo J, Delcán JL. Utilidad de las nuevas técnicas de imagen, segundo armónico y contraste en la visualización del borde endocárdico. Análisis de la reproducibilidad en la valoración de la contracción segmentaria. Rev Esp Cardiol 2000; 53: 1459-1466
43. Hundley WG, Kizilbash AM, Afridi I, Franco F, Peshock RM, Grayburn PA. Administration of an intravenous perfluorocarbon contrast agent improves echocardiographic determination of left ventricular volumes and ejection fraction: comparison with cine magnetic resonance imaging. J Am Coll Cardiol 1998; 32: 1426-1432
44. Hundley WG, Kizilbash AM, Afridi I, Franco F, Peshock RM, Grayburn PA. Effect of contrast enhancement on transthoracic echocardiographic assessment of left ventricular regional wall motion. Am J Cardiol 1999; 84:1365-1369
45. Nanda NC, Wistran DC, Karlsberg RP, Hack TC, Smith WB, Foley DA, Picard MH, Cotter B. Multicenter evaluation of SonoVue for improved endocardial border delineation. Echocardiography 2002; 19:27-36
46. Senior R, Anderson O, Caidahl K, Carlens P, Herregods MC, Jenni R, Kenny A, Melcheeer A, Svedenhag J, Vanoverschelde JL. Enhanced left ventricular endocardial border delineation with an intravenous injection of SonoVue, a new echocardiographic contrast agent: A European multicenter study. Echocardiography 2000; 17: 705-711
47. Grayburn PA, Mulvagh S, Crouse L. Left ventricular opacification at rest and during stress. Am J Cardiol 2002; 90 (suppl): 21J-27J
48. Stratton JR, Lighty GW Pearlman AS, Ritchie JL. Detection of left ventricular thrombus by two-dimensional echocardiography: sensitivity, specificity and causes of uncertainty. Circulation 1982; 66:156-166.
49. Reilly JP, Tunick PA, Timmermans RJ, Stein B, Rosenzweig BP, Kronzon I. Contrast echocardiography clarifies un-interpretable wall motion in intensive care unit patients. J Am Coll Cardiol 2000; 35: 485-490
50. Yong Y, Wu D, Fernández V, Kopelen HA, Shimoni S, Nagueh SF, Callahn JD, Bruns DE, Shaw LJ, Quiñones MA, Zoghbi WA. Diagnostic accuracy and cost-effectiveness of contrast echocardiography on evaluation of cardiac function in technically very difficult patients in the intensive care unit. Am J Cardiol 2002; 15: 711-718
51. National Heart, Lung and Blood Institute. Morbidity from Coronary Heart Disease in the United States.

National Heart, Lung and Blood institute Data Fact Sheet. Bethesda (MD): 1990
52. Porter TR, Xie F, Kricsfeld A, Chiou A, Dabestani A. Improved endocardial border resolution during dobutamine stress echocardiography with intravenous sonicated dextrose albumin. J Am Coll Cardiol 1994; 23: 1440-1443
53. Rainbird AJ, Mulvagh Sl, Oh JK, Mc Cully RB, Klarich KW, Shub C, Mahoney DW, Pellika PA. Contrast dobutamine stress echocardiography: clinical practice assessment in 300 consecutive patients. J Am Soc Echocardiogr 2001; 14:378-385
54. Shaw LJ, Monaghan MJ, Nihoyannopolous P. Clinical and economic outcomes assessment with myocardial contrast echocardiography. Heart 1999; 82 (suppl3): III16-III21
55. Kaul S, Senior R, Dittrich H, Raval V, Khattar R, Lahiri A. Detection of coronary artery disease with myocardial contrast echocardiography: comparison with 99mTcsestamibi single photon emission computed tomography. Circulation 1997; 96(3):785-792
56. Mor-Avi V, Caiani EG, Collins KA, Korcarz CE, Bednarz JE, Lang RM. Combined assessment of myocardial perfusion and regional left ventricular function by analysis of contrast enhances power modulation images. Circulation 2001; 104: 352-357
57. Gibbons RJ, Balady GJ, Bricker JT, Chaitman BR, Fletcher GF, Froelicher VF, Mark db, Mc Callister BD, Moss An, O'Reilly MG, Winters WL Jr. ACC/AHA 2002. Guideline update for exercise testing: a report of the American College of Cardiology/ American Heart Association Task Force on Practice guidelines (committee on exercise testing) 2002
58. Villanueva FS. Myocardial contrast echocardiography in acute myocardial infarction. Am J Cardiol 2002; 90(suppl): 38J-47J
59. Cain P, Khoury V, Short L, Marwick TH. Usefulness of quantitative echocardiographic techniques to predict recovery of regional and global left ventricular function after acute myocardial infarction. Am J Cardiol 2003; 91: 391-396
60. Lepper W, Hoffman R, Kamp O, France A, Cock CC, Kohl HP, Seesawed GT, Dahl JV, Janssens U, Voci P, Visser CA, Hanrath P. Assessment of myocardial reperfusion by intravenous myocardial contrast echocardiography and coronary flow reserve after primary percutaneous transluminal coronary angiography in patients with acute myocardial infarction. Circulation 2000; 101; 2368-2374
61. Latiffe S, Higashiyama A, Masugata H, peters B, Strachan M, Kwan OL, DeMaria AN. Contrast echocardiography can assess risk area and infarct size during coronary occlusion and reperfusion: experimental validation. J Am Coll Cardiol 2002; 39:1546-1554
62. Zoghbi WA. Evaluation of myocardial viability with contrast echocardiography. Am J Cardiol 2002; 90(suppl): 65J-71J
63. Balcells E, Powers ER, Lepper W, Belcik T, Wei K, Ragosta M, Sarnady H, Lindner JR. Detection of myocardial viability by contrast echocardiography in acute infarction predicts recovery of resting function and contractile reserve. J Am Coll Cardiol 2003; 41: 827-833

Chapter 4
Quantification Methods in Contrast Echocardiography

María J. Ledesma-Carbayo • Norberto Malpica • Andrés Santos
Miguel Angel García Fernández • Manuel Desco

Introduction

Ultrasonographic contrast agents in echocardiography are a rapidly developing research field. Several new acquisition techniques particularly suited to the acquisition of contrast images have been made available in the last few years, although the clinical usefulness of most of them is still under evaluation.

The two main goals for the use of these agents are the enhancement of the boundary between myocardial tissue and blood, and the analysis of myocardial perfusion.

The enhancement of the endocardial border observed after contrast administration [1] increases the conspicuity of the images and improves the results provided by the algorithms oriented to the assessment of ventricular wall motion. It also enables the use of more advanced semiautomatic quantitative procedures, which demand the highest image quality.

The second application mentioned is the direct assessment of myocardial blood flow and flow reserve. Provided this assessment was clinically reliable it would play a crucial role for the determination of the functional impact of the coronary artery disease. To date, the results have been interpreted mainly visually, either qualitatively or establishing semiquantitative scores. However, the use of true quantitative techniques, based on parametric models, is of increasing interest because of its higher objectivity.

Despite the numerous advances in acquisition and postprocessing techniques attained in the past years, it is remarkable that clinical acceptance remains low. Some reasons for this reportedly slow incorporation [2] into the routine practice may be the complexity of the methodology, the difficulty of the visual interpretation of the results and the lack of standardized quantification procedures and cut-off values agreed upon for the different parameters. It is even debatable whether the quantitative values provided by the various existing software packages (supplied either by scanner manufacturers or third-party companies) are totally equivalent. At present, many clinical studies still rely on an essentially qualitative interpretation of the images, while the most advanced mathematical approaches seem to lack sound clinical validation, confirmed by independent publications.

Acquisition of Contrast Studies

The acquisition protocol determines the quantification algorithms that can be applied to the dataset. The quantification algorithm must be suited to the contrast administration method (infusion or bolus) and to the particular imaging technique used (triggered, real-time, intermittent imaging, etc.). It is thus appropriate to briefly describe some concepts related to the acquisition protocol as far as they condition the quantitative analysis.

Contrast Administration Techniques

Bolus administration consists of a rapid injection (about 30 s) of a small amount of contrast agent, usually non-diluted. It is done through an intravascular line and is usually followed by a saline solution flush (about 5 ml) to push the bolus further into the blood stream. Direct intracoronary injection is a variant of this technique, mostly used in experimental studies.

Bolus administration saves time and is relatively easy to perform. It has been indicated for applications such as endocardial border detection and, in some cases, qualitative myocardial perfusion rest studies. Drawbacks of this technique are the short time available to acquire the data and its lower reproducibility reported in comparative studies [2]. Quantitative measurements of timings and high-peak video density may potentially mitigate these problems (see paragraph "Bolus Analysis).

The alternative administration technique, known as continuous infusion, is often achieved by means of a mechanical pump that performs a slow delivery of a diluted solution of the contrast agent. It offers several advantages, such as a longer period for imaging acquisition, a video intensity well within the optimum detection range, and a lower shadowing effect due to attenuation artefact. On the other hand, it is more difficult to perform and the stability of the contrast solution along the infusion becomes a critical issue, since changes in contrast concentration may affect the shape of the input function altering the quantification results. Despite these disadvantages, continuous infusion is clearly the preferred method for myocardial perfusion studies, particularly when performing quantitative analysis [3,4].

Imaging Techniques

The last decade has been extremely productive combining contrast agent properties and imaging techniques. Initially, fundamental imaging was applied in contrast echocardiography basically after direct intracoronary injection of the agent, observing a noticeable left ventricular cavity opacification and, to some extent, myocardial changes in video intensity. The combination of fundamental imaging and Doppler echocardiography provided a better framework to improve cardiovascular flow measurements. However, harmonic imaging, in some cases combined with Doppler echocardiography, provided the greatest improvement toward a proper myocardial perfusion quantification [5, 3].

From that time, a boom of different acquisition techniques took place, taking advantage of a deeper knowledge of the interaction between microbubbles and the ultrasonic wave. When microbubbles are exposed to ultrasound pressure they change in size until they begin to resonate, even leading to a bubble disruption if the peak pressure is over 1 MPa [2]. The behavior is directly related to the peak pressure (related to the incident ultrasound transmit power), that can be controlled through the mechanical index parameter. Peak tissue pressure and its effect on microbubbles are usually measured through a parameter known as 'mechanical index' (MI), equal to the peak negative pressure divided by the square root of the frequency. This parameter reflects the normalized energy to which a target is exposed, usually defined at 1 MHz. Microbubbles present linear oscillations for MI below 0.1, nonlinear oscillation for MI between 0.1 and 1.0 and disruption for MI above 1.0. According to this parameter, it is customary to classify the different acquisition methods as *destructive*, those that use high MI, and *nondestructive* when low MI is applied.

Discrimination between the signal corresponding to the microbubbles from that of the tissue can be performed by exploiting different consequences of the nonlinear behavior of the microbubbles. One approach is based on the fact that nonlinear interactions produce backscatter signals with higher power in signal harmonics. A second approach makes use of the phase shift with respect to the transmitted signal produced in the backscatter signal by the nonlinear oscillations. Most of the current acquisition methods send successive ultrasound pulse packets with different properties, either in amplitude or phase. Pulse processing consists of adding successive responses in such a way that the linear response of tissues is cancelled, selecting the nonlinear response of the contrast agent. Among these methods we can distinguish *multiple-pulse methods* and *single-pulse methods*. Multiple-pulse methods send several pulse packages for every scan line; line response is the result of the processing of these multiple pulses. Single-pulse methods combine single-pulse response of consecutive lines to cancel tissue signal. These methods, reviewed in [6], are globally called *nonlinear hamonic imaging methods* and can be used either with high or low mechanical index.

Table 4.1 summarizes some commercially available imaging techniques from those described in the previous paragraphs, indicating their most common brand name.

It may be interesting to indicate which techniques are more adequate depending on the type of quantitative assessment intended. In this sense, as indicated before, two main types of studies can be defined: those aiming at tracking the endocardial wall border and those that pursue a direct quantification of myocardial perfusion.

Table 4.1. Correspondence between major imaging methods and some commercially available techniques, indicating whether they use high or low mechanical index (MI)

Methods	Brand names	MI
Fundamental imaging		High
Harmonic imaging	Second Harmonic Imaging	High
	Ultraharmonic Imaging[a]	High
Doppler harmonic imaging	Color Power Angio[b]	High
	Power Harmonic Imaging[a]	High
	Power Doppler[b]	High
Single-pulse transmission	CCI[b] (Cadence Coherent Contrast Imaging)	Low/High
Multiple pulse transmission	CPS[b] (Cadence Contrast Pulse Sequencing Technology)	Low/High
	Power Modulation[a]	Low/High
	Coded Harmonic Agio[c]	Low/High
	Power Pulse Inversion[d]	Low/High
	Power Harmonic Imaging[a]	Low/High

[a]Philips/Agilent; [b]Siemens Acuson; [c]General Electric; [d]Philips/ATL

Quantitative Myocardial Border Tracking

Studies to be analyzed for quantitative border tracking have been mainly acquired with bolus administration of a nondiluted contrast agent, usually acquiring only one cycle [7]. However, it has also been proposed to use continuous infusion in order to attain a more controlled environment allowing one to acquire several views [8]. Concerning imaging techniques, harmonic imaging or Doppler harmonic imaging are recommended [9, 7, 2], although other methods, such as continuous imaging with low mechanical index, have also been used to assess motion and perfusion at the same time [10].

Quantitative Myocardial Perfusion

It is impossible to establish only one acquisition technique suitable for quantitative assessment of myocardial perfusion, since most of the imaging techniques, administration methods, and acquisition parameters have been used to this purpose, leading to the existence of multiple combinations of protocols. This fact, combined with the machine and contrast agent dependence, affects the repeatability of the results very negatively, giving rise to a certain confusion in the literature.

Harmonic imaging has been proven to be superior to fundamental imaging for myocardial perfusion [5]. Recentely, nonlinear methods combining multiple pulses have been reported as the preferred methods [11]. Regarding administration techniques, both bolus and continuous infusion allow application of quantification algorithms, although usually the latter is the preferred method [3, 4, 11]. The most common acquisition protocols are the following:

1. Triggered imaging using high MI after a bolus administration. Perfusion can be quantified by applying a gamma model (see paragraph "Bolus Analysis").
2. Continuous imaging (real-time imaging) combined with nonlinear harmonic multiple pulse cancellation methods and low mechanical index. These methods require continuous infusion. Acquisition consists of a high MI burst to disrupt most of the agent in the ventricular cavity, followed by multiple low MI pulses that allow sampling of the reperfusion process from which one or more curves are drawn that can be analyzed according to an exponential model (see paragraph "Reperfusion Model").
3. Intermittent imaging. This acquisition protocol uses an incremental time triggering combined with nonlinear harmonic multiple pulse cancellation methods and high MI. The basis of this acquisition method is the strong, brief nonlinear echo produced when bubbles disrupt. First, a prolonged high MI burst is applied to destroy all the agent present in the cavity and myocardium. Triggers are then programed to be produced incrementally in time to obtain the refilling curve. As in the previous case, quantification of the results is also based on a reperfusion exponential model (see paragraph "Reperfusion Model").

Contrast-Enhanced Endocardial Border Detection Quantification

The assessment of regional myocardial wall function has always been an important and unresolved issue since the introduction of echocardiography as a diagnostic tool. Many cardiac pathologies are characterized by developing regional wall motion abnormalities, especially in early stages of the disease, in spite of well preserved indices of global performance. Abnormal regional wall motion is an early finding in many cardiac pathologies and has a critical importance in terms of an early diagnosis of the disease process.

Global and regional wall motion have been commonly assessed qualitatively by visual examination of the endocardial displacement and wall thickening of each myocardial segment. Although the American Society of Echocardiography proposed standardized protocols for acquisition and scoring of stress echocardiography [12], a significant interinstitutional disagreement on regional analysis interpretation was reported [13]. More objective quantitative methods are warranted to homogenize the interpretation of these studies.

The automated assessment of cardiac motion has been intensively pursued in the last decade [14]. Lately, most of the efforts are being made in cardiac magnetic resonance imaging, and more specifically in tagged magnetic resonance, which are currently the reference modalities to estimate cardiac motion [15]. While new ultrasound techniques provide higher image quality, increasing attention is being paid to the automatic processing of echocardiographic sequences [16-18].

An automatic tracking of the endocardial border may allow for a more objective evaluation of stress echocardiography and an easier calculation of global function parameters, such as ventricular volume and ejection fraction. These automatic algorithms may clearly benefit from contrast echocardiography, since the latter noticeably enhances the tissue–blood interface, [1, 19], particularly when combined with the new nonlinear harmonic acquisition technique. It is currently recommended for clinical use in global functional examination and stress echocardiography when conventional ultrasound imaging is suboptimal [7].

The simplest approach for quantitative left ventricular global function assessment based on border tracking uses a manual contour delineation in systolic and diastolic frames, allowing computation of ejection fraction-related parameters. The use of contrast agents may allow for the use of semiautomatic thresholding techniques to define the endocardial border [10].

Contrast echocardiography may also allow one to extend the conventional color kinesis to a broader group of patients, providing a very good visualization together with a quantification of the endocardial excursion magnitude and timing [20].

The technique known as 'acoustic quantification' (AQ, Philips-Agilent) produces a rough segmentation of cardiac structures by thresholding the backscatter signal from conventional ultrasound studies. Slight changes in AQ configuration allow its use for the quantification of contrast studies [21] providing a more reliable automatic endocardial delineation.

More advanced image processing methods are based on mathematical tools known as 'active' or 'deformable' models. These models, which can be used to generate a completely automatic segmentation of the sequences, consist in geometrical curves that evolve towards the image edges. The algo-

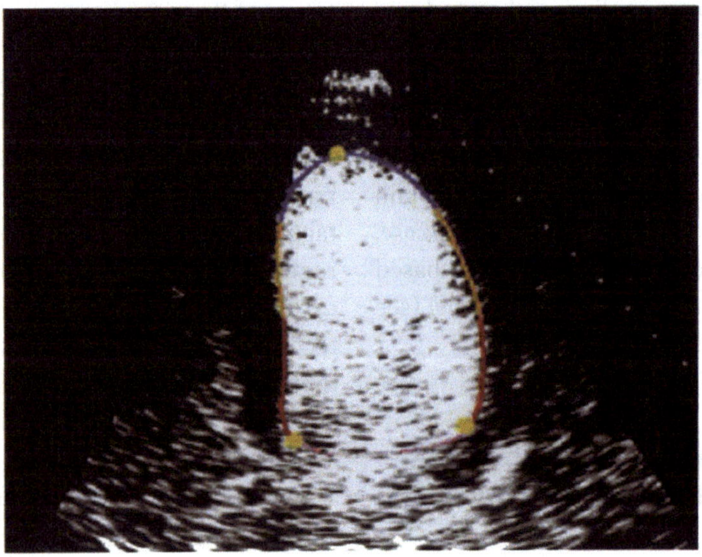

Fig. 4.1. Tracking of endocardial border in contrast-enhanced two-dimensional sequences. The tracked contour is presented as a color overlay

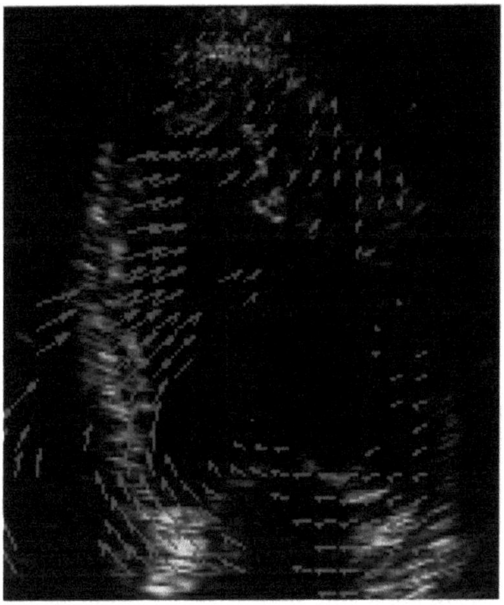

Fig. 4.2. Dense myocardial displacement field in a patient with hypokinetic function of the lateral wall and the basal and distal septum segments

rithms operate iteratively, changing the shape and dimensions of the borders until converging to the real structure edges. Prior constraints can be added to adapt the deformable model to a particular shape [17]. The contours obtained after tracking the whole sequence can be processed to generate global functional parameters and regional endocardial excursion (Fig. 4.1). These methods can be extended to three-dimensional imaging (3D+T) to obtain global three-dimensional measurements [22].

Another approach is to track all the image pixels, providing a dense myocardial displacement field that represents the magnitude and direction of the movement for every pixel in the image [18]. Although this method has only been tested in noncontrast harmonic imaging for wall motion assessment, it also has clear potential applications in contrast echocardiography (Fig. 4.2)[1].

This type of method may provide not only an assessment of the heart motion but also the possibility to compensate that movement, producing artificially still sequences, much more appropriate for obtaining functional information with contrast echocardiography. This issue is explored further in a later section (see paragraph "Effect on the Cardiac Motion").

Contrast Quantification for Myocardial Perfusion Assessment

A reliable assessment of the myocardial perfusion is one of the most ambitious goals of contrast echocardiography. Nevertheless, it is quite evident that, as in other imaging techniques such as nuclear medicine or cardio MRI (magnetic resonance imaging), the simple visualization of differences in video intensity between cardiac segments is not enough to provide objective, reliable and repeatable measurements.

Under some reasonable assumptions, quantitative measurements of video intensity are related to the contrast agent concentration in different myocardial regions. Thus, the video intensity information in contrast studies may be used to obtain a spatial assessment of myocardial perfusion, applying adequate models and quantification algorithms.

Myocardial perfusion assessment by means of contrast agents does not provide a high

[1] Studies in figures 2 to 10 have been processed with the CUSQ® software package, developed by the authors and distributed by SIEMENS-ACUSON.

spatial resolution, limiting the sensitivity in cases of small defects. However, several studies support that a good quantitative assessment improves the accuracy, even to a degree comparable to that of SPECT studies [11].

Basic Quantification

The most simple approach to contrast echocardiography quantification consists of taking video intensity measurements on regions of interest (ROI) defined in single frames or image sequences (cineloops) .

Single-Frame Quantification

Once a suitable image in a sequence has been selected, the video intensity in different points or regions in the myocardium can be measured. Typically, a region-of-interest (ROI) is defined and the maximum and/or mean intensity of the pixels within the ROI is computed. ROIs could be placed within a single segment or perfusion territory. The advantage of working with ROIs instead of individual pixels is that the averaging minimizes the effect of the noise (statistical error, scatter, artifacts).

As the change in signal strength due to the contrast is usually small, its detection is hindered by the noise; the application of subtraction techniques may increase the signal-to-noise ratio. Subtraction assumes that the acquired signal is composed of the addition of signal caused by the contrast agent and 'background' information or noise. If this second component is identified, it can be subtracted. This is usually achieved by acquiring several images before the contrast appearance and subtracting the average value of these images. Obviously, it is necessary to acquire all the images at the same moment in the cardiac cycle, or alignment methods have to be applied (see paragraph "Effect on the Cardiac Motion").

It is also possible to define linear ROIs or 'profiles' and to draw a graph of intensities along the line. In this way, spatial variations of intensity (variations of perfusion) along the line can be easily visualized. These profiles do not have to be straight lines, since the user can define any curve as desired (Fig. 4.3).

Single-frame quantification provides a way of determining relative perfusion values between different myocardial regions, although it is an oversimplistic method that cannot deal with movement or time evolution information. When this information is required, sequences or cineloops of images have to be analyzed.

Sequence Quantification

The interpretation of image intensity data as a function of time provides functional information of clinical relevance. A sequence or cineloop of images can be analyzed by obtaining a time curve of the evolution of video intensity in different ROIs or in every pixel. Usually, mean intensity within the ROI, after background subtraction, is displayed as a function of time. ROIs are defined as in single-image analysis, but in this case, their position in the myocardium should be corrected along the sequence (see paragraph "Effect on the Cardiac Motion" for automatic or semiautomatic ROI repositioning) (Fig. 4.4).

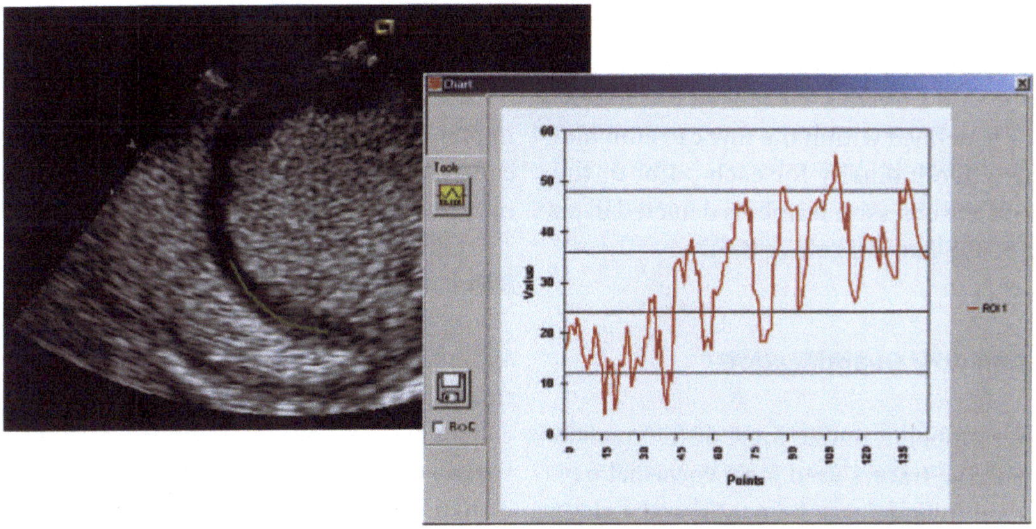

Fig. 4.3. Video intensity along a profile drawn within the myocardium

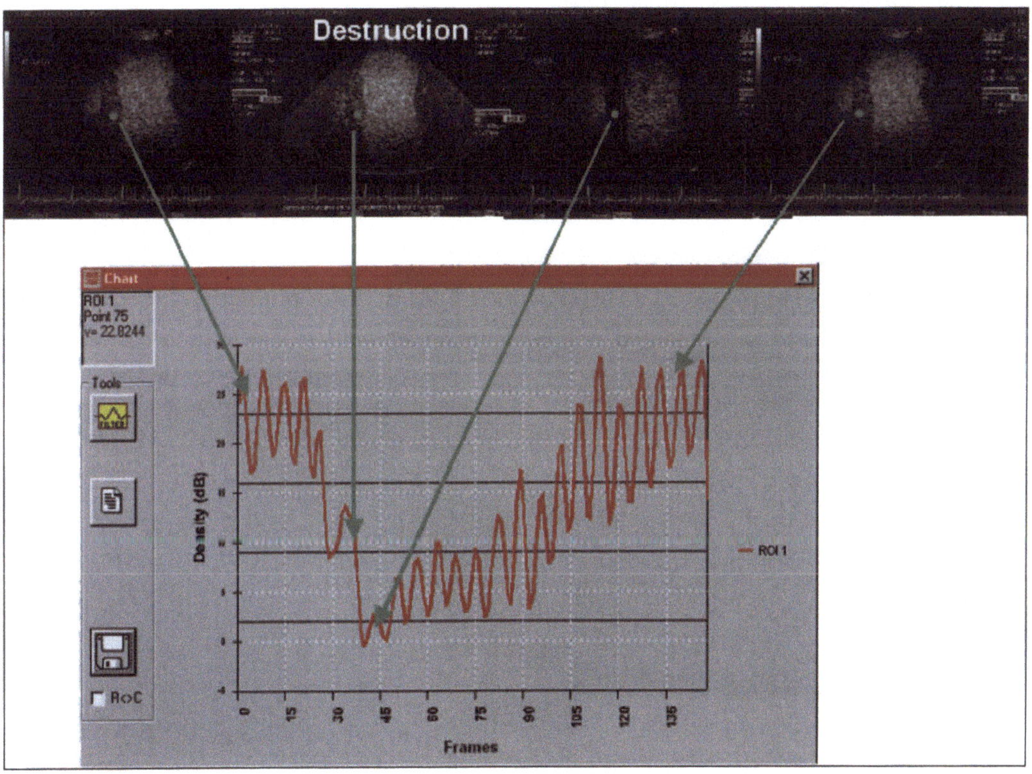

Fig. 4.4. Evolution of the video intensity along time in a ROI drawn within the myocardium The *second frame* corresponds to the moment when a high MI burst is applied From that moment on, reperfusion of the myocardial tissue takes place and can be quantified applying a proper mathematical model

Another way of visualizing spatial and temporal information together is the creation of a curved or calculated M-mode: a line is defined within the myocardium and the video intensity for each point in the curve at successive frames is depicted in an M-mode-like image (Fig. 4.5).

Parametric Quantification

Microbubbles, unlike most of the nuclear medicine tracers used for myocardial perfusion imaging, can be considered strictly intravascular, as they remain in the intravascular space during their transit through the myocardium [2]. For this reason, quantitative information about myocardial blood flow and/or myocardial blood volume can be obtained by applying well-known mathematical models derived from indicator dilution principles [23].

Two main models are applicable, depending on whether the administration of the contrast agent was performed with bolus injection or continuous infusion.

Bolus Analysis

Visual analysis of the video intensity variations after a bolus injection is difficult and cannot provide objective parameters. Quantitative analysis to obtain information related to the blood flow in the myocardium can be performed applying classical mathematical methods.

For this kind of analysis, end-systolic images are acquired from each cardiac cycle from just before contrast injection until its disappearance [3]. Prior to the contrast

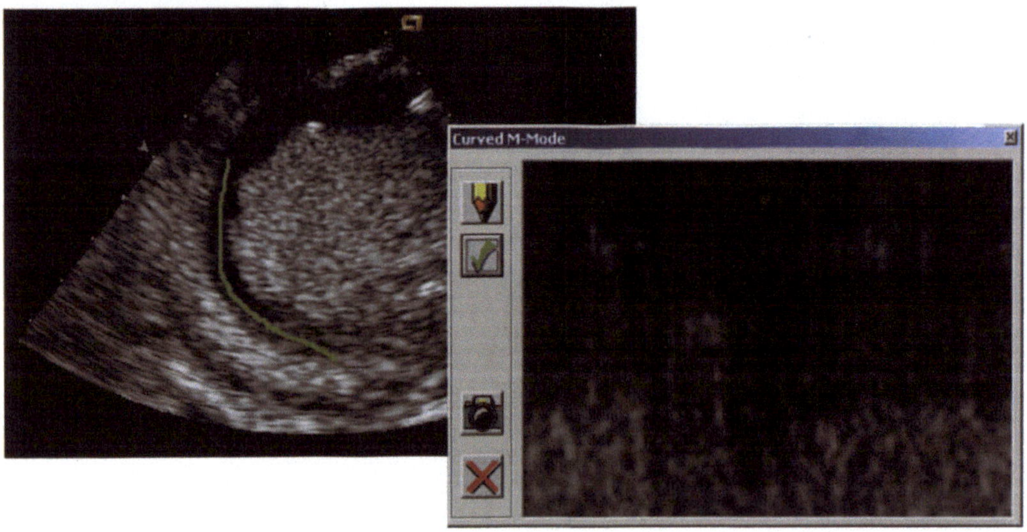

Fig. 4.5. Curved M-mode. A curve is drawn in a frame and exported to all the remaining frames of the sequence (allowing repositioning). The calculated M-mode image visually represents the changes in video intensity along time

appearance, four to six images are acquired and averaged for background subtraction [24]. Time intensity plots from background-subtracted video intensity are then fitted to a gamma-variate function [3, 25]:

$$y = A\,t\,e^{-\alpha t} \qquad (1)$$

where A is a scaling factor, t is time and α is a parameter related to the transit rate of the tracer (Fig. 4.6).

From this model, the following parameters can be obtained:

- Peak video intensity ($A/\alpha\varepsilon$), proportional to the volumetric flow.
- Time-to-peak, $1/\alpha$, time from the beginning of the curve to the maximum intensity.
- Mean transit time (MTT) of the bolus, the average time that the contrast agent takes to travel through the volume under analysis. It corresponds to the center of gravity of the curve, which only coincides with the time of the maximum in symmetrical curves. It is calculated as the first moment of the concentration time intensity plot, approximately equal to $2/\alpha$ (Fig. 4.6).

The mean transit rate (reciprocal of MTT) of a tracer through a sample of myocardial tissue is proportional to the flow-to-volume ratio. Its changes, thus, reflect changes in the regional blood flow if the coronary blood volume is constant or the variations in blood volume if the flow is constant.

The accuracy of the relation between the MTT parameter and myocardial flow has been validated in experimental models and clinical perfusion studies. For example, Wei et al. [3] present a comparison with radiolabeled microsphere myocardial blood flow measurements, showing that a mild to mod-

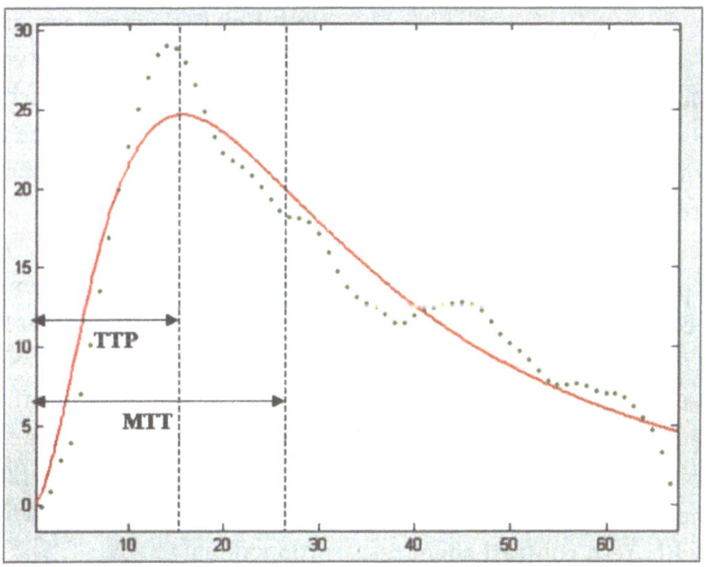

Fig. 4.6. Gamma-variate function (*red*) fitted to a real perfusion curve (*green dots*). Time-to-peak and mean transit time parameters are represented

erate stenosis (<85% lumen diameter narrowing) on an epicardial coronary artery can be detected by identifying the decrease in myocardial blood volume distal to the stenosis.

The gamma-variate function presumes that the system behaves like a two-compartment model and that the bolus entering the myocardial bed is perfect, in the sense of following a mathematical delta function (infinitely short). The lack of detailed knowledge about the shape of the input function, among other technical difficulties, limits the accuracy and usefulness of this technique in clinical practice. Other more complex models able to take into account an imperfect input function have been tested, although their accuracy has not shown to be significantly superior to that of the gamma model [3]. Continuous infusion using reperfusion models is an alternative that offers several advantages, as will be discussed in the next section.

Reperfusion Model

As seen in paragraph "Imaging Tecniques", microbubbles react in different ways to the ultrasonic pulses depending on the mechanical index. This property of the microbubble behavior can be used to measure blood reperfusion in the myocardium. A burst of high-MI pulses sent during a continuous infusion of the contrast agent destroys all the microbubbles, allowing one to record the replenishment of the myocardial tissue [26] as blood with fresh contrast agent reenters the cardiac wall. Two different acquisition techniques are being used to study reperfusion: continuous (real-time) imaging and intermittent imaging.

Images can be acquired in two different ways: (a) triggered mode, in which only one image per cycle is acquired, generally at end-diastole, and (b) continuous or real-time mode, in which images are acquired continuously at a relatively high frame rate. Continuous or real-time imaging makes use of a high-energy (high MI) ultrasound pulse that destroys all the microbubbles and then continuously acquires images using low MI pulses that do not destroy the microbubbles. This allows the increasing degree of myocardial reperfusion to be recorded as an increase of opacification or video intensity.

The mathematical analysis of the data is based on a single-compartment model with an input considered as a step function [25]. The model is defined by a differential equation $dC(t)/dt = \beta[G(t) - C(t)]$, which describes the change in myocardial concentration C(t) within a mixing chamber of volume V with a flow-to volume ratio β, under a certain input function G(t). Solving the equation when the input is a step function leads to an exponential solution of the following form:

$$y = A(1 - e^{-\beta t})$$

where y is the videointensity value, β is the video intensity increase rate, and A is the asymptotic value of video intensity after complete replenishment (value of the plateau) (Fig. 4.7). The slope at the origin ($t = 0$) is $A\beta$. It can be shown [26] that, according to the model, the blood flow (f) must be proportional to $A\beta$.

A different acquisition technique known as 'intermittent imaging' has also been used

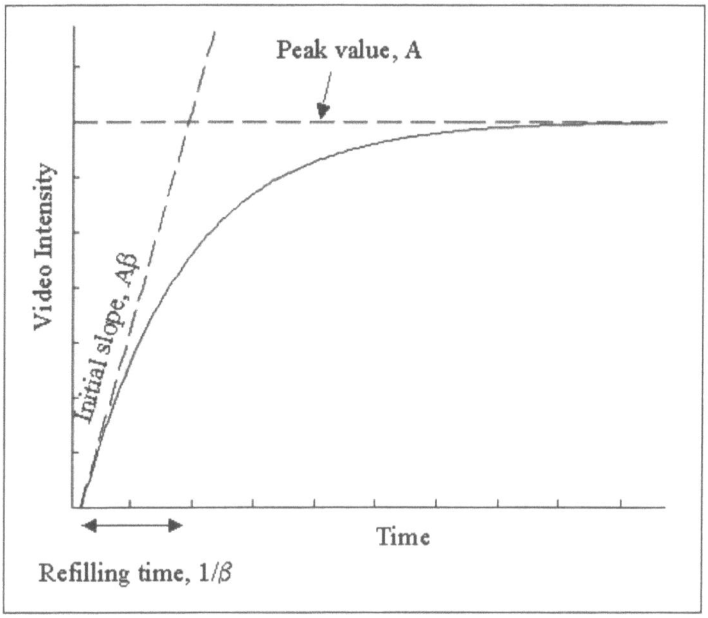

Fig. 4.7. Exponential model with parameters A, β and Aβ indicated

for reperfusion assessment. With this technique, every image is acquired by using high-MI ultrasonic pulses, thus destroying all the microbubbles every time. To measure reperfusion, the time interval between pulses (pulsing interval, PI) is increased in each acquisition to allow a higher amount of contrast to reenter the field at each repetition. Wei et al. [26] proposed a two-piece linear model for the resulting curve: a linear increase in intensity until reaching a constant plateau. However, the video intensity versus pulsing interval curve is also adjusted to an exponential model as in the previous case. The justification for this is that nonuniformities in the ultrasound beam shape and bubble destruction lead to a more 'rounded' curve that can be heuristically approximated by an exponential. An alternative reason to fit an exponential curve may simply be to accept the same compartmental model as in the previous case, since intermittent imaging could be considered a particular case of the continuous curve, sampled at a lower (and perhaps irregular) rate.

In the case of continuous imaging, a cyclic variation of signal intensity can be observed, due to heart beating. This high-frequency variation has been analyzed in some reports, although systolic/diastolic ratios do not seem to be related to regional functional parameters [27, 28]. For this reason, to obtain a correct fitting when using real-time imaging, it is very convenient to perform a previous low-pass filtering of the curve.

The quantification procedure involves the same steps in both acquisition modes:

1. Acquisition of frames following bubble destruction.

2. Regions of interest are placed within the myocardium and repositioned along the sequence, either manually or using some automatic procedure.
3. Time curves are obtained for each region.
4. The curves are low-pass filtered, particularly in the case of real-time acquisition.
5. The parameters of the model are obtained after adjusting the curve to an exponential function by any of the mathematical algorithms available.

Figure 4.8 shows an image of a sequence with two ROIs defined. On the right, the time curves corresponding to the regions are displayed, showing the fitted exponential models. Notice the different degrees of reperfusion (values of A) and replenishment rates (described by β) corresponding to regions with normal and reduced perfusion.

Masugata et al. [29] studied the values of the reperfusion parameters under graded coronary stenosis, and showed that β and Aβ correlated well with the degree of stenosis, while A alone did not.

A comparison between real-time and intermittent triggered imaging for the quantification of coronary stenosis and transmural perfusion gradient was reported by Masugata et al. [30] using an open-chest model in dogs. They showed that for the quantification of altered myocardial blood flow these methods are equivalent, both visually and quantitatively. With both imaging modalities, the product of Aβ shows a good correlation with myocardial blood flow measured with fluorescent microspheres, higher than that found using parameters A or β alone. The asymptotic plateau of video intensity was found to be lower with real-time imaging, requiring a higher amount of

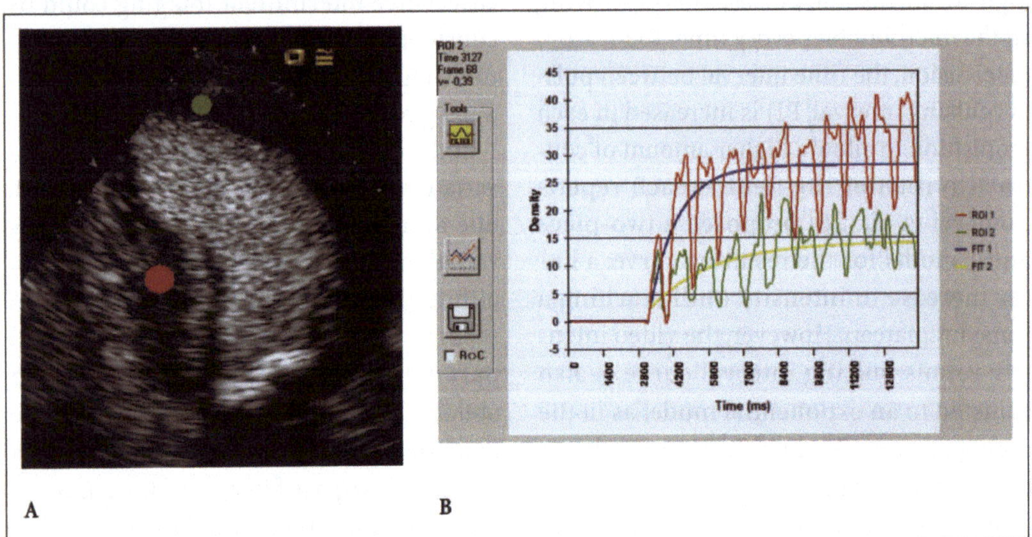

Fig. 4.8. A Two regions of interest in different myocardial segments (real-time acquisition) **B** Corresponding time intensity curves and fitted exponential models for both ROIs. The *green* ROI corresponds to a hypoperfused segment

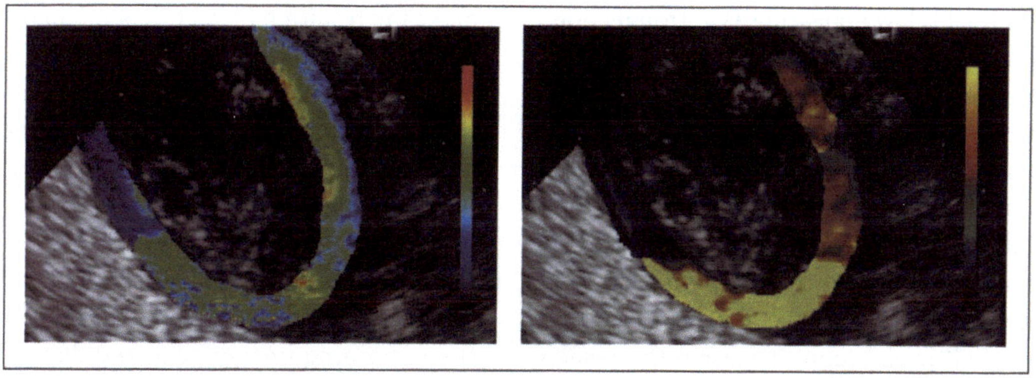

Fig. 4.9. Parametric images obtained from a mini-pig (open-chest experimental model) with reduction of the LAD coronary artery flow. Sequence was acquired with continuous infusion and real-time ECG-gated acquisition mode (CCI, Siemens-Acuson) and quantified according to an exponential model. Parameters A (*left*) and β (*right*) are overlaid in color over the first image after bubble destruction. Ischemic region shows significantly smaller A and β in comparison with the normally perfused segments

contrast to obtain the same intensity values.

A new and more attractive way of presenting these data ('parametric imaging') is being progressively introduced. It consists in obtaining time curves for all the pixels in the image instead of working only with a few number of separate ROIs [31]. Any parameter of the model (A, β, Aβ, time to peak) can then be computed for any pixel, showing their value as a color overlay in the parametric image, as shown in Fig. 4.9. Parametric imaging requires a very good alignment of all the images in the sequence (see paragraph "Effect of the Cardiac Motion").

Limitations of the Quantification Methods

Accuracy of the quantification methods as a myocardial perfusion assessment tool is impaired by several factors, whose knowledge is critical to improving reliability in the future. Some of them may apply to all quantification techniques, while others are only relevant for model-based methods.

One problem common to all the techniques is the possible lack of linearity between video intensity and the concentration of the contrast agent. Although all the quantification techniques assume a linear relationship between regional video intensity and the concentration of the contrast agent, this is just an approximation, not fully justified in most imaging systems [23]. Two different processes are involved in this assumption: the nature of the backscatter signal depending on the microbubble concentration and the representation of this received signal as an image. Relative changes in contrast agent concentration produce variations of the ultrasound backscatter signal, also affected by scattering and absorption mechanisms during its propagation. The effect of these problems is less important when the concentration of contrast is low, appearing as a strongly nonlinear saturation effect at higher concentrations [25]. In the sonographer, the representation of the received signal as an image is generated through a look-up table (LUT) that maps signal intensity onto video intensity (either gray level or color); this map may be (and frequently is) strongly nonlinear. To achieve a better dynamic range it is common to present the results on a scale in decibels that implies a logarithmic translation. This cause of nonlinearity is not supposed to be a problem for the quantitative analysis as it can be mathematically corrected if the look-up table is known.

Another factor that affects all the quantification methods is that intensity values may differ greatly among subjects or even among repetitions of the experiment, as a consequence of the depth-dependent attenuation of reflected sound waves. This is generally overcome by using relative measurements obtained by normalizing the video intensity of the myocardium with respect to that of the cavity.

Methods based on the reperfusion parametric quantification model have some specific limitations that may degrade the goodness-of-fit to the theoretical exponential curve:

a. Uncertainty about the position of the initial point. The initial point for curve fitting should be selected in a moment with minimum contrast. However, depending on the specific sonographer and acquisition parameter settings, a different degree of microbubble destruction is achieved [26]. Noise in this initial part of the curve can make the resulting fit very dependent on the particular initial point chosen. Another possibility is to add a constant term (y_0) to the exponential model, to account for this nonzero initial value, obtaining the following model:

$$y = A(1 - e^{-\beta t}) + y_0$$

Other authors [31] make use of a precontrast image that is subtracted from all the remaining images acquired during reperfusion. This method, however, assumes a correct realignment of all frames with the precontrast image.

b. Curve filtering. The time curve is usually low-pass filtered before adjustment to the exponential model. The type and degree of filtering can affect the adjustment and modify the value of the parameters obtained from the model.

c. Validity of the exponential model. Throughout the quantification process it is assumed that the reperfusion process is accurately modeled by an exponential function. This is only an approximation, and the reliability of the parameters obtained is obviously limited by the goodness-of-fit of the model to the real reperfusion process. The behavior of the contrast agent during its passage through the myocardium is more complex than the model presumes. The microbubbles do not seem to pass unimpeded through the microcirculation and hence their behavior does not follow a straight compartmental model [25].

All these limitations may introduce inaccuracies in the actual values of the parameters, as obtained after the exponential fitting. The problem is particularly severe when trying to compare values obtained with different acquisition settings or using different quantification software packages. It is, however, less worrying in comparative studies carried out with the same setting.

Finally, another source of error, also common to all the quantification techniques, is that due to the movement of the transducer, respiration, etc., there may be a displacement of the images along the sequence. This is especially severe when using real-time acquisition, as the position of the structures changes continuously along the heart cycle. This particularly difficult problem is addressed in the next section.

Effect of the Cardiac Motion

As already mentioned in this chapter, in most of the applications of myocardial contrast quantification, heart motion constitutes a significant source of error which needs to be corrected. The complete sequence of images or at least the ROIs must be carefully aligned to obtain accurate time curves for model fitting or to create parametric images representing a certain feature for every pixel. If it is done manually (usually with ROIs), the operator must revise the whole cineloop to validate that the position of the ROI is correct in every frame. For some applications, the only concern is that the region does not include at any moment bright values from the neighboring cavities [32]. In studies aiming at the detection of small perfusion defects or when slight differences are expected, a finer alignment must be carried out. This is the case, for example, in studies that try to calculate endocardial/epicardial perfusion ratios [30].

Although most studies still rely on a manual alignment to properly position the ROIs [33], an increasing number of attempts at using automatic alignment or tracking tools is being observed [34]. These automatic methods can be divided into two main groups, those using algorithms to reposition individual ROIs, and registration-based approaches, in which the whole images are realigned.

Algorithms in the first group track local intensity in a pixel-to-pixel (or small neighborhoods) basis, seeking for correspondences between local gray level patterns. Among these techniques, reviewed in [35], the most representative are 'optical flow' and 'block matching' methods. Some global smoothness constraint is normally added to impose spatial coherence in the displacement field, to avoid big changes in the displacement amplitude and direction in a small neighborhood. These methods have long been proposed in conventional echocardiography as an alternative to Doppler imaging to estimate tissue motion [36] or to assess myocardial deformation [37]. We have evaluated several local block matching algorithms as a tool to track a ROI along the sequence in contrast echocardiography. Results have proven accurate enough for clinical purposes and computation times may allow for real-time processing (Fig. 4.10).

The second approach retrieves the displacement vectors for every point in the image finding the deformation field between every pair of images, in a process commonly denoted as alignment or registration. These

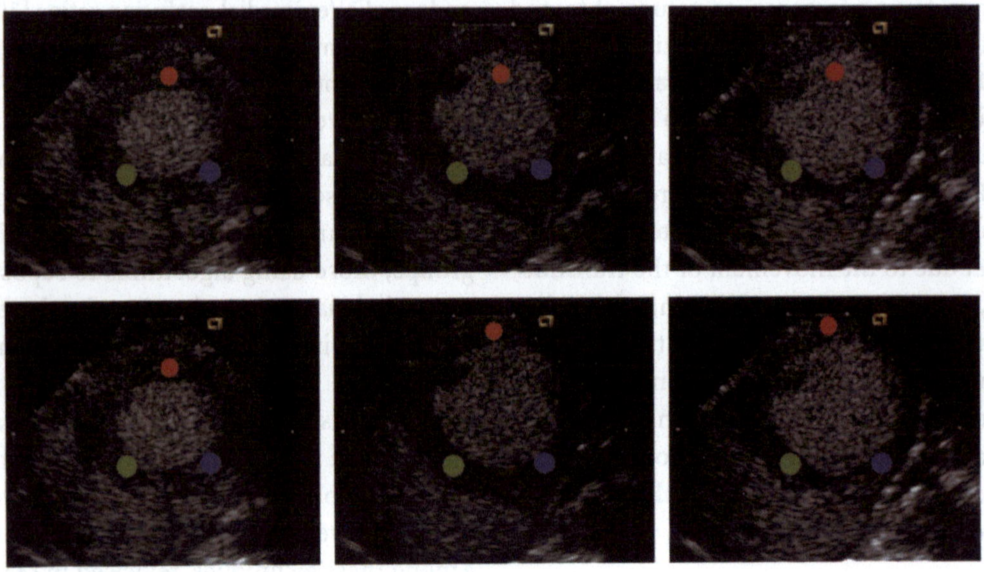

Fig. 4.10. Three frames of a sequence on which three ROIs have been defined. *Upper row* shows the position of the ROIs without any tracking. *Lower row* shows the position after automatic tracking

methods take into account all the pixels in the image (or the object of interest) in a global manner, obtaining all the displacements at the same time. The smoothness and spatial coherence is therefore automatically imposed within the deformation definition.

The deformation computed for any pair of images provides an incremental displacement between them, obtained by minimizing the difference in intensity between the two images while iteratively adjusting the deformation parameters. The intensity similarity measurements more commonly used are cross-correlation or least-squares differences. The alignment process is repeated for all the consecutive pairs of images in the cardiac cycle sequence and the incremental displacements are added together to compute the accumulated displacement for every point in the image. Once known, the deformation field can be applied either to compute trajectories (or derived parameters: velocity, acceleration, strain, etc.) or to actually deform the images making them match each other [18, 24, 38]. The nature of the deformation depends on the acquisition technique; with triggered methods, normally rigid transformations (translation and rotation) are enough. This is the approach used in [24]. With real-time methods, nonrigid transformations are needed due to the elastic nature of the myocardium [18, 38].

An advantage of whole-image registration is that once the complete sequence is correctly aligned, all the pixels can be studied, enabling an easy calculation of parametric images.

Future Trends

Myocardial contrast echocardiography has evolved from the initial experiments using intra-arterial injections and fundamental imaging to a more productive environment, employing intravenous administration, more advanced acquisition techniques that noticeably enhance the image, and a quantitative interpretation of the results. The possibility of generating parametric images, that leads to results more similar to those classically obtained by other image modalities, such as nuclear medicine or cardio MRI is remarkable. However, a reliable use of parametric imaging requires a solution to the problem of movement. As mentioned in this chapter, some mathematical approaches to this issue are yielding very promising results, although clinical validation will require more time. Nevertheless, we must take into account that these movement-correction techniques are only an approximation, since the movement of the heart takes place in 3D while the correction works strictly in-plane. Only a 3D acquisition would provide a complete dataset that would allow for an exact compensation of the displacement of the structures under analysis. The feasibility of perfusion analysis using 3D echocardiography is stressed in some recent studies [39]. One of the problems of working in 3D is the difficult visualization of the data; Yao et al.[40] proposed a bull's-eye view to present perfusion defects. Three-dimensional echocardiography technology is not yet mature, although great advances both in acquisition and in quantification methods are expected in the near future.

Another interesting approach would be to integrate the information provided by different methods of analysis, particularly myocardial perfusion assessment and wall motion analysis. This could increase the sensitivity and specificity of myocardial contrast echocardiography.

Finally, it should be underlined that the difficult introduction of these techniques into routine practice depends mainly on the lack of standardized procedures, both for the acquisition and for the quantitative analysis. If manufacturers and users reached an accord on at least some well-tested procedures, it would be easier to collect multicentre data to establish clinical indications, sensitivity and specificity in different pathologies and clinical situations.

References

1. Cohen JL, Cheirif J, Segar DS, Gillam LD, Gottdiener JS, Hausnerova E, Bruns DE (1998) Improved left ventricular endocardial border delineation and opacification with OPTISON (FS069), a new echocardiographic contrast agent. Results of a phase III Multicenter Trial. J Am Coll Cardiol 32:746-752
2. Becher H, Burns P (2000) Handbook of Contrast Echocardiography. Springer-Verlag Berlin Heidelberg
3. Wei K, Jayaweera AR, Firoozan S, Linka A, Skyba DM, Kaul S (1998) Basis for detection of stenosis using venous administration of microbubbles during myocardial contrast echocardiography: bolus or continuous infusion? J Am Coll Cardiol 32:252-260
4. Lindner JR, Villanueva FS, Dent JM, Wei K, Sklenar J, Kaul S (2000) Assessment of resting perfusion with myocardial contrast echocardiography: theoretical and practical considerations. Am Heart J 139:231-240

5. Marwick TH, Brunken R, Meland N, Brochet E, Baer FM, Binder T, Flachskampf F, Kamp O, Nienaber C, Nihoyannopoulos P, Pierard L, Vanoverschelde JL, van der Wouw P, Lindvall K (1998) Accuracy and feasibility of contrast echocardiography for detection of perfusion defects in routine practice: comparison with wall motion and technetium-99m sestamibi single-photon emission computed tomography. The Nycomed NC100100 Investigators. J Am Coll Cardiol 32:1260-1269
6. Vannan MA, Kuersten B (2000) Imaging techniques for myocardial contrast echocardiography. Eur J Echocardiogr 1:224-226
7. Mulvagh SL, DeMaria AN, Feinstein SB, Burns PN, Kaul S, Miller JG, Monaghan M, Porter TR, Shaw LJ, Villanueva FS (2000) Contrast echocardiography: current and future applications. J Am Soc Echocardiogr 13:331-342
8. Weissman NJ, Cohen MC, Hack TC, Gillam LD, Cohen JL, Kitzman DW (2000) Infusion versus bolus contrast echocardiography: a multicenter, open-label, crossover trial. Am Heart J 139:399-404
9. Rubin DN, Yazbek N, Garcia MJ, Stewart WJ, Thomas JD (2000) Qualitative and quantitative effects of harmonic echocardiographic imaging on endocardial edge definition and side-lobe artifacts. J Am Soc Echocardiogr 13:1012-1018
10. Mor-Avi V, Caiani EG, Collins KA, Korcarz CE, Bednarz JE, Lang RM (2001) Combined assessment of myocardial perfusion and regional left ventricular function by analysis of contrast-enhanced power modulation images. Circulation 104:352-357
11. von Bibra H, Bone D, Niklasson U, Eurenius L, Hansen A (2002) Myocardial contrast echocardiography yields best accuracy using quantitative analysis of digital data from pulse inversion technique: comparison with second harmonic imaging and harmonic power Doppler during simultaneous dipyridamole stress SPECT studies. Eur J Echocardiogr 3:271-282
12. Schiller NB, Shah PM, Crawford M, DeMaria A, Devereux R, Feigenbaum H, Gutgesell H, Reichek N, Sahn D, Schnittger I, et al. (1989) Recommendations for quantitation of the left ventricle by two-dimensional echocardiography. American Society of Echocardiography Committee on Standards, Subcommittee on Quantitation of Two-Dimensional Echocardiograms. J Am Soc Echocardiogr 2:358-367
13. Hoffmann R, Lethen H, Marwick T, Arnese M, Fioretti P, Pingitore A, Picano E, Buck T, Erbel R, Flachskampf FA, Hanrath P (1996) Analysis of interinstitutional observer agreement in interpretation of dobutamine stress echocardiograms. J Am Coll Cardiol 27:330-336
14. Fedele F, Trambaiolo P, Magni G, De Castro S, Cacciotti L (1998) New modalities of regional and global left ventricular function analysis: state of the art. Am J Cardiol 81:49G-57G.
15. Clarysse P, Han M, Croisille P, Magnin IE (2002) Exploratory analysis of the spatio-temporal deformation of the myocardium during systole from tagged MRI. IEEE Trans Biomed Eng 49:1328-1339
16. Marwick TH (2002) Quantitative techniques for stress echocardiography: dream or reality? Eur J Echocardiogr 3:171-176
17. Jacob G, Noble JA, Kelion AD, Banning AP (2001) Quantitative regional analysis of myocardial wall motion. Ultrasound Med Biol 27:773-784
18. Ledesma-Carbayo MJ, Kybic J, Desco M, Santos A, Unser M (2001) Cardiac motion analysis from ultrasound sequences using non-rigid registration. In: Niessen WJ, Viergeber MA (eds) MICCAI. Springer Verlag, Berlin, pp 889-896
19. Crouse LJ, Cheirif J, Hanly DE, Kisslo JA, Labovitz AJ, Raichlen JS, Schutz RW, Shah PM, Smith MD (1993) Opacification and border delineation improvement in patients with suboptimal endocardial border definition in routine echocardiography: results of the Phase III Albunex Multicenter Trial. J Am Coll Cardiol 22:1494-1500
20. Takeuchi M, Yoshitani H, Miyazaki C, Haruki N, Otani S, Sakamoto K, Yoshikawa J (2003) Color kinesis during contrast-enhanced dobutamine stress echocardiography. Circ J 67:49-53
21. Spencer KT, Bednarz J, Mor-Avi V, DeCara J, Lang RM (2002) Automated endocardial border detection and evaluation of left ventricular function from contrast-enhanced images using modified acoustic quantification. J Am Soc Echocardiogr 15:777-781
22. Papademetris X, Sinusas AJ, Dione DP, Duncan JS (2001) Estimation of 3D left ventricular deformation from echocardiography. Med Image Anal 5:17-28
23. Mor-Avi V, Akselrod S, David D, Keselbrener L, Bitton Y (1993) Myocardial transit time of the echocardiographic contrast media. Ultrasound Med Biol 19:635-648
24. Jayaweera AR, Sklenar J, Kaul S (1994) Quantification of images obtained during myocardial contrast echocardiography. Echocardiography 11:385-396
25. Jayaweera AR, Edwards N, Glasheen WP, Villanueva FS, Abbott RD, Kaul S (1994) In vivo myocardial kinetics of air-filled albumin microbubbles during myocardial contrast echocardiography. Comparison with radiolabeled red blood cells. Circ Res 74:1157-1165
26. Wei K, Jayaweera AR, Firoozan S, Linka A, Skyba DM, Kaul S (1998) Quantification of myocardial blood flow with ultrasound-induced destruction of

microbubbles administered as a constant venous infusion. Circulation 97:473-483
27. Janerot-Sjoberg B, von Schmalensee N, Schreckenberger A, Richter A, Brandt E, Kirkhorn J, Wilkenshoff U (2001) Influence of respiration on myocardial signal intensity. Ultrasound Med Biol 27:473-479
28. Bekeredjian R, Hansen A, Filusch A, Dubart AE, Da Silva KG, Jr., Hardt SS, Korosoglou G, Kuecherer HF (2002) Cyclic variation of myocardial signal intensity in real-time myocardial perfusion imaging. J Am Soc Echocardiogr 15:1425-1431
29. Masugata H, Peters B, Lafitte S, Monet G, Ohmori K, DeMaria AN (2001) Quantitative assessment of myocardial perfusion during graded coronary stenosis by real-time myocardial contrast echo refilling curves. J Am Coll Cardiol 37:262-269
30. Masugata H, Lafitte S, Peters B, Strachan GM, DeMaria AN (2001) Comparison of real-time and intermittent triggered myocardial contrast echocardiography for quantification of coronary stenosis severity and transmural perfusion gradient. Circulation 104:1550-1556
31. Linka AZ, Sklenar J, Wei K, Jayaweera AR, Skyba DM, Kaul S (1998) Assessment of transmural distribution of myocardial perfusion with contrast echocardiography. Circulation 98:1912-1920
32. Lafitte S, Higashiyama A, Masugata H, Peters B, Strachan M, Kwan OL, DeMaria AN (2002) Contrast echocardiography can assess risk area and infarct size during coronary occlusion and reperfusion: experimental validation. J Am Coll Cardiol 39:1546-1554
33. Di Bello V, Pedrinelli R, Giorgi D, Bertini A, Talini E, Mengozzi G, Palagi C, Nardi C, Dell'Omo G, Paterni M, Mariani M (2002) Coronary microcirculation in essential hypertension: a quantitative myocardial contrast echocardiographic approach. Eur J Echocardiogr 3:117-127
34. García-Fernández MA, Bermejo J, Pérez-David E, López-Fernández T, Ledesma MJ, Caso P, Malpica N, Santos A, Moreno M, Desco M (2003) New techniques for the assessment of regional left ventricular wall motion. Echocardiography (in press)
35. Barron JL, Fleet DJ, Beauchemin SS (1994) Performance of optical flow techniques. Int J Computer Vision 12:43-77
36. Hein IA, O'Brien WD (1993) Current time-domain methods for assessing tissue motion by analysis from reflected ultrasound echoes - A review. IEEE Trans Ultrason, Ferroelec, Freq Contr 40:84-102
37. Mailloux GE, Langlois F, Simard PY, Bertrand M (1989) Restoration of the velocity field of the heart from two dimensional echocardiograms. IEEE Trans Med Imag 8:143-153
38. Noble JA, Dawson D, Lindner J, Sklenar J, Kaul S (2002) Automated, nonrigid alignment of clinical myocardial contrast echocardiography image sequences: comparison with manual alignment. Ultrasound Med Biol 28:115-123
39. Camarano G, Jones M, Freidlin RZ, Panza JA (2002) Quantitative assessment of left ventricular perfusion defects using real-time three-dimensional myocardial contrast echocardiography. J Am Soc Echocardiogr 15:206-213
40. Yao J, De Castro S, Delabays A, Masani N, Udelson JE, Pandian NG (2001) Bulls-eye display and quantitation of myocardial perfusion defects using three-dimensional contrast echocardiography. Echocardiography 18:581-588

Chapter 5

Clinical Application of Quantitative Analysis in Myocardial Contrast Echocardiography

Luciano Agati • Gianni Tonti • Gianni Pedrizzetti

After many years of study and research, the non-invasive assessment of myocardial perfusion by the intravenous injection of echocontrast agents has become a clinical reality [1-6]. The fast technological progress of echocardiographic imaging and the approval of some first- and second-generation contrast agents such as *Levovist* (Schering), *SonoVue* (Bracco Imaging), *Optison* (Amersham Health), *Definity* (Bristol-Myers Squibb) *Imagent* (Alliance Pharmaceutical Corp., San Diego, CA), for use in humans in Europe and the USA explains the growing interest in this new methodology.

To date, intravenous myocardial contrast echocardiography (MCE) seems to be one of the most cost-effective techniques for assessing microvascular dysfunction in patients with coronary artery disease [7, 8]. Compared to radionuclide myocardial imaging, which detects regional differences in left ventricular perfusion and is dependent on cellular metabolism for radionuclide uptake, MCE is strictly dependent on microvascular integrity and allows the evaluation of nutrient myocardial blood flow that actually feeds dysfunctioning segments [9].

MCE has been particularly used in patients with acute myocardial infarction (AMI) since it is a low-cost bedside technique with the potential to be widely available [10]. TIMI myocardial perfusion grade, Doppler flow wire, magnetic resonance imaging and nuclear myocardial perfusion imaging have also been used to assess microvascular integrity after reperfusion therapy; however, none of them has been implemented in routine diagnosis of acute coronary syndromes because they are either invasive and more expensive or not easily available in most hospitals and in this particular setting.

The use of intracoronary and intravenous MCE in patients with AMI has allowed the clinical demonstration of no-reflow phenomenon, showing that about one-third to one-fourth of patients with AMI had an inadequate tissue perfusion despite angiographically successful coronary recanalization [11, 22].

Considering that the emerging pathophysiological paradigm of acute coronary syndromes centres on the role of activated platelets and links the epicardial manifestation of plaque disruption to the impairment of microvascular function, MCE may provide definitive evidence on the protective role of the new antiplatelets drugs, in particular glycoprotein IIb/IIIa inhibitors, against microvascular damage in patients with AMI.

The no-reflow extent soon after reperfusion is a good predictor of irreversible left ventricular (LV) dysfunction at follow-up [11, 24]. Conflicting data exist on changes of microvascular perfusion in the convalescent stage after AMI [25]. Different studies indicated that ischaemic microvascular damage may be reversible or progressive after coronary reflow. We and others [14, 15] have demonstrated, by MCE, that either ischaemic microvascular damage or LV dysfunction may recover in the late stage of AMI. These observations confirm the presence of "microvascular stunning". However, the degree of perfusion and functional improvement varies among patients. This improvement may continue for up to 7 months. In our experience, the degree of MCE reflow at 2–3 weeks after AMI is highly predictive of LV function recovery up to 6 months after AMI. Thus, in patients surviving AMI, the predischarge MCE analysis of the extent of residual perfusion within the infarct zone is a simple and useful method to better distinguish still viable from necrotic myocardial regions.

The relationship between MCE residual perfusion into the infarct zone and inotropic reserve has been deeply investigated [26-29]. However, recent MCE studies have suggested a beneficial role of microvascular integrity on post-infarction LV remodelling, independent of the effective functional recovery [30, 31]. This hypothesis is in keeping with the paradigm that thrombolysis after AMI increases survival without improving LV function.

Imaging Methods for MCE

Two imaging modalities, intermittent and real-time imaging, are currently used to detect microbubbles in the myocardium. At sufficiently high acoustic pressures, ultrasounds destroy microbubbles (stimulated acoustic emission) producing a strong signal that can be easily detected using the intermittent imaging modality, whereas at low acoustic pressures microbubbles resonate producing a weak harmonic signal that can be detected using real-time imaging [5, 6] (Figs. 5.1–5.3).

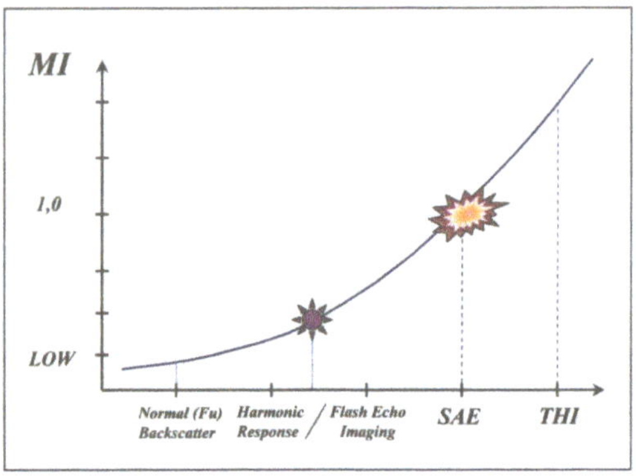

Fig. 5.1. Relationship between ultrasound energy and bubble behavior. *MI* mechanical index; *SAE* stimulated acoustic emission

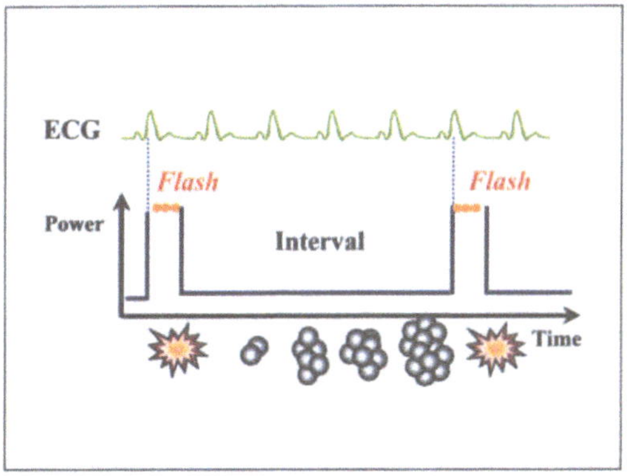

Fig. 5.2. Intermittent imaging

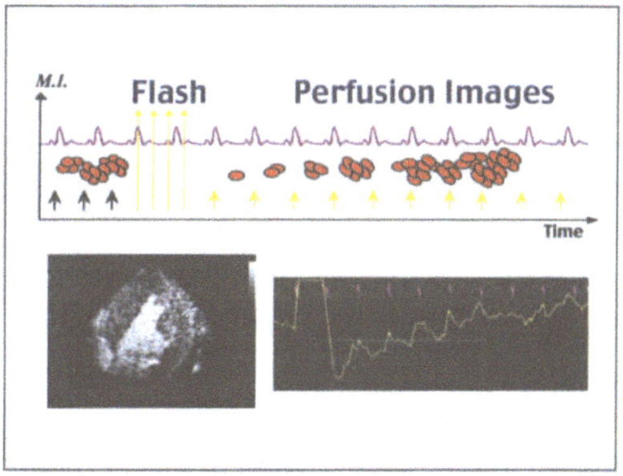

Fig. 5.3. Real-time imaging

Intermittent Imaging

To obtain a reliable myocardial opacification by destructive methods, contrast agents with a thin shell and a low persistent gas should be used. The reduced solubility and the high molecular weights of gases used for "second-generation" contrast agents make it harder to differentiate them from tissue when a microbubble destruction imaging technique is used [32-34].

Levovist®, which is a galactose-based echo-enhancing "first-generation" contrast agent highly responsive to ultrasound, is currently the most widely used agent for intermittent imaging. When mixed with water, it results in microbubbles of air covered by a thin layer of palmitic acid. Almost all microbubbles within the myocardium are "acoustically destroyed" by a single sweep of ultrasound resulting in a high and rapid Doppler signal.

The higher the transmitted power, the more bubbles are destroyed resulting in a sudden increase in returning signal amplitude. The faster the bubbles disappear, the easier it is to separate that effect from cardiac motion which also produces a changing signal. Several parameters affect microbubble dissolution, including their composition, amplitude and frequency of insonation [5, 6]. To ensure complete microbubble destruction after a single ultrasound sweep during continuous contrast media infusion and to avoid motion artefacts, the amount of ultrasound exposure may be enhanced by increasing the frame rate and mechanical index (MI). Further, the higher PRF (3.2–6.2 kHz) should be used since frequency of insonation affects dissolution rate [5, 6, 32-34].

Real-Time Imaging

To assess the replenishment curves, the "flash" method is currently used [35]. After a few frames (5–9) at high energy using a mechanical index as high as possible, all the bubbles are destroyed; switching to low MI (0.09–0.15), a signal produced from bubble resonation may be followed until a complete refilling is reached. For these imaging modalities only second-generation contrast agents are used.

A new second-generation echocontrast agent, SonoVue™, has been recently approved and is now introduced in the European market. SonoVue™ is a new echo-contrast agent made of microbubbles stabilized by phospholipids and containing sulphur hexafluoride [36]. The introduction of SonoVue® in phase III clinical trials coincided with the introduction of real-time perfusion imaging in clinical practice. At present, SonoVue® is one of the most promising contrast agent when used with low MI techniques because of the following characteristics: it is highly responsive to ultrasound energy, it is easily destroyed at high energy, and the harmonic signal at low energy is strong.

MCE: Quantitative Analysis

In a narrow range, myocardial video intensity (VI) reflects linearly the concentration of microbubbles in the region analysed. Myocardial bubble concentration is mainly dependent on three factors: (a) myocardial blood volume (MBV), (b) the fraction of the MBV within the ultrasound beam that is filled with microbubbles, and (c) the concentration of microbubbles in the blood [5]. Thus, for quantitative analysis, continuous contrast infusion is mandatory to maintain the blood concentration of bubbles constant. Higher doses of contrast produce far-field attenuation, whereas lower doses preclude an adequate myocardial opacification. A fine balance must be achieved between good myocardial opacification and the least amount of shadowing, by adjusting the rate of contrast infusion.

After the flash in real-time imaging, or increasing the pulse intervals using intermittent imaging, myocardial VI progressively increases with time until the MBV within the entire ultrasound beam is filled reaching a plateau, at which time VI reflects MBV. At this point, the signal detected in the myocardium is a corollary of the blood volume of myocardial capillaries. The rate of change of VI from baseline to plateau represents microbubble velocity (MV). As Wei et al. [37] showed, for each segment, plots of signal intensity versus time or pulsing intervals may be constructed and fit an exponential function $y = A \times (1-e^{-\beta t})$ where A is the plateau or VI peak and β is the rate constant that determines the rate of increase in VI. A is a measure of myocardial blood volume, β is a measure of myocardial blood flow velocity and the product $A \times \beta$ is a measure of myocardial blood flow.

Since the myocardial blood flow should be reduced (in the infarct area), the rate of destruction of contrast may exceed its replenishment in this zone if a shorter intermittent imaging is used [14]. For this reason, end-systolic trigger intervals should be increased. During these prolonged trigger intervals, particular attention should be paid to maintaining the same scan plan by reducing the patient's breathing. All these problems are completely avoided using real-time imaging.

When steady-state is achieved, myocardial VI is influenced by both MV and MBV. Unfortunately, myocardial VI also depends on several other factors such as cardiac output, acoustic impedance of the chest wall, and in particular the homogeneity of the ultrasound field. If the acoustic pressure within the ultrasound field is inhomogeneous, bubbles destruction/resonation occurs and hence myocardial VI may vary between different beds in different views. To avoid this pitfall, the ratio between the VI of the segment and the brightest normokinetic segment of the same view should be used. Alternatively, myocardial opacification may be normalized for the signal intensity of the left ventricular blood pool and expressed in percentage.

For quantitative purposes, digital or radiofrequency data have been used instead of video signal since the latter contains only part of the information available in the digital data. The limited dynamic range of the video signal (20–30 dB vs >50 dB in digital) may mask contrast effects in the lowest and highest range of signal intensities. For these reasons quantitative analysis of digital data results in improved diagnostic accuracy as compared to qualitative analysis of video signal [38].

Finally, since myocardial regions with prior myocardial infarction have a higher VI during harmonic imaging at baseline, quantitation may be helpful to appreciate small increases in VI after microbubble injection. In these patients, for qualitative assessment, color-coded images should be preferred over gray-scale since the human eye can discern only a few shades of gray but it can discriminate between thousands of colors.

Software for Quantitative Analysis

For an adequate quantification of the contrast signal it is crucial to follow the systo-diastolic motion of the heart walls. The heart shows not only inherent movement but also displacements due to respiration. Moreover, the physician performing the examination can move the probe itself during data acquisition. For these reasons, if the signal from the wall is detected using a region of interest (ROI) placed at a fixed location, the ROI frequently falls on other structures (i.e., left or right ventricular cavities or outside the heart). Thus, to quantify the wall-related properties it is important to verify that the selected ROI will remain inside the tissue in all the images of the sequence, otherwise information that does not pertain to the tissue is included and the analysis is corrupted. Using this method, the sequence should be reviewed frame by frame and the ROI is manually moved when it falls outside the tissue. This approach is extremely time consuming (in real-time imaging up to 200 frames for each ROI should be reviewed). Some software applications (based on standard edge detection or on cross-correlation alignment) may automatically carry out this procedure. However, in most cases these techniques are not able to guarantee the accuracy of the results since they incorporate no information about the structure and the geometry, and the wall detection is still manually verified.

Conversely, if the wall is continuously tracked, the right signal originating from the tissue is detected and quantitative parameters of regional perfusion may be correctly analyzed.

We developed a new revolutionary method for quantitative analysis of destruction/replenishment curves based on automatic loop processing by an advanced tracking technique. The software (AMID®) is able to continuously track the myocardial wall and analyze the time evolution of the VI in correspondence with the detected wall. MCE images have to be digitally stored in a magneto-optical disk. At least ten cardiac cycles after the flash should be stored in the optical disk to be able to follow the entire replenishment phase. The loops are then automatically processed. The central points (axis) of the myocardial region are determined by an advanced image processing technique that allows recognition of the coherence of the image in a space-time (three-dimensional) domain; in the same manner, the width of the myocardium is defined by a rigorous statistical approach that defines the dispersion of coherence of this previously found center. Such a technique defines the position and thickness of the wall at each instant. The ROI becomes a moving one and the analysis is not restricted to a group of points fixed in space, which may fall outside of the real ROI at some instants, but rather to points that continuously identify and follow the correct tissue area.

Once the myocardium region is systematically determined, at each instant, the signal intensity of the points that belong to such areas is averaged and a smooth myocardial signal intensity is obtained without the introduction of any artificial smoothing procedure. This signal is then analyzed. In the case of a real-time analysis, the signal presents systo-diastolic oscillations that are preferably eliminated a priori to better quantify the purely refilling properties. This can be done by a moving average filtering, commonly with a Gaussian window, with the width calculated by the heartbeat frequency.

The flash period is automatically determined, and then a nonlinear fit to the single exponential function is performed in two steps. A tentative value of the parameters is estimated by explicit formulas; the peak is estimated from the average of the highest values in the signal, and the corresponding refilling time is obtained from an integral condition. Starting from these parameters, a least square error minimization procedure, based on the simplest method, will eventually converge to the optimal peak and refilling time of the exponential fitting function.

The entire procedure is automatically done by the software (AMID®); human intervention is limited to the initial definition (drawing) of a polygon that contains the myocardium at any time. Errors are essentially related to the image quality (Fig. 5.4).

Using this software, VI plots may be generated for each myocardial segment from 4-, 3-, and 2-chamber views at baseline and during hyperemic stimulation, and regional coronary flow reserve (CFR) can be calculated.

One of the problems frequently observed in a correct definition of replenishment curves, either in intermittent or in real-time imaging, is the value of VI in the first frame after the flash. If after the flash VI in the myocardial wall is not zero or near zero (i.e., if bubbles are not totally destroyed, or if tissue brightness is appreciable), and, to a greater extent, if the value of the brightness does not appear homogeneous in the entire myocardium, a mathematical correction is necessary. Two conditions can be responsible for the nonzero brightness:

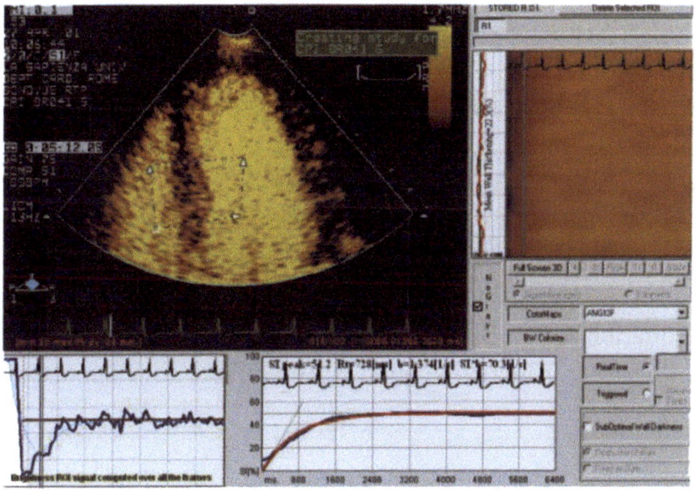

Fig. 5.4. AMID® software

a) ***Temporal Shift.*** In the first frame, contrast medium has not been totally destroyed. In this case the software can analyze the refilling curve starting from a nonzero level of intensity. It assumes that we are only observing a final feature of the refilling curve, and we are not able to see the starting point. Thus the refilling curve starts from a virtual time, $t0<0$ coming before the beginning of the observation. The correction performed by the software is shown in Fig. 5.5. Mathematically the simple exponential curve $y = A\ x\ (1-e^{-\beta t})$ is substituted by $y = A\ x\ (1-e^{-\beta(t\ t0)})$ that originates at $t=t_0$ instead of $t=0$. This correction can be applied when raw data are available: since the signal of the contrast is separated from that coming from the wall, the nonzero value of brightness is imputable to the residual presence of contrast agent and not to the wall.

b) Intensity Shift. Working on video data, if we are sure that all the contrast has been destroyed in the first frame of the sequence, the nonzero starting point can only be related to the wall brightness (the gray level gain is too high). In such cases we have to assume that the value we read is equivalent to the zero density of contrast and the software performs an "*intensity shift*". The value of signal intensity is proportionally scaled on the y axis assuming the intensity value of the first frame as the starting point for the

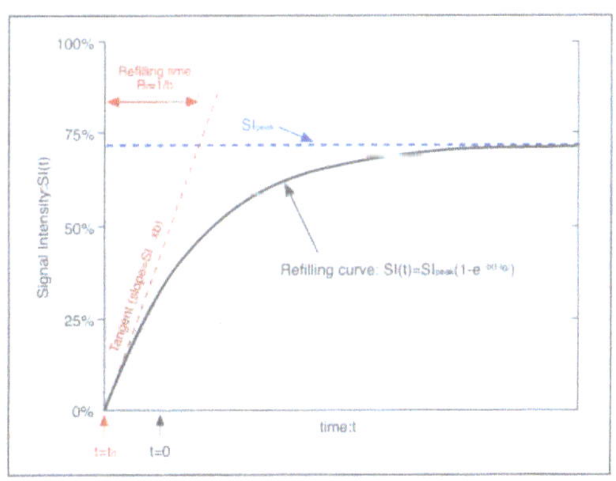

Fig. 5.5. Temporal shift. Refilling curve is not zero at $t=0$ since contrast bubbles are not totally destroyed after the flash

best-fit procedure. The procedure is shown in Fig. 5.6 and corresponds to the corrected exponential curve $y = s_0 + B \times (1 - e^{-\beta t})$.

The two choices (temporal or intensity shift) are almost equivalent. When they are applied to the same analysis, they yield the same parameter. The different peak intensity obtained (A and B) is related according to the following equation $A = s_0 + B$; the refilling slope then varies accordingly.

The quantitative analysis of the segmental curves of replenishment by means of dedicated software is a fundamental evolution in contrast imaging. However, this approach is time consuming (for a single patient, the tracing, analysis and comparison of 16 segments is required) and not immediately comparable with the most common methods of perfusion imaging (i.e., SPECT and PET).

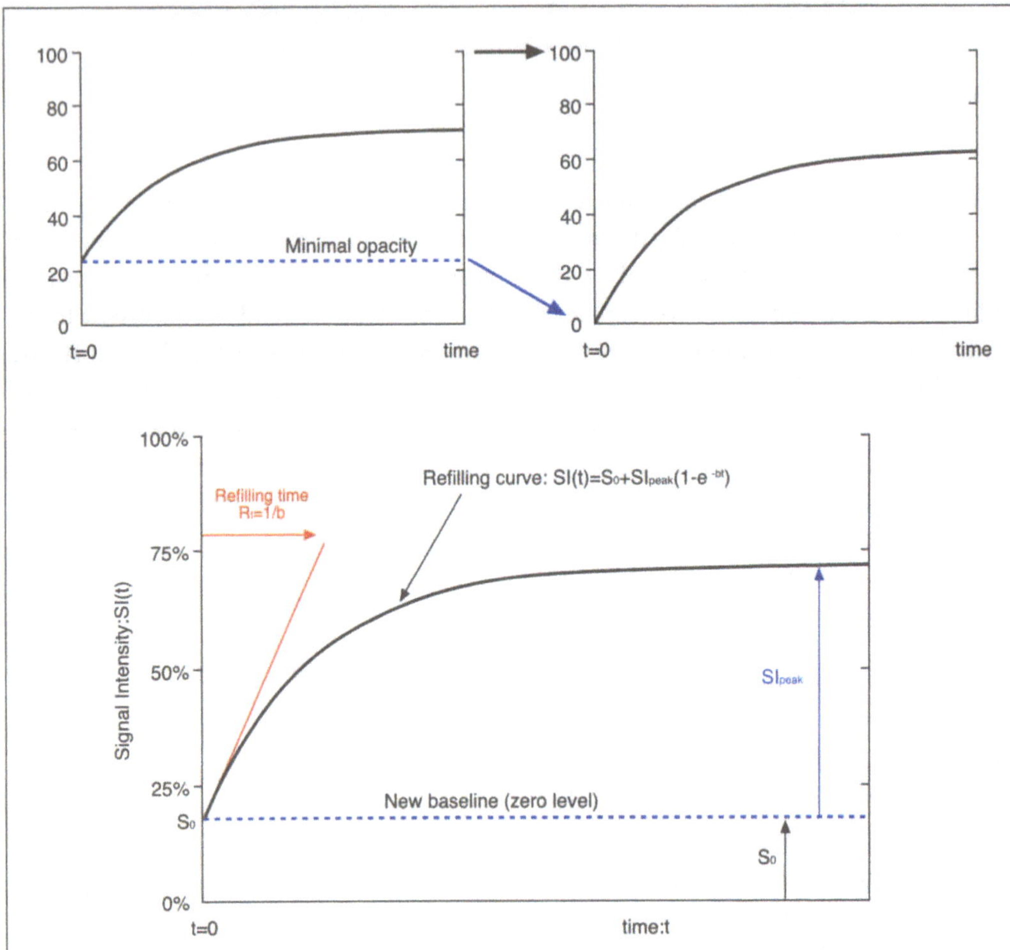

Fig. 5.6. Intensity shift. Rescaling of the minimum brightness to zero since video intensity recorded at *t*=0 is not due to contrast agent

Parametric Imaging

An innovative method for obtaining quantitative images of microcirculatory flow is the parametric approach. By this method, the spatial distribution of parameters related to perfusion are shown in an image format. Parametric images may be derived from any series of images using mathematical models. A mathematical research is necessary to design physiological models. The key consideration is the stability and robustness of the algorithms used to fit data at each point in space. Unfortunately, in some regions the signal-to-noise ratio is reduced because of the three-dimensional nature of the data. It is therefore necessary to use a fitting algorithm able to provide meaningful results under all circumstances.

Further complications arise in the analysis of time series of two-dimensional images where the differences from the baseline are significant with a strongly nonhomogeneous distribution. In such cases, the spatial and temporal correlations may be best studied using a data reduction strategy. Major problems in the analysis of myocardial data are related to the relevance of wall displacements. Standard techniques of image processing are able to calculate the brightness for every pixel of the image: therefore it is simple to reconstruct the intensity–time behavior of bubbles in relation to fixed coordinates in a space domain. But when in a temporal sequence the pixels of the ROI continuously change their coordinates, it is necessary to track the ROI to extract the numerical data. A possible solution to this problem can be found in the detection of the moving tissue and in the artificial re-alignment, instant by instant, of the anatomical structures in a representative (sys/dia, or average) position. In this way, the analysis of the data is analogous to one on fixed space coordinates, and an accurate parametric representation, with single images, of property that changes continuously in space and time domain is provided.

The method of wall tracking developed by our group (previously described in more details) detects the position of the ventricular wall all along the cardiac cycle. Once the ventricular wall is detected for each frame, a mid-wall line is automatically computed and all the frames are aligned. As a consequence of the systo-diastolic change of the left ventricle in width and in length, the size of the individual frames is rescaled to an "average size" to achieve good alignment. In this way, pixels that are homologous (i.e., correspond to the same anatomical region) are correctly superimposed in the 3-D matrix of the loop. From the 3-D matrix, it is very easy to obtain synthetic images for each MCE-derived parameter (β, refilling time, peak intensity, SI x β, time averaged brightness) using a color code (Figs. 5.7, 5.8).

Clinical Application of Quantitative Analysis

Myocardial Infarction

Kloner et al. [39] showed that with myocardial infarction, myocyte loss is accompanied by a loss of microvasculature, thus MCE detection of a perfusion defect may be evidence of a lack of tissue viability. In partic-

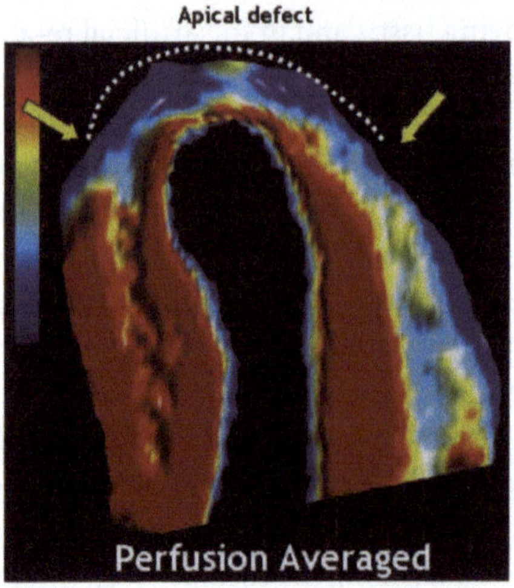

Fig. 5.7. Parametric imaging. Averaged perfusion in a patient with acute myocardial infarction and apical contrast defect

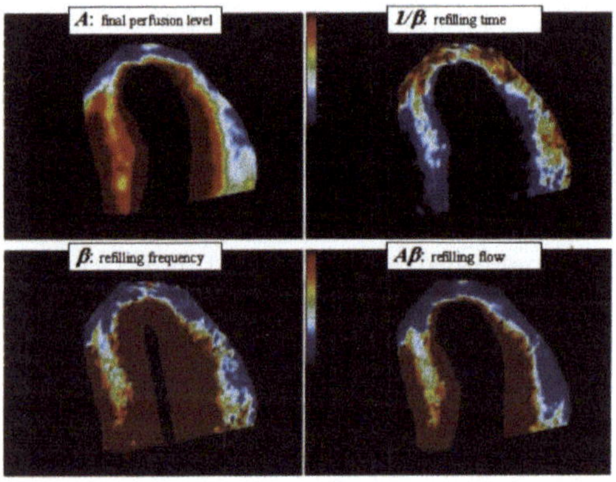

Fig. 5.8. Parametric imaging in a patient with acute myocardial infarction and apical contrast defect

ular, poor myocardial opacification within a myocardial region could result from either reduced myocardial velocity (MBF) or reduced MBV (i.e., myocardial infarction). In patients with postischemic left ventricular dysfunction, if both MCE-derived quantitative parameters are reduced, myocardial viability is unlikely. Conversely, if MV is decreased and MBV is normal, myocardial viability is more likely.

A recent elegant study in patients with postischemic LV dysfunction [40] aimed at assessing the histological correlates of MCE-derived quantitative parameters confirms that hypothesis. The study shows that peak contrast effect (A), an index of MBV, correlates with microvascular density and capillary area and inversely with collagen content. Conversely, the rate of increase of contrast intensity (β), an index of MBV, and the product A x β, an index of MBF, are reduced in the presence of high collagen content and low microvascular density. In segments with intact microvasculature, a wide range of myocardial blood velocity and flow was observed; however, both parameters are significantly higher in segments with recovery. Thus, although peak signal intensity is a simple and useful parameter of viability, velocity indices may more accurately predict myocardial hibernation.

Coronary Artery Disease

In patients without myocardial infarction, unlike with SPECT imaging, it is quite rare to observe a reversible perfusion defect with MCE. Quantitative analysis during hyperemic stimulation is mandatory since, on visual assessment, myocardial regions may appear normally opacified [41]. Preliminary data showed a satisfactory correlation between intracoronary Doppler flow wire parameters and MCE-derived flow reserve parameters during hyperemic stimulation [42-45]. In particular, the latter technique has potential advantages since coronary flow reserve as assessed by intracoronary Doppler flow-wire is dependent on a number of factors other than microvascular integrity. Conversely, MCE provides information on the myocardial volume and flow of a given region allowing the assessment of the absolute amount of myocardium at risk.

Several studies using either intermittent imaging at increasing trigger intervals or real-time perfusion imaging demonstrated that each coronary lesion may be characterized by a peculiar curve during vasodilator testing [46-49]. Different patterns, on qualitative and quantitative assessment, may be summarized as follows:

a. Normal rise of peak intensity and homogeneous opacification in normal coronary artery.
b. Reduced rate of rise and preserved peak intensity with homogeneous opacification in non-flow-limiting stenosis.
c. Reduced rate of rise and peak intensity with homogeneous opacification in flow-limiting stenosis.
d. Patchy opacification in mixed defect in myocardial regions with partially infarcted tissue.
e. Mostly absence of myocardial opacification in myocardial scar.

Conclusions

In conclusion, intravenous MCE is becoming a useful tool in clinical decision making as well as in research on patients with coronary artery disease. We expect the quality of MCE images to improve further in the near future introducing third-generation contrast agents and new transducers able to work at higher harmonics.

Quantitative analysis has a potential to play a crucial role in the assessment of coronary stenosis significance and in discovering myocardial hibernation. In the near future we expect to have quantitative software directly available on the echocardiography machine to be able to assess the contrast refilling on-line from digital data. Finally, quantitation may have an educational purpose helping to evaluate the quality of contrast insonation and the reliability of contrast injection.

References

1. Burns PN, Powers JE, Hope Simpson D. Brezina A, Kolin A, Chin CT. Harmonic Power Mode Doppler using microbubble contrast agents: an improved method for small vessel flow imaging. *Proc IEEE UFFC* 1995:1547-50
2. Burns PN, Wilson SR, Muradali D, Powers JE, Fritzsch T. Intermittent US harmonic contrast enhanced imaging and Doppler improves sensitivity and longevity of small vessel detection. *Radiology* 1996, 201, 159-63
3. Becher H, Tiemann K, Schlief R, Luderitz B, Nanda. Harmonic power Doppler contrast echocardiography: preliminary clinical results. *Echocardiography* 1997:14:637-42
4. Porter TR, Xie F, Kricsfeld D, Ambruster RW. Improved myocardial contrast with second harmonic transient response imaging in humans using intravenous perfluorcarbon-exposed sonicated dextrose albumin. J Am Coll Cardiol 1996; 27:1497-501
5. Lindner JR, Villaneuva FS, Dent JM, Sklenar J, Kaul S Assessment of resting perfusion with myocardial contrast echo: theoretical and practical considerations. Am Heart J 2000;139:231-40
6. Agati L, Funaro S, Veneroso G, Volponi C, De Maio F, Madonna MP, Fedele F. Non-invasive assessment of myocardial perfusion by intravenous contrast echocardiography. *Ital Heart J* 2001;2:6:403-407
7. Firschke C, Lindner JR, Wei K, Goodman NC, Skyba DM, Kaul S. Myocardial perfusion imaging in the

setting of coronary stenosis and acute myocardial infarction using venous injection of a second-generation echocardiographic contrast agent. Circulation 1997; 96:959-67
8. De Jong N. Imaging methods for MCE: what to expect in near future. Eur J Echocardiography. 2002,3:245-306
9. Kaul S, Senior R, Dittrich H, Raval U, Khatter R, Lahiri A. Detection of coronary artery disease with myocardial contrast echocardiography: comparison with 99m Tc-sestamibi single photon emission tomography. *Circulation* 1997;96:785-92
10. Agati L, Funaro S, Veneroso G, Volponi C, Tonti G. Clinical utility of contrast echocardiography in the management of patients with acute myocardial infarction. *Eur Heart J* 2002, 4 (suppl C) C27-C34
11. Ito H, Tomooka T, Sakai N, et al. Lack of myocardial perfusion immediately after successful thrombolysis. A predictor of poor recovery of left ventricular function in anterior myocardial infarction. Circulation 1992; 85:1699-705.
12. Kenner MD, Zajac EJ, Kondos GT, et al. Ability of no-reflow phenomenon during an acute myocardial infarction to predict left ventricular dysfunction at one-month follow-up. Am J Cardiol 1995; 76:861-8.
13. Agati L. Microvascular integrity after reperfusion therapy. Am Heart J 1999; 138:76-79
14. Agati L, Voci P, Bilotta F, et al. Influence of residual perfusion within the infarct zone on the natural history of left ventricular dysfunction after acute myocardial infarction: a myocardial contrast echocardiographic study. J Am Coll Cardiol 1994; 24:336-42.
15. Ragosta M, Camarano G, Kaul S, et al. Microvascular integrity indicates myocellular viability in patients with recent myocardial infarction. New insights using myocardial contrast echocardiography. Circulation 1994; 89:2562-9.
16. Ito H, Okamura A, Iwakura K, et al. Myocardial perfusion patterns related to thrombolysis in myocardial infarction perfusion grades after coronary angioplasty in patients with acute anterior wall myocardial infarction. Circulation 1996; 93:1993-9.
17. Lim YJ, Nanto S, Masayauma et al. Myocardial salvage; its assessment and prediction by the analysis of serial myocardial contrast echocardiograms in patients with acute myocardial infarction. Am Heart J 1994; 128:649-56
18. Agati L, Voci P, Hickle P et al: Tissue-type plasminogen activator versus primary coronary angioplasty: impact on myocardial tissue perfusion and regional function 1 month after uncomplicated myocardial infarction. J Am Coll Cardiol 1998; 31:338-43
19. Porter TR, Li S, Oster R, Deligonul U: The clinical implications of no reflow demonstrated with intravenous perfluorcarbon containing microbubbles following restoration of Thrombolysis in Myocardial Infarction (TIMI 3) flow in patients with acute myocardial infarction. *Am J Cardiol*, 1998; 82(10):1173.7
20. Agati L, Funaro S, Volponi C. Intravenous contrast echocardiography with harmonic angio for the assessment of myocardial salvage after thrombolytic therapy in acute anteroseptal myocardial infarction: comparison with clinical markers of successful reperfusion. *Circulation* 2000,102, Suppl II-748
21. Agati L, Funaro S, Veneroso G, Bilotta F. Assessment of no-reflow phenomenon after acute myocardial infarction using Harmonic Angio and intravenous pump infusion of Levovist: comparison with intracoronary contrast injection. *J Am Soc Echo* 2001;14:773-81
22. Lepper W, Hoffmann R, Kamp O, Franke A, de Cock CC, Kuhl HP, Sieswerda GT, vom Dahl J, Jansen U, Voci P, Visser C, Hanratah P. Assessment of myocardial reperfusion by intravenous MCE and coronary flow reserve after primary PTCA in patients with AMI. Circulation 2001;101:2368-74
23. Ito H, Maruyama A, Iwakura K et al. Clinical implications of the "no reflow" phenomenon. A predictor of complications and left ventricular remodeling in reperfused anterior wall myocardial infarction. Circulation 1996; 93:223-28.
24. Sakuma T, Hayashi Y, Sumii K et al: Prediction of short- and intermediate-term prognoses of patients with acute myocardial infarction using myocardial contrast echocardiography one day after recanalization. J Am Coll Cardiol 1998; 32:890-897
25. Ito H, Iwakura K, Maruyama T, et al. Temporal changes in myocardial perfusion patterns in patients with reperfused anterior wall myocardial infarction. Circulation 1995; 91:656-62
26. Agati L, Voci P, Luongo R, et al. Combined use of dobutamine echocardiography and myocardial contrast echocardiography to predict recovery of regional dysfunction after coronary revascularization in patients with recent myocardial infarction. Eur Heart J 1997; 18:771-9
27. Agati L, Autore C, Iacoboni C et al: The complex relation between myocardial viability and functional recovery in chronic left ventricular dysfunction. Am J Cardiol 1998; 81(12A):33G-35G
28. Bolognese L, Antoniucci D, Rovai D et al. Myocardial contrast echocardiography versus dobutamine echocardiography for predicting functional recovery after acute myocardial infarction treated with

primary coronary angioplasty. J Am Coll Cardiol 1996; 28:1677-83
29. Main ML, Magalaski A, Morris BA, Coen MM, Skolnick DG, Good TH. Combined assessment of microvascular integrity and contractile reserve improves differentation of stunning and necrosis after acute anterior wall myocardial infarction. J Am Coll Cardiol 2002;40:1079-84
30. Bolognese L, Cerisano G, Buonamici P et al: Influence of infarct-zone viability on left ventricular remodeling after acute myocardial infarction. Circulation 1997; 96:3353-59
31. Agati L, Funaro S, Volponi C, Veneroso G, Autore C. Influence of microvascular damage on left ventricular remodeling after acute myocardial infarction. *J Am Coll Cardiol* 2001, 37, Suppl A 390A
32. Irvine T, Wanitkun S, Powers J, Shiota T, Kenny A, Sahn DJ. Acoustically stimulated transient power scattering explains enhanced detection of the very low velocities in myocardial capillaries by power Doppler imaging: an in vitro study. J Am Soc Echocardiogr, 1999; 12(8):643-9
33. Pelberg RA, Wei K, Kamiyama N, Sklenar J, Bin J, Kaul S. Potential advantage of flash echocardiography for digital subtraction of B-mode images acquired during myocardial contrast echocardiography. J Am Soc Echocardiogr 1999; 12:85-93
34. Albrecht T, Urbank A, Mahler M, Bauer A, Dorè CJ, Blomley MJK, Cosgrove DO, Schlief R. Prolongation and optimization of Doppler enhancement with a microbubble US contrast agent by using continuous infusion: preliminary experience. Radiology 1998; 207:339-47
35. Tiemann K, Lohremeier S, Kuntz S, Koster J, Pohl C, Burns P, Porter T, Nanda N, Luderitz B, Becher H. Real-time contrast echo assessment of myocardial perfusion at low emission power. Echocardiography 1999; 16,799-809
36. Schneider M, Arditi M, Barrau M, Brochot J, Broillet A, Ventrone R, Yan F, BR1: A new ultrasonographic contrast agent based on sulfur hexafluoride-filled microbubbles. Invest Radiol 1995; 30:451-457
37. Wei K, Jayaweera A, Firoozan S, Linka A, Skyba D, Kaul S. Quantification of myocardial blood flow with ultrasound-induced destruction of microbubbles administered as a continuous venous infusion. Circulation 1998; 97:473-83
38. Von Bibra H, Bne D, Niklasson U, Eurenius L, Hansen A. MCE yields best accuracy using quantitative analysis of digital data from pulse inversion technique: comparison with second harmonic imaging and harmonic power Doppler during simultaneous dipyridamole stress SPECT studies. Eur J Echocardiography. 2002,3:271-283
39. Kloner RA, Rude RE, Carlson N, Maroko PR, De Boer LWV, Braunwald E: Ultrastructural evidence of microvascular damage and myocardial cell injury after coronary artery occlusion: which comes first ? Circulation 1980;62:945-52.
40. Shimoni S, Frangogiannis NG, Aggeli CJ, Shan K, Quinones MA, Espada R, Letsou GV, Lawrie GM, Winters WL, Readron MJ, Zoghbi WA. Microvascular structural correlates of MCE in patients with CAD and LV dysfunction. Circulation 2002;106: 950-56
41. Agati L, et al: Dipyridamole myocardial contrast echocardiography in patients with single vessel coronary artery disease: perfusion, anatomic and functional correlates. Am Heart J 1994; 128:28-35.
42. Agati L, Autore C, Funaro S, Veneroso G, Dagianti A, Lamberti A, Fedele F. Non-invasive assessment of myocardial perfusion using Harmonic Angio and intravenous pump infusion of Levovist®: Preliminary results in patients with acute myocardial infarction. Am J Cardiol 2000; 86 (suppl) 28G-30G)
43. Agati L, Funaro S, Veneroso G, Madonna MP, De Maio F, Celani F, Iacoboni C, Adorisio R, Fedele F. Use of MCE in identifying patients with failed reperfusion after thrombolysis in acute myocardial infarction: comparison with TIMI myocardial perfusion grade and clinical markers of reperfusion. JACC (Suppl) 2003 in press
44. Agati L, Iacoboni C, De Maio F, Funaro S, Madonna MP, Celani F, Adorisio R, Benedetti G, Fedele F. Tissue level perfusion after primary or rescue coronary angioplasty in acute myocardial infarction. A myocardial contrast echocardiography study. JACC (suppl) 2003 in press
45. Wei K, Ragosta M, Thorpe J, Coggins M, Moos S, Kaul S. Noninvasive quantification of coronary blood flow reserve in humans using myocardial contrast ecicardiography. Circulation 2001;103:2560-65
46. Masugata H, Cotter B, Peters B et al: Assessment of coronary stenosis severity and transmural perfusion gradient by myocardial contrast echocardiography. Circulation 2000; 102:1427-35
47. Heinle SK, Noblin J, Best PM et al: Assessment of myocardial perfusion by harmonic power Doppler imaging at rest and during adenosine stress. Circulation 2000; 102:55-62
48. Andrassy P, Zielinska M, Busch R, Schomig A, Firschke C. Myocardial blood volume and the amount of viable myocardium early after mechanical reperfusion of acute myocardial infarction: prospective study using venous contrast echocardiography. Heart 2002;87:350-55
49. Masugata H, Peters B, Lafitte S et al: Quantitative assessment of myocardial perfusion during graded coronary stenosis by real time myocardial contrast echo refilling curves. J Am Coll Cadiol 2001; 37: 262-69

Chapter 6
Contrast Echocardiography for Left Ventricular Opacification

Partho Sengupta • Bijoy K. Khandheria

Accurate assessment of left ventricular (LV) function is of paramount importance in clinical cardiology. Although the LV contraction and relaxation occur in a complex three-dimensional format, changes in two-dimensional regional and global LV geometry during a cardiac cycle provide a reliable estimate of the overall LV function. This information is obtained comprehensively during real-time two-dimensional echocardiography by quantifying the extent of wall thickening, endocardial motion and serial changes in LV sizes and volumes. Accurate echocardiographic interpretation, however, necessitates a proper delineation of the blood–endocardial interface and is not found adequately in a significant proportion (10%–20%) of patients referred for routine echocardiographic evaluation in clinical practice [1]. Suboptimal image quality in these patients results from a variety of factors including obesity, lung disease or chest wall deformities, thereby obviating an optimal application and utilization of cardiac ultrasound. Alternate techniques have emerged in the last decade for improving the diagnostic yield of echocardiography in such patients and include modalities like tissue harmonic imaging, contrast echocardiography and Doppler imaging for myocardial motion [2-7]. This chapter highlights the concepts and application of intravenous contrast for LV opacification, its clinical utility and relative merits in assessing structural and functional abnormalities of the left ventricle.

Concepts and Technique

Gas bubbles interact complexly with incident ultrasound beams. Ultrasonic waves not only get reflected at the gas–liquid interface but are also modified in amplitude and frequency due to rapid bubble oscillations [8, 9]. The ultrasound beam therefore encounters a wider scattering and frequency modulation with contrast agents than red-blood cells and hence echoes returning from bubbles effectively delineate the blood pool–endocardial interface [8, 9].

Harmonic Imaging

Echoes returning from bubble are resultant of both linear and nonlinear oscillations. Unequal alternate expansion and contraction of bubbles during nonlinear oscillations result from insonation at resonant frequency and lead to generation of harmonics which are at multiples of the insonating frequency [10]. By using filtering algorithms, the harmonics can be selectively enhanced for improving the echocardiographic appearance of the contrast. When the receiver is tuned to receive double the incidental frequency it is called "first harmonics". The signal-to-noise ratio for bubbles can be further improved by using subharmonics (1/2 insonation frequency) or ultraharmonics (1.5 f). Harmonics are also produced from tissues and significantly alter the gray-scale image quality in a significant number of patients [11]. However, endocardial border visualization could remain inadequate despite the use of harmonic imaging in some patients. The combined use of harmonics with contrasts in such patients could be more useful for delineating the endocardial border since production of harmonics is more significant for contrasts.

Power Doppler Imaging

The property of contrast bubbles in scattering ultrasonic waves more effectively than red blood cells can also be used for improving the Doppler signal strength and over the years has been used for enhancing the Doppler signals of tricuspid regurgitation. This property of contrast is used in power Doppler imaging for selective enhancement of contrast signal by displaying the strength of Doppler signal rather than Doppler velocity [12]. Spatial information provided by this mode is inferior to conventional B-mode imaging for quantifying regional cardiac anatomy. However, its ability to differentiate the contrast-enhanced ventricular cavity from myocardial wall, principally by using variables like motion velocity and phase changes, makes it an attractive alternative when underlying myocardial acoustic properties are suboptimal.

Power Modulation and Pulse Inversion

Power modulation and pulse inversion modes are designed specifically for selectively enhancing microbubble scatter while suppressing the reflections from cardiac structures [13]. The returning waves from the contrast bubbles are a mixture of linear (fundamental) and nonlinear frequency and can be further modified by sequentially alternating the phase or amplitude of ultrasound signal (pulse inversion and power modulation) [13, 14]. By adding the returning signals, fundamental frequencies of opposite polarities cancel each other out while the non-linear frequencies from bubbles are enhanced. This technique is extremely useful for continuous assessment of LV function like that required during stress echocardiography and for real-time myocardial perfusion imaging.

Contrast Agents

Contrast echocardiography began with the use of agitated saline solutions, but these did not pacify the left side of the heart since they were filtered into the pulmonary circulation. LV opacification was achieved with the use of agents that were small and stable enough to traverse the pulmonary circulation. These first-generation agents included air bubbles stabilized by encapsulation (sonicated Albumin) or by adherence to microparticles (Levovist) [15-17]. Subsequently, air was replaced with low-solubility fluorocarbon gases (second-generation agents – Optison, SonoVue) which improved the persistence of the contrast effect for prolonged contrast imaging [18, 19]. Third-generation agents use polymer shell and low-solubility gases and produce more intense contrast but are not yet commercially available. Trials comparing the relative efficacy of different agents have been performed. Two phase 3 clinical trials used second-generation agents – Echogen (Sonus Parmaceuticals, Botell, WA) and Optison (Amersham Health, Princeton, NJ) – and compared them with sonicated albumin (Albunex) [20, 21]. In the first study, endocardial border delineation improved in 88% of patients with Echogen and only in 45% of cases with Albunex [20]. In the second study, endocardial border definition improved in 93% of patients with Optison and only 75% of patients with Albunex [21]. Recently, a multicentric trial evaluated the efficacy of SonoVue (Bracco Diagnostics Inc., Princeton, NJ) and compared it with Albunex and agitated saline. Complete LV opacification was seen in 34%–87% of cases receiving SonoVue compared to 0%–16% of Albunex receiving patients [22]. These studies clearly establish the superiority of second-generation agents and are currently recommended for enhancing the delineation of endocardial borders in patients with sub-optimal images.

Performing a Contrast Study

Contrast Administration

Special care is taken while performing a contrast study to avoid undue destruction of the contrast bubble. The agent is prepared immediately before administration and withdrawn into a syringe with simultaneous application of a vent to avoid bubble disruption by pressure changes. Use of gentle agitation helps in obtaining a uniform distribution of the agent, which is administered through a large peripheral vein, usually the antecubital vein. LV opacification can be adequately achieved by injecting very small doses (<1 ml) of second-generation contrast as IV bolus followed by rapid infusion of saline through a three-way canula [7]. Prolonged imaging needed for assessment of regional myocardial function during stress echocardiography or for assessing myocardial perfusion, however, may require a slow continuous infusion.

Imaging

Although contrast studies can be evaluated using fundamental imaging, with wide availability of harmonic imaging, contrast imaging is currently performed only when tissue harmonics fail to adequately delineate endocardial borders [7-23]. The initial mode is either a harmonic B-mode or pulse inversion (ATL). Echocardiographic settings are optimized with low transmit energy (mechanical index <0.6 for harmonic or <0.3 for pulse inversion imaging), slightly reduced gain for reducing echoes originating from the myocardium, low to medium dynamic range, medium to high compression, medium line density with persistence disabled and focus set in left ventricle below the mitral valve [23]. Examination is performed first with apical views followed by parasternal views since intense opacification of the right ventricle in initial frames can obviate adequate ultrasonic wave penetration in parasternal views.

If harmonic B-mode imaging is inadequate, power Doppler imaging of the left ventricle can be performed. The settings include a mechanical index of 1.0, display mode with either color Doppler (standard color variance mode or a unidirectional map) or a standard power Doppler map, highest level of pulse-repeating frequency, highest line density, and medium sensitivity with persistence disabled [23]. However, application of this Doppler technique is limited by low frame rates (typically 10-15 frames/s compared to 50 or more frames/s for harmonic B-mode). Its use for analysis of regional wall motion is obviated by frequent occurrence of motion artifacts. However, its advantage in being highly sensitive in detecting small amounts of contrasts results in minimal requirement of contrast agents for adequate LV opacification.

Clinical Applications *(Figs. 6.1-6.3)*

LV Volumes and LV Ejection Fraction

Improved visualization of the LV endocardium by using echocardiographic contrast leads to increased accuracy and reduced variability in manually traced LV volumes and ejection fraction estimates [3]. Hundley et al. compared the efficacy of contrast enhanced echocardiography for calculating LV functions with cine magnetic resonance imaging (MRD) in 40 patients referred for routine echocardiographic evaluation of LV ejection fraction [24]. There was an excellent correlation between MRI and contrast echocardiography (R=0.92) for assessment of LV ejection fraction. Contrast echocardiography was superior to standard echocardiography in classifying the degree of LV dysfunction and was particularly useful in subjects with two or more adjacent endocardial segments not visualized at baseline.

Harmonic imaging when used alone is superior to fundamental imaging for delineating LV endocardial border. However, tissue harmonic imaging when used alone could overestimate the thickness of the myocardial wall and underestimate the LV volumes and ejection fraction [25]. Nahar et al. compared LV ejection fraction obtained by four different echocardiographic modalities – fundamental imaging, harmonic imaging and harmonic with contrast imaging – in 50 patients with technically difficult echocardiograms [26]. Three echocardiographers measured the biplane two-dimensional echocardiographic LV ejection fraction independently and were blinded to radionuclide angiography.

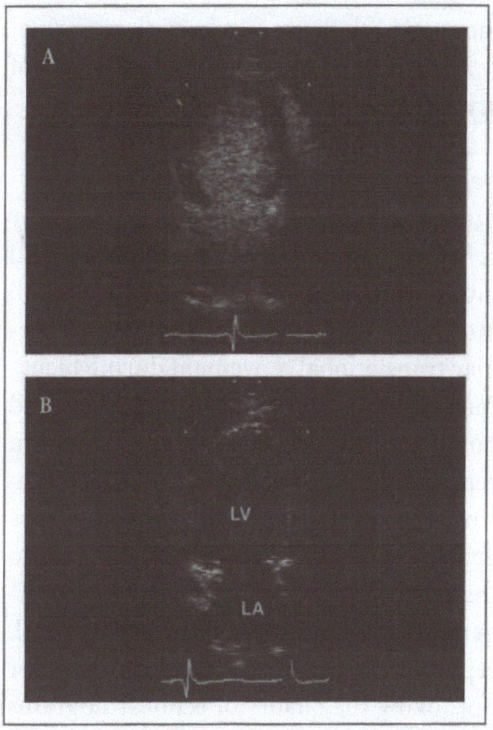

Fig. 6.1. A Opacification of the left ventricle allows delineation of the walls of the ventricle. SonoVue was the agent used in this case. **B** Two-dimensional echocardiographic image showing poor delineation of the walls making analysis of the regional wall motion or even systolic function difficult

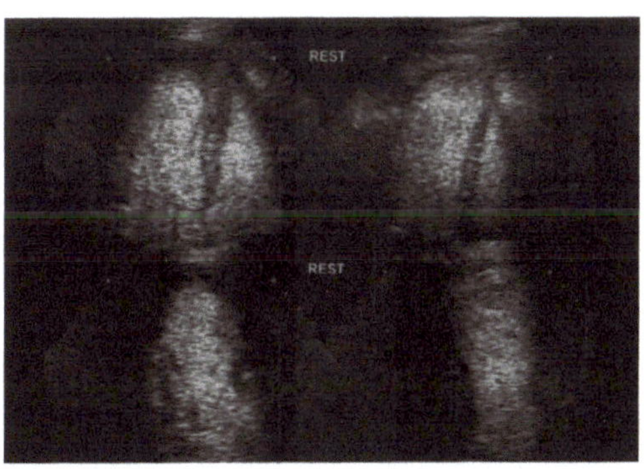

Fig. 6.2. Contrast-enhanced images showing the left ventricle (Four-chamber view on the *top right* and *left*, and two-chamber view on the *bottom right* and *left*). The ventricular walls are well delineated, and permit analysis of the global and regional systolic function

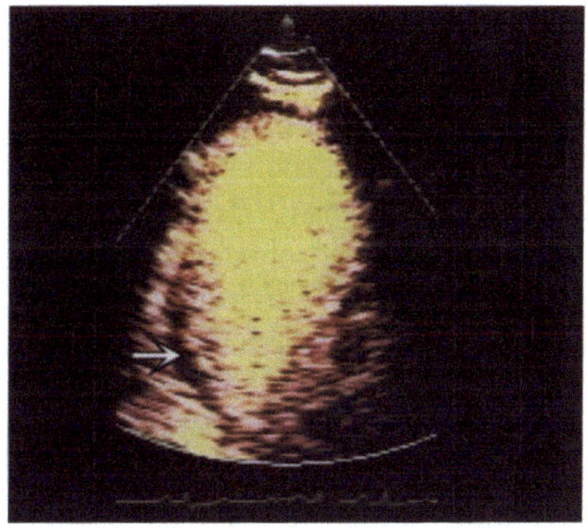

Fig. 6.3. Contrast-enhanced left ventricular cavity demonstrating the walls. *Arrow* is pointing towards an area of perfusion defect. This patient had coronary artery disease of significance in the circumflex territory

Although the correlation between radionuclide angiography and different echocardiographic techniques improved incrementally with the addition of each technique, the best correlations (R= 0.95-0.96) were observed for the combination of contrast with harmonic imaging.

Despite the endocardial border delineation being enhanced with contrast, the acoustic interface between the low-intensity blood pool and high-intensity myocardial wall is minimized, thereby making automatic endocardial border detection by traditional acoustic quantification techniques unusable. One approach is to use intermittent triggered imaging for quantifying the end-systolic and end-diastolic frames and manually outlining the endocardial borders to calculate the LV volumes [27]. However, this approach needs careful image acquisition with patients holding their breath for 5–10 s. Slight variations in scanplane could introduce large errors in LV volume estimation. Low frame rates further limit the ability to visualize cardiac dynamics and assess ventricular function. Efforts for bridging the gap and streamlining new tools for quantitative analysis of LV volumes and ejection fraction are underway. Recently, a modified acoustic quantification technique was shown to effectively define the blood–endocardial interface in contrast-enhanced images [28, 29]. LV measurements with this automated technique were in close agreement with those obtained by manually tracing the end-diastolic and end-systolic borders.

Regional Wall Motion at Rest

Studies have reported the incremental utility of using intravenous contrast for improving reader confidence in interpretation of wall motion during transthoracic echocardiography [3-30]. Hundley et al. studied 420 myocardial segments in 35 patients referred for evaluation of LV function [31]. Regional wall motion was assessed from apical 2-chamber and 4-chamber views in a 12-segment model before and after administration of IV contrast and compared to findings on MRI. Classification of normal versus abnormal segments improved following administration of contrast and its use was at its best in identifying wall motion in lateral and anterior walls. In these regions, correct identification of endocardium and differentiation of normal versus abnormal motion improved from 78% to 98% and 65% to 88% respectively, and altered the overall wall motion assessment in seven (20%) patients. A marked improvement was noted also in the extent of interobserver agreement on both the presence of an abnormal wall motion and its qualitative assessment of severity.

Regional Wall Motion During Stress

The accuracy of stress echocardiography rests on correct interpretation of wall motion abnormalities. Excessive chest wall motion during hyperventilation and cardiac translational movement during tachycardia alter image quality during stress, and non-diagnostic echocardiograms have been reported in 30% patients [32]. Interpretation of exercise and dobutamine stress echocardiograms was initially shown to improve with the administration of first-generation contrast agents. Porter et al. reported the use of sonicated Albumin for improving the quality of echocardiograms during dobutamine stress echocardiography [33]. Improved endocardial resolution was seen in 93% of patients with inadequate baseline images and 95% of patients with sub optimal images at peak stress. Subsequent studies revealed that contrast was particularly helpful in visualization of the basal lateral, basal anterior, and apical segments. Further improved results have been reported with the use of native tissue harmonic imaging in combination with second-generation contrast agents. Malhotra et al. evaluated the use of Optison in 200 patients undergoing dobutamine stress echocardiography [34]. Native tissue harmonic imaging provided clear visualization of segments in 65% of patients, and when native tissue harmonic imaging was combined with contrast administration this improved to 96%. Recent introduction of pulse inversion and power modulation techniques have led to use of these techniques for giving combined assessment of regional wall motion and myocardial perfusion during stress echocardiography. Mor-Avi et al. in a recent experiment reported successful use of contrast echo for simultaneous real-time assessment of myocardial perfusion and regional LV function [35]. The availability of this information promises to improve the accuracy of echocardiographic diagnosis of coronary artery disease.

Contrast Echocardiography in the Intensive Care Unit Setting

Use of transthoracic echocardiography in critically ill patients is often limited by suboptimal images resulting from mechanical ventilation, use of bandages, lung disease, subcutaneous emphysema, chest tubes, inadequate cooperation and inability to position patients in the left lateral decubitus position [36]. Kornbluth et al. evaluated the benefits of performing transthoracic echocardiography incrementally with fundamental tissue harmonic imaging and harmonic imaging combined with intravenous Optison in 50 consecutive mechanically ventilated patients in ICU [37]. A total of 850 segments were either poor or not seen and 78% of these improved to good or excellent quality with contrast echocardiography versus 23% with tissue harmonics. Conversion of nondiagnostic to diagnostic imaging occurred in 85% of patients with contrast echocardiography versus 15% of patients with tissue harmonics. Recently, Yong et al. compared harmonic imaging alone or in combination with contrast to transesophageal echocardiography (TEE) in 32 patients in ICU who were considered technically difficult (> 50% of segments not visualized from any view) [38]. An excellent or adequate endocardial delineation could be achieved in 13% of segments with fundamental imaging, 34% with harmonic imaging and 87% with contrast, which was equivalent to that obtained by a TEE (87% vs 90%, p = NS). Agreement with TEE in exact wall motion interpretation improved from fundamental (48%) to harmonic (58%) and was maximum with contrast imaging (70%). Similarly, the estimation of LV ejection fraction was possible in 31% of segments with fundamental imaging, 50% with harmonic imaging and 97% with contrast, later correlating best with ejection fraction evaluated by TEE ($R = 0.92$). Scine TEE is relatively invasive, uncomfortable, requires sedation and carries a small but definite risk of complications; harmonic imaging with contrast is a relatively safe alternative to obtain incremental information in critically ill patients.

Detection of LV Thrombi

Transthoracic echocardiography is currently used as a standard technique for detection of LV thrombus and, provided the echocardiographic image is optimal, it has a sensitivity ranging from 92% to 95% and specificity approaching 95% [39, 40]. The diagnosis is at times difficult because of near-field clutter, reverberation artifacts, a false tendon or poor endocardial border delineation. Recently, intravenous contrast has been used for improving the diagnostic yield of transthoracic echocardiography in detecting mural thrombi. Thanigraj et al. evaluated the use of two-dimensional echocardiography for detecting LV thrombus in 409 patients [41]. With the use of fundamental or second harmonic imaging an optimal image quality for making a conclusive diagnosis was seen in 219 (54%) cases. Additional contrast studies were performed in 48 of the remaining 190 patients with a nondiagnostic test. Of these, 43 (90%) had diagnostic tests, with thrombi being detected in 11 additional cases and being absent in the remaining 32 cases. Since the majority of patients with LV thrombus need long-term anticoagulant therapy, use of contrast echocardiography for improving the diagnostic accuracy of this condition seems clinically justified.

Other Clinical Uses of LV Contrast Opacification

Contrast echocardiography has been shown to be useful in identifying structural abnormalities of the left ventricle particularly in identifying patients with an apical variant of hypertrophic cardiomyopathy, LV aneurysms and pseudo-aneurysms and noncompaction of LV myocardium [6, 23, 42]. Enhancement of Doppler signals from pulmonary veins could also be used to assess the pattern of diastolic LV filling and used as an estimate for diastolic dysfunction [23].

Pitfalls and Troubleshooting

Several technical problems may limit proper delineation of endocardial borders during contrast echocardiography. For example, if the contrast dose is not adequate in a given gray-scale, tissue signals in the LV may not be distinguishable from the contrast signals. This is called an "anticontrast effect" and can be avoided by injecting a slightly larger dose of contrast [23, 43]. However, with excess contrast dose, particularly with an intravenous bolus administration, large concentration of contrast near the apex may scatter and absorb the ultrasonic beams completely in the near fields thereby preventing penetration into deeper regions. Attenuation is particularly problematic in parasternal windows where dense opacification of the right ventricle may obviate visualization of the left ventricle. This can be prevented by using apical views where the attenuation is lowest and usually subsides by waiting for contrast washout. Excessive acoustic power may cause destruction of bubbles near the apex making it difficult to visualize the near fields. Reducing acoustic power so that mechanical index is less than 0.6 can alleviate this problem [23, 43].

Several artifacts may limit regional wall motion analysis during real-time imaging. This includes apical swirling resulting from nonuniform mixing of contrast agents or systolic fading caused by microbubble compression [23, 43]. Gating the images to the electrocardiograph can resolve this problem but at the cost of not seeing wall motion in real time. During power Doppler imaging, movement of myocardial tissue may also produce Doppler signals. This can be avoided by using a high-pass filter. However, rapid myocardial wall motion during breathing and coughing or exaggerated cardiac motion during physical or dobutamine stress result in wall motion velocities which exceed the filter limits. These wall motion artifacts can be easily recognized as colored flashes occuring over epi- or pericardial layers and can be avoided by properly altering the pulse repeating frequency, filtering algorithms, or by using a slightly different scanplane [23]. Another problem that can be encountered with the use of power Doppler is myocardial blooming. The ultrasound beam used to form an image is not of a precise width but tapers in intensity at its edges. When ultrasound encounters a strong scatter near the edge of the beam, it is interpreted as bigger than its actual anatomical size. This is particularly noticeable in colored images in which arrival of contrast in the myocardium causes color to bleed into the myocardium. This can be taken care of by either adjusting the contrast dose, altering the receiver gains, or by decreasing the length of color detection system so that more lines can be read in a shorter time [23].

Cost-Effectiveness and Clinical Utilization

Contrast echocardiography has been shown to be cost-effective since it improves laboratory efficacy and obviates the need for additional testing [44]. It is particularly advantageous in intensive care units and is 3% and 17% more cost-effective than TEE in determining regional and global left ventricular function in critically ill patients [38]. Despite its benefits and wide research interest, its clinical utilization has been hindered. One of the reasons for this has been the need for a certain degree of technical expertise that is critical for optimal performance and interpretation of contrast echocardiograms. The American Society of Echocardiography currently recommends trained (level 2 or 3) physicians, cardiac sonographers and laboratory staff for establishing an effective system of performing contrast echocardiography [1]. Contrast echocardiograms can be performed in out-patient departments, but need trained staff for intravenous catheter placement and contrast administration. In addition, a wider dissemination and utilization of contrast techniques is possible when uniform reimbursement policies are made for using contrast in appropriate subjects as and when required.

Summary and Future Directions

Intravenous contrast agents provide enhanced objective assessment of regional and global LV structure and function in patients with suboptimal echocardiography images. They are best utilized incrementally with native tissue harmonic B-mode imaging and several studies have validated their efficacy in improving diagnostic yield and operator confidence in interpreting either resting or stress images. Harmonic power Doppler imaging for real-time color-coded contrast imaging with or without newer automatic border detection algorithms is a powerful alternative for rapid and accurate quantification of regional and global LV functions. Despite its efficacy, the optimal way to perform contrast studies deserves meticulous attention to avoid misinterpretation of artifacts. These are likely to be circumvented in the future by technical developments that will provide more precise bubble information and parallel other improvements in digital techniques for regional and global LV function assessment. Quantification of LV volumes and function by using contrast with real-time three-dimensional echocardiography is attractive and has the distinct advantage of avoiding misalignment of image planes (fore-shortening). With the evolution of more and more such alternatives, better clinical algorithms will be developed, tailored to the needs of each individual case. Wider dissemination of contrast knowledge coupled with growth in clinical information and technical skills could perhaps virtually eliminate a "technically difficult echocardiogram".

References

1. Mulvagh SL, DeMaria AN, Feinstein SB, Burns PN, Kaul S, Miller JG, Monaghan M, Porter TR, Shaw LJ, Villanueva FS. Contrast echocardiography: current and future applications. J Am Soc Echocardiogr. 2000; 13:331-42
2. Fedele F, Trambaiolo P, Magni G, De Castro S, Cacciotti L. New modalities of regional and global left ventricular function analysis: state of the art. Am J Cardiol. 1998;81:49G-57G
3. Grayburn PA, Mulvagh S, Crouse L . Left ventricular opacification at rest and during stress. Am J Cardiol. 2002;90:21J-27J
4. Lang RM, Mor-Avi V, Zoghbi WA, Senior R, Klein AL, Pearlman AS.The role of contrast enhancement in echocardiographic assessment of left ventricular function. Am J Cardiol. 2002;90:28J-34J
5. Mulvagh SL, Foley DA, Belohlavek M, Seward JB. Image enhancement by noncontrast harmonic echocardiography. Part I.Qualitative assessment of endocardial visualization. Mayo Clin Proc. 1998;73:1062-5
6. Senior R. Left ventricular contrast echocardiography: role for evaluation of function and structure. Echocardiography. 2002;19:615- 20.
7. Stewart MJ. Contrast echocardiography. Heart 2003;89:342-8
8. Lindner JR.Contrast echocardiography. Curr Prob Cardiol 2002;27:454-519
9. Wei K, Skyba DM, Firshke C, Lindner JR, Jayawera AR, Kaul S. Interaction between microbubbles and ultrasound in vitro and in vivo observation. J Am Coll Cardiol 1997; 29:1081-8
10. Kasprzak JD, Paelinck B, Ten Cate FJ, Vletter WB, de Jong N, Poldermans D, Elhendy A, Bouakaz A, Roelandt JR. Comparison of native and contrast-enhanced harmonic echocardiography for visualization of left ventricular endocardial border. Am J Cardiol. 1999;83:211-7
11. Caidahl K, Kazzam E, Lidberg J, Neumann Andersen G, Nordanstig J, Rantapaa Dahlqvist S, Waldenstrom A, Wikh R. New concept in echocardiography: harmonic imaging of tissue without use of contrast agent. Lancet. 1998;352:1264-70
12. Mor-Avi V, Bednarz J, Weinert L, Sugeng L, Lang RM. Power Doppler imaging as a basis for automated endocardial border detection during left ventricular contrast enhancement. Echocardiography. 2000;17:529-37
13. Caiani EG, Lang RM, DeCara J, Bednarz JE, Weinert L, Korcarz CE, Collins KA, Mor-Avi V. Objective assessment of left ventricular wall motion from contrast-enhanced power modulation images. J Am Soc Echocardiogr. 2002;15:118-28
14. Vancon AC, Fox ER, Chow CM, Hill J, Weyman AE, Picard MH, Scherrer-Crosbie M.Pulse inversion harmonic imaging improves endocardial border visualization in two-dimensional images:comparison with harmonic imaging. J Am Soc Echocardiogr. 2002;15:302-8
15. Crouse LJ, Cheirif J, Hanly DE, Kisslo JA, Labovitz AJ, Raichlen JS, Schutz RW, Shah PM, Smith MD. Opacification and border delineation improvement in patients with suboptimal endocardial border definition in routine echocardiography: results of the Phase III Albunex Multicenter Trial. J Am Coll Cardiol. 1993 1;22:1494-500
16. Lindner JR, Dent JM, Moos SP, Jayaweera AR, Kaul S. Enhancement of left ventricular cavity opacification by harmonic imaging after venous injection of Albunex. Am J Cardiol. 1997;79:1657-62
17. Firschke C, Koberl B, von Bibra H, Horcher J, Schomig A. Combined use of contrast-enhanced 2-dimensional and color Doppler echocardiography for improved left ventricular endocardial border

delineation using Levovist, a new venous echocardiographic contrast agent. Int J Card Imaging. 1997; 13:137-44
18. Bokor D.Diagnostic efficacy of SonoVue. Am J Cardiol. 2000;86:19G-24G
19. Cohen JL, Cheirif J, Segar DS, Gillam LD, Gottdiener JS, Hausnerova E, Bruns DE. Improved left ventricular endocardial border delineation and opacification with OPTISON (FS069), a new echocardiographic contrast agent. Results of a phase III Multicenter Trial. J Am Coll Cardiol. 1998 Sep;32(3):746-52
20. Grayburn PA, Weiss JL, Hack TC, Klodas E, Raichelen JS, Vannan MA, Klein AL, Kitzman DW, Chrysant SG, Cohen JL, et al. Phase III multicentric trial comparing the efficacy of 2% dodecofluoropentane emulsion (Echogen) and sonicated 5% human albumin (Albunex) as ultrasound contrast agents in patients with suboptimal echocardiograms. J Am Coll Cardiol 1998;32:230-6
21. Cohen JL, Cherif J, Segar DS, Gillam LD, Gottdiener JS, Hausnerova E, Burns DE. Improved left ventricular endocardial border delineation and opacification with OPTISON (FS069), a new echocardiographic contrast agent. Results of a phase III multicentric trial. J Am Coll Cardiol 1998; 32:746-52
22. Nanda NC, Wistran DC, Karlsberg RP. Hack TC, Smith WB, Foley DA, Picard MH, Cotter B. Multricenter evaluation of Sonovue for improved endocardial border delineation. Echocardiography 2002;19:27-36
23. Becher H, Burns PN. Assessment of left ventricular functions by contrast echo. In: Becher H, Burns PN. Handbook of contrast echocardiography. LV function and myocardial perfusion. Berlin: Springer-Verlag, 2000:48-81
24. Hundley WG, Kizilbash AM, Afridi I, Franco F, Peshock RM, Grayburn PA. Administration of an intravenous perfluorocarbon contrast agent improves echocardiographic determination of left ventricular volumes and ejection fraction: comparison with cine magnetic resonance imaging. J Am Coll Cardiol. 1998 ;32:1426-32
25. Hirata K, Watanabe H, Beppu S, Muro T, Teragaki M, Yoshiyama M, Takeuchi K, Yoshikawa J. Pitfalls of echocardiographic measurement in tissue harmonic imaging: in vitro and in vivo study. J Am Soc Echocardiogr. 2002;15:1038-44
26. Nahar T, Croft L, Shapiro R, Fruchtman S, Diamond J, Henzlova M, Machac J, Buckley S, Goldman ME.Comparison of four echocardiographic techniques for measuring left ventricular ejection fraction. Am J Cardiol. 2000;86:1358-62
27. Hirooka K, Yasumura Y, Tsujita Y, Hanatani A, Nakatani S, Miyatake K, Yamagishi M. An enhanced method for left ventricular volume and ejection fraction by triggered harmonic contrast echocardiography. Int J Cardiovasc Imaging.2001;17:253-61
28. Spencer KT, Bednarz J, Mor-Avi V, DeCara J, Lang RM. Automated endocardial border detection and evaluation of left ventricular function from contrast-enhanced images using modified acoustic quantification. J Am Soc Echocardiogr. 2002;15:777-81
29. Yu EH, Skyba DM, Sloggett CE, Jamorski M, Iwanochko RM, Dias BF, Rakowski H, Siu SC.Determination of left ventricular ejection fraction using intravenous contrast and a semiautomated border detection algorithm. J Am Soc Echocardiogr. 2003; 16:22-8
30. Vlassak I, Rubin DN, Odabashian JA, Garcia MJ, King LM, Lin SS, Drinko JK, Morehead AJ, Prior DL, Asher CR, Klein AL,Thomas JD.Contrast and harmonic imaging improves accuracy and efficiency of novice readers for dobutamine stress echocardiography. Echocardiography. 2002 Aug;19(6):483-8
31. Hundley WG, Kizilbash AM, Afridi I, Franco F, Peshock RM, Grayburn PA. Effect of contrast enhancement on transthoracic echocardiographic assessment of left ventricular regional wall motion. Am J Cardiol. 1999; 84:1365-8, A8-9
32. Marwick TH, Nemec JJ, Pashkow FJ, Stewart WJ, Salcedo EE. Accuracy and limitations of exercise echocardiography in a routine clinical setting. J Am Coll Cardiol 1992; 19:74-81
33. Porter TR, Xie F, Kricsfeld A, Chiou A, Dabestani A. Improved endocardiaal border resolution during dobutamine stress echocardiography with intravenous sonicated dextrose albumin. J Am Coll Cardiol 1994; 23:1440-3
34. Malhotra V, Nwogu J, Bondmass MD, Bean M, Bieniarz T, Tertell M, Conliss M, Devries S.Is the technically limited echocardiographic study an endangered species? Endocardial border definition with native tissue harmonic imaging and Optison contrast: a review of 200 cases. J Am Soc Echocardiogr. 2000; 13:771-3
35. Mor-Avi V, Caiani EG, Collins KA, Korcarz CE, Bednarz JE, Lang RM.Combined assessment of myocardial perfusion and regional left ventricular function by analysis of contrast-enhanced power modulation images. Circulation. 2001 17;104:352-7
36. Yong Y, Wu D, Fernandes V, Kopelen HA, Shimoni S, Nagueh SF, Callahan JD, Bruns DE, Shaw LJ, Quinones MA, Zoghbi WA. Diagnostic accuracy and cost-effectiveness of contrast echocardiography on evaluation of cardiac function in technically very

difficult patients in the intensive care unit.Am J Cardiol. 2002; 89:711-8
37. Kornbluth M, Liang DH, Brown P, Gessford E, Schnittger I.Contrast echocardiography is superior to tissue harmonics for assessment of left ventricular function in mechanically ventilated patients.Am Heart J. 2000;140:291-6
38. Yong Y, Wu D, Fernandes V, Kopelen HA, Shimoni S, Nagueh SF, Callahan JD, Bruns DE, Shaw LJ, Quinones MA, Zoghbi WA. Diagnostic accuracy and cost-effectiveness of contrast echocardiography on evaluation of cardiac function in technically very difficult patients in the intensive care unit. Am J Cardiol. 2002; 89:711-8
39. Visser CA, Kan G, David GK, Lie KI, Durrer D. Two-dimensional echocardiography in the diagnosis of left ventricular thrombus: a prospective study of 67 patients with anatomic validation. Chest 1983; 83:22832
40. Stratton JR, Lighty GW Jr, Pearlman AS, Ritchie JL. Detection of left ventricular thrombus by two dimensional echocardiography: sensitivity, specificity, and cause of uncertainity. Circulation 1982;66:156-66
41. Thanigaraj S, Schechtman KB, Perez JE.Improved echocardiographic delineation of left ventricular thrombus with the use of intravenous second-generation contrast image enhancement. J Am Soc Echocardiogr.1999;12:1022-6
42. Ward RP, Weiner L, Spencer KT, Furlong KT, Bednarz J, DeCara J, Lang RM. Quantitative diagnosis of apical cardiomyopathy using contrast echocardiography. J Am Soc Echocardiogr 2002;15:316-22
43. Kaul S. Instrumentation for contrast echocardiography. Am J Cardiol 2002; 90:8J-14J
44. Shaw LJ. Impact of contrast echocardiography on diagnostic algorithms: pharmacoeconomic implications. Clin Cardiol 1997; 20:139-48

Chapter 7
Coronary Flow Reserve and Myocardial Contrast Echocardiography

Luis Moura • Miguel Angel García Fernández • José Luis Zamorano

Although there are several diagnostic techniques available for assessing coronary function, the quantification of coronary flow (CF) and coronary flow reserve (CFR) by angiography using an intracoronary Doppler flow wire is usually invasive. Recently, there have been several advances in echocardiography, not only in the direct visualization of the coronary arteries, but also in measuring CF and CFR. In this chapter, the current state of myocardial contrast echocardiography will be revisited, as well as the measurement of CF and CFR by transthoracic echocardiography (TTE) and transesophageal echocardiography (TEE), with special emphasis on recent advancements in ultrasound contrast-enhanced agents.

CF and CFR: Physiological Aspects

Coronary resistance is determined not only by the "tone" of the arteries, but also by the extrinsic compression of the coronary arteries by myocardial muscle during systole. The coronary blood flow has the peculiarity of having a two-phase characteristic pattern and the blood supply to the myocardium takes place fundamentally during diastole (Fig. 7.1). The ratio between diastolic and systolic coronary flow velocity is higher than 1.5 in the left coronary artery and its branches. In the right coronary artery (RCA), this diastolic blood flow is less predominant, probably due to the small systolic resistance in the right coronary side [1].

The left internal mammary artery (LIMA) without anastomosis has a pattern of systolic flow, the native coronary arteries have a two-phase pattern with predominant diastolic flow, and bypass graft with LIMA has a two-phase pattern, although the diastolic component is undoubtedly less intense than in the native coronary arteries. The ratio of diastolic and systolic blood flow velocity in coronary bypass grafts of the LIMA is smaller in the proximal portion than in the distal segment [2, 3]. However, the flow in coronary artery bypass grafts of the saphena vein shows a predominant diastolic component along the

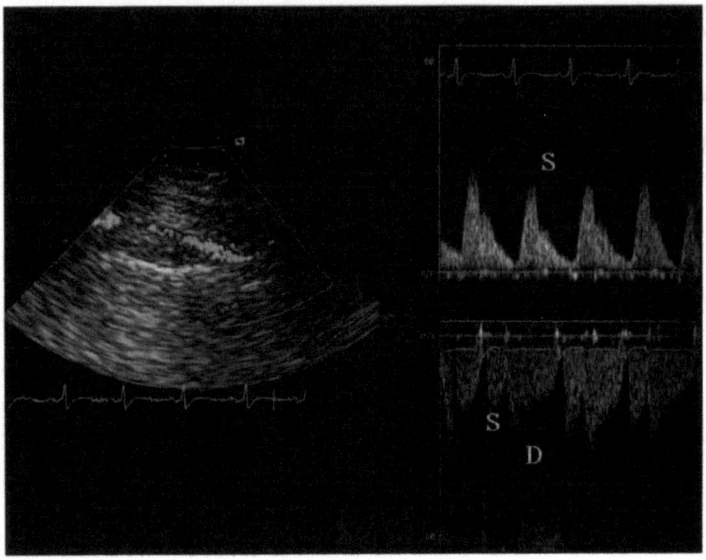

Fig. 7.1. *Right:* LAD mid-segment analysis. *Top left:* Arterial flow with a systolic wave (*S*). *Bottom left:* Two-phase coronary flow with predominant diastolic wave (*D*)

whole vessel, and the flow velocity is also lower in the saphena bypass grafts than in those of the LIMA in all segments studied [2].

Characteristics of CF in CAD

In the presence of coronary stenosis, we observed a decrease of the maximum flow velocity distal to the stenosis, when compared with flow velocity obtained in proximal segments of the same artery and in distal segments of other healthy coronary arteries. Specifically, we found a decrease of the maximum diastolic flow velocity, with relative preservation of the systolic component; thus, the predominant diastolic component in coronary artery disease becomes less clear, and a predominant systolic component may exist. From another point of view, there is a decrease in the hyperemic response in the presence of coronary stenosis compared to that obtained in normal coronary arteries [4, 5].

CFR: Definition

The severity of a lesion is evaluated in relation to the severity of stenosis of the lumen; however, there is only a modest relationship between functional and clinical repercussion of the disease, because the functional repercussions of a coronary lesion cannot be known solely by the data obtained with angiography. Under normal conditions, coronary blood flow can be increased several times above resting levels in situations that increase myocardial oxygen demand. The concept of CFR, therefore, is the capacity of the basal coronary flow to increase under situations of maximum myocardial requirements. Moreover, coronary flow is measured under basal conditions and after vasodilator coronary stress, i.e. CFR is the ratio between CF obtained after vasodilator stress and CF at basal conditions. Thus, the measurement of CFR has the advantage of offering a combination of anatomical and functional information [6, 7].

Using an intracoronary Doppler flow wire, it has been proved that the CF may increase over five to six times in the presence of normal levels of aortic pressure [8, 9]. Although the CFR is modestly correlated with the anatomical severity of the stenosis [10], the CF increases less under pharmacological vasodilators than normal coronary arteries [11, 12]. Furthermore, the CFR correlates well with the severity of myocardial perfusion defects [13], as well as having prognostic value [14, 15]. Kern et al. have demonstrated that "limited" coronary lesions (severity of the stenosis between 40% and 70%) with normal translesional physiology have a good natural prognosis, evaluated according to the need for future revascularization [15].

Therefore, the concept of CFR adds functional information to the opposing anatomical angiographic issues that acquire special relevance in lesions with "limited" severity. This physiological information, however, should also be interpreted within the clinical context of the patient [16].

CFR: Conditional Factors

Firstly, the CFR can be decreased with significant coronary artery stenosis. However, when there is a stenosis, the decrease in blood flow is compensated, under basal conditions, by a decrease of the coronary microcirculation resistance. However, although this mechanism usually compensates the CF under basal conditions, it may not be sufficient when the stenosis is very severe; additionally, the basal vasodilatation of the microcirculation limits its capacity to reduce the resistance when the metabolic demands of the myocardium increase, requiring a reduction of the CFR. Secondly, there are factors that can modify the CFR which have no relation with the severity of the coronary stenosis.

In coronary arteries with significant stenosis, the CF increases less with pharmacological vasodilators than in normal coronary arteries. The CFR is decreased when a lumen stenosis exists, the value of the CFR being inversely related with the severity of the stenosis [7]. A coronary stenosis of at least 60% is required to decrease the CFR [17].

Wilson et al. obtained an excellent correlation between CFR measured by intracoronary Doppler flow guide wire and the stenosis diameter, i.e. the percentage of area reduction and the absolute value of the minimum section area. In this study, all the lesions with a diameter ≤ 50% and area ≤ 70% had a normal CFR, i.e. higher than 3.5. The lesions with a diameter higher than 60% and an area superior to 80% both had a CFR smaller than 3.5. The values of CFR in lesions with a diameter of 50%–60% and an area of 70%–80% overlapped with the normal value of 3.5 of the CFR [18]. The CFR correlates modestly with the anatomical severity of the stenosis [10], because there may be other issues besides stenosis severity that might influence the CFR [19-23]. The value of the CFR depends on the following variables:

1. The perfusion coronary pressure and, therefore, the arterial pressure. Small changes in the arterial pressure may result in a significant modification of the flow during the maximum vasodilatation in normal coronary arteries.
2. The basal level of coronary flow. A basal increment of the coronary flow reduces the values obtained by the measurement of CFR. The basal CF is a function of metabolic demands. However, basal CF can also be increased, in the presence of recent myocardial ischemia, which acquires relevance when the CFR values are analyzed after a percutaneous transluminal coronary angioplasty (PTCA).
3. The pressure–flow ratio during maximum vasodilatation. The CFR changes with heart rate, contractility, preload and blood viscosity.

Tachycardia affects the CFR increasing the metabolic demands and reducing the relative time of diastole. Some conditions that affect the coronary microcirculation can also decrease the CFR, such as diabetes, left ventricular hypertrophy, myocardial infarction, syndrome X and hematological diseases [24]. For example, the CFR value would be the same for a coronary stenosis of 80% in an artery that supplies a normal ventricle and for a coronary stenosis of 50% that operates in a position of the curve with a less favorable relation pressure-flow [25].

Techniques for Measuring CFR

The CFR is calculated by dividing CF after coronary vasodilatation and CF under basal conditions. Therefore, most of the existing techniques to measure CFR involve the measurement of CF, or at least the velocity of CF, under basal conditions and after a vasodilatatory coronary pharmacological therapy. An ideal agent for studying CFR should produce a rapid hyperemic response and have a very short half life. In Europe, dipyridamole and adenosine are probably the most widely used vasodilatatory coronary agents in noninvasive studies of CFR. Traditionally, CF and CFR have been quantified by coronary angiography and intracoronary Doppler. Although widely validated, these techniques have the disadvantage of being invasive. Furthermore, they have the limitation of not evaluating the differences between basal vasodilatation before and after PTCA, which may interfere in the measurement of the CFR after PTCA. Moreover, the noninvasive study of CF and CFR achieved has special interest. Among the noninvasive techniques for measuring CFR are radioisotopic techniques, although these are indirect forms of measuring the CF [26, 27].

Echocardiography has also attempted, from the beginning, to visualize the coronary arteries, as well as to measure the CF and CFR, so as to reliably detect coronary stenosis. At first once the coronary artery was visualized, echocardiography could hypothetically detect a stenosis via three mechanisms:

1. Direct or indirect (calcified areas) visualization of stenosis.

2. Color Doppler, detecting aliasing areas and turbulence secondary to increased CF velocity in the coronary stenosis.
3. Measuring CF by pulse wave (PW) Doppler; velocity modifications of coronary basal flow as a decrease of CFR after coronary vasodilatatory stress can theoretically detect coronary stenosis.

TTE in the Study of Coronary Anatomy and CF

From the inception of echocardiography, the visualization of the coronary arteries has been attempted more or less successfully. In 1976, Weyman visualized the left main coronary artery by transthoracic echocardiography (TTE) [28]. Initially, the visualization of proximal segments of the coronary arteries by TTE was used to detect aneurysms in patients with Kawasaki disease [29-32] and in some children with congenital heart disease [33]. The initial success of echocardiography was extended to the visualization of the coronary arteries in adults, as well as in direct or indirect detection of coronary stenosis.

Evaluation of Anatomy and Flow of the Native Coronary Arteries

There are multiple studies that have tried to visualize the coronary arteries by TTE [28, 34-63]. These studies agree in pointing out a high percentage (between 58% and 90%) of visualization of the left main coronary artery and the proximal segment of the RCA (up to 91% of cases), while the other arteries are visualized in a smaller proportion of patients. Thus, the left anterior descending coronary artery (LAD) is visualized in between 47% and 86% of cases and the circumflex coronary artery (LCx) in 30% of cases.

Douglas et al. demonstrated that with modifications (angulations and rotations) in the standard windows, images of important segments of the epicardial vessels can be obtained, suggesting the potential use of echocardiography in coronary stenosis detection [44].

In some cases, it is possible to detect the existence of disease of the left main coronary artery by detecting calcifications in this vessel [34, 37-42]. Although the left main coronary artery and the proximal portion of the RCA can be visualized by TTE in a high percentage of patients, the measurement of Doppler flow in those areas has been technically difficult.

Even for the evaluation of the LAD by TTE, this proximal segment is located too far from the transducer for appropriate visualization. However, the middle segment of this artery is visualized in a significant proportion of patients [35, 36, 43, 56, 57].

In the study of Presti et al., appropriate visualization of the LAD was made in 90 patients (70% of those studied) by short-axis parasternal window [36]. Coronary angiography was performed on all patients so as to assess the diagnostic value of TTE in detecting disease of the proximal LAD. Of those patients, 27 had normal angiographic coronary arteries and 18 were considered normal according to an echocardiographic study. In 33 patients with significant stenosis and in 11 of the 12 patients with no significant stenosis, the artery was considered diseased by TTE. Finally, 18 patients had coronary disease, but without involvement of the proximal LAD, and in 15 of these patients the echocardiographic study showed that there was disease of the LAD. Therefore, in this study TTE had a sensitivity of 98% and a specificity of 67% in detecting the proximal LAD. There were 24 patients in whom echocardiographic study had predicted proximal LAD disease which was not confirmed in the coronary angiograph; however, 12 of them had disease of the distal segments of this artery.

Moreover, when using Doppler studies for the diagnosis of LAD disease, a decrease of the quotient between diastolic and systolic velocity in basal conditions indicates coronary stenosis. In the study of Watanabe et al., 113 patients were studied with coronary angiography and high-frequency TTE, with detection of LAD coronary flow in 81% of patients (9). In this study, a quotient between diastolic and systolic velocities lower than 1.6 had a sensitivity and a specificity of 84% and 82%, respectively, in detecting significant disease of the LAD (94% and 81% for a quotient mean velocity lower than 1.5).

TTE in the Study of Coronary Anatomy and CF

Transesophageal echocardiography (TEE) allows a greater proximity of the transducer to the coronary arteries, which allows the use of a higher frequency transductor resulting in better quality images [64, 65]. TEE has proved to be useful in visualizing the coronary arteries in a significant proportion of patients, especially for the left main coronary artery that can be visualized in 75%–100% of cases. Visualization of the proximal segment of the LAD and LCx is possible in 50% of cases, although in some studies this proportion has been higher [66-90]. Memmola et al. studied 160 patients by TEE, with the left main coronary artery, the LAD and LCx being visualized in 94%, 78% and 82% of patients, respectively [78]. The proportion of patients in which visualization of the proximal segment of the RCA is possible varies between 13% and 100%, depending on the study series [66, 70, 75, 77]. Yamagishi et al. visualized the lumen of the left main coronary artery and the LAD in 77% of cases, the LCx in 54% and the RCA in 26% [75].

Analysis of CF by TEE

With TEE, the visualization of the CF by color Doppler is also possible in some patients, as well as the measurement of its velocity and the CFR using pulse wave (PW) Doppler. The Yamagishi's group visualized the flow of the left main coronary artery and LAD by color Doppler in 89% of cases [70]. PW Doppler with TTE shows a two-phase pattern with diastolic predominance, similar to the one obtained by intravascular echocardiography and by TTE. In the Yamagishi et al. study, the flow of the proximal LAD was visualized in 77% of cases, the diastolic peak velocity being 40 ± 14 cm/s [68, 70, 75]. The flow of the RCA was visualized in 26% of patients, but it was not possible to evaluate the flow of the LCx. In the study of Iliceto et al., it was possible to measure CFR in the proximal segment of the LAD by TTE in 70% of cases [74].

Analysis of CFR by TEE

TEE also allows the measurement of CFR by studying the flow of the coronary sinus [90-92] or by evaluating segmental contractility during dobutamine stress echocardiography [93]. The ability of TEE to visualize the coronary arteries and detect, with color Doppler and PW Doppler, the CF and measure CFR, makes this technique useful in the detection of significant coronary stenosis. In the study of Iliceto et al., the CFR was 3.2 ± 0.9 and more than 2 in all subjects without stenosis of the LAD, and 1.5 ± 0.5 in patients with significant stenosis of the LAD, being more than 2 in only one of the six cases [74]. Yamagishi et al., studied 20 patients with left main coronary artery disease and 32 control subjects, obtaining appropriate images of the left main coronary artery in 85% of patients (17/20) and in 94% of controls (30/32) [75].

Coronary stenosis was visualized clearly in 12 of the 17 patients. In 26 of the 30 control subjects, the absence of stenosis was clearly noted, while it was observed in the other four images that simulated stenosis in the middle segment of left main coronary artery. Thus, the sensitivity and the specificity of disease detection in the left main coronary artery were 71% and 87%, respectively. In the same study, the sensitivity and specificity increased with the use of color Doppler; hence, color Doppler had a sensitivity and specificity in detection of left main coronary disease of 94% and 90%, respectively. The CF velocity could be measured by PW Doppler in 10 patients and in 21 controls; in the former, the velocity of CF in the stenosis was 116 ± 28 cm/s, compared with 29 ± 12 cm/s in the control group.

Although TEE may provide more quality images of the coronary arteries, this technique also has some limitations in the evaluation of coronary stenosis. First, it is a semi-invasive technique. Moreover, the LCx and RCA cannot be studied in most of the patients. In the case of the LCx, the angle between CF and the ultrasound is not adapted in most of the cases; in the case of the RCA, the position of the sample volume is not very stable as is the case with the LAD [68-70, 74]. There are some limitations regarding the LAD; although visualization is possible in a significant proportion of patients, it is limited to the more proximal segment of the vessel [66, 72, 76]. For this reason, some authors have suggested the combination of TTE and TEE for the appropriate study of the LAD (on the proximal segment and the segment that circulates for the interventricular anterior groove) [50]. The diagnostic value of TEE in detecting significant disease of the LAD is limited by its low sensitivity and specificity making this technique of little clinical utility.

Utility of Contrast-Enhanced Agents in the Study of CF

The idea of developing echocardiographic signal with microbubble administration is more than 30 years old [94]. With contrast agents able to pass freely through the pulmonary microcirculation and therefore to flow to the arterial blood, there has emerged an interest in the study of the coronary arteries by echocardiography, not only for their visualization but especially for the possibility of accurately detecting the existence of coronary stenosis (Fig. 7.2).

Mulvagh et al. validated the noninvasive measurement of CFR in dogs [95]. They studied the animals using both intracoronary Doppler and TTE second harmonic imaging, after intravenous injection of AF0145. CFR was measured by dividing the integral of velocity under basal conditions and after adenosine administration. CF morphology obtained by TTE was similar to the one obtained with the invasive method. The CFR values were similar for both techniques (3.3 ± 1.0 by TTE and 3.6 ± 1.2 with intracoronary Doppler), with an excellent correlation between both measurements ($r = 0.95$). Moreover, Mulvagh emphasized the ability of the second harmonic, correlated with intravenous administration of contrast, to detect CF reliably. This technique has also been validated by other groups [96, 97]. Caiati et al. measured CFR by intracoronary Doppler and TTE after the administration of Levovist in 17 patients, obtaining an excellent correlation between both measurements ($r = 0.88$) [98]. Since the CF velocity is also excellently cor-

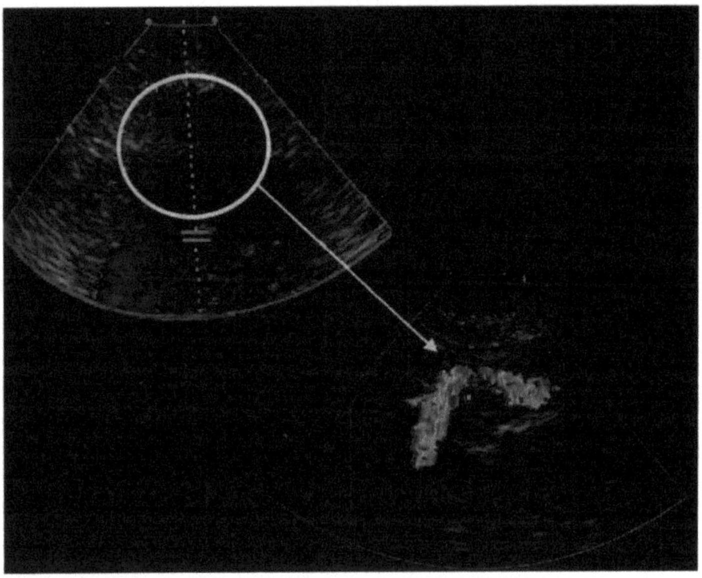

Fig. 7.2. Coronary flow analysis under basal conditions (*top*); blood flow registration was impossible. After intravenous administration of Levovist the signal of coronary flow was increased showing the LAD apical segment flow

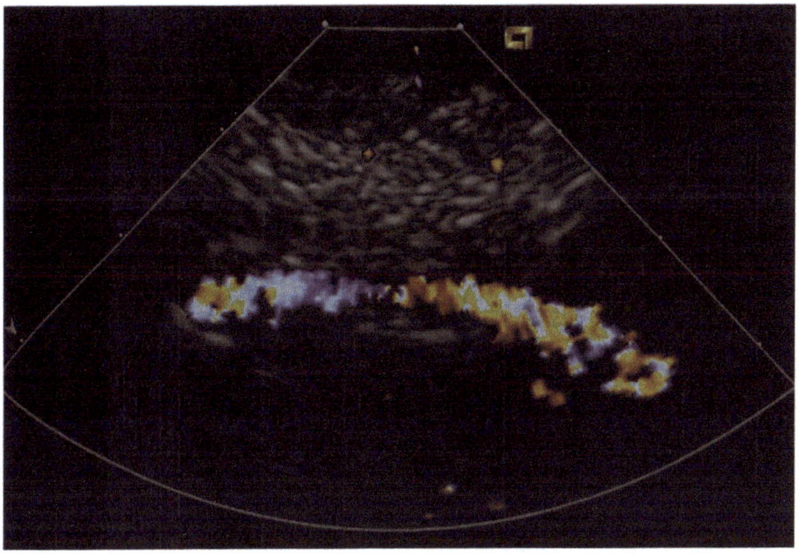

Fig. 7.3. Same LAD mid-segment analysis as in Fig. 7.2, after intravenous injection of contrast

related with the CF, the CFR measured as a quotient of CF velocities has an excellent correlation with CFR measured as a quotient of the absolute values of CF [97].

The improvement in the Doppler signal obtained by administration of contrast-enhanced agents makes noninvasive detection of coronary stenosis with TTE or TEE more reliable. Iliceto et al. studied CF in 35 patients using TEE (color Doppler and PW Doppler), comparing these methods before and after administering different doses of Levovist [98]. These authors demonstrated that the administration of Levovist increases the number of patients in which the flow is detected with better quality and it also increases the signal of the PW Doppler (Fig. 7.3).

Caiati et al. studied 31 patients using TEE, at basal conditions and after the administration of Levovist, before performing a coronary angiography procedure [99]. In 16 of the 31 patients, they demonstrated significant disease of the LAD with coronary angiography, and none of the patients had disease of the left main coronary artery. The longitude of the LAD visualized was 7 ± 5 mm in basal conditions and 18 ± 6 mm after the injection of contrast. When considering an increment of more than 50% among both samples as a diagnostic criterion of stenosis of the LAD, 15 of the 16 stenoses were detected (sensitivity 93%) and none of the patients without disease (specificity 100%). The sensitivity and specificity for the detection of LAD disease were 25% and 100% for Doppler in basal conditions and 19% and 100% for bidimensional echocardiography, respectively. On the other hand, one could locate the stenosis with accuracy in most of the patients, with a difference of less than 2 mm between TEE after contrast administration and coronary angiography, except in two patients. These authors concluded that contrast-enhanced TEE can be useful in the diagnosis of LAD stenosis.

Some good results have been obtained in noninvasive detection of LAD disease using TTE. However, some limitations persist: CFR cannot be validated if measured at the level of the stenosis. To avoid this, in patients with relatively high baseline velocity (> 50cm/s), it is recommended to take a second reference sample, in a different portion of the artery. In a certain number of cases, the angle was quite large (30°), causing underestimation of the true velocity. However, for the purpose of CFR evaluation, the absolute velocity value was not needed because CFR is a quotient of two velocities. Lastly, occlusion or distal disease in the LAD can result in false-negative cases, probably because of the detection of flow in branches of the artery or in the artery prior to stenosis.

The infusion of contrast-enhanced agents has also been useful in the evaluation of coronary bypass grafts of the internal mammary artery using TEE [100]. Therefore, in spite of the limitations, intravenous infusion of contrast-enhanced agents can be useful for noninvasive detection of significant stenosis of the LAD, improving the results obtained by TTE and TEE. This is of special interest in patients with left bundle branch block (LBBB) or when reevaluating the CF after trombolitic therapy in patients with acute myocardial infarction. On the other hand, this noninvasive technique can help diagnose clinical conditions without coronary disease but impaired CFR, such as microvascular angina, hypertrophic cardiomyopathy, arterial hypertension and others.

Recent Approaches to the Detection and Quantification of Coronary Artery Disease Using MCE

As mentioned previously, advances in the last 10 years have enabled the widespread use of myocardial contrast echocardiography (MCE) for assessing myocardial perfusion. This assessment is critical in evaluating the severity of coronary artery disease and the efficacy of pharmacologic, mechanical, or surgical interventions. MCE measures myocardial blood flow (MBF) by investigating flow velocity and myocardial blood volume. Although there are potential limitations in the use of MCE for determining MBF, its use is feasible in the experimental laboratory and in the clinical environment.

Because the microvascular rheology of the microbubbles used for MCE is similar to that of red blood cells (RBC) [101, 102], MCE has been shown to be able to noninvasively and accurately quantify MBF velocity [103].

The measurement of MBF in absolute terms (i.e., in milliliters per minute per gram) has become increasingly important in the evaluation of patients with coronary artery disease (CAD). Until recently, these measurements could only be obtained in humans by use of positron emission tomography (PET) [104, 106]. However, clinical application of this approach has been hampered by the limited availability and the cost of PET scanners, as well as by their inability to evaluate regional contractile function.

MCE is a relatively new technique that uses microbubbles to produce myocardial opacification [107]. Although assessment of myocardial perfusion by MCE has been used for many years, its widespread application to patients with CAD was limited by the need to inject the microbubbles into the aorta or directly into the coronary arteries. During the past 5 years, three major advances have enabled the echocardiographic detection of CAD and the quantification of MBF after intravenous injections of microbubbles:

1. The development of second-generation microbubbles containing nondiffusible, high molecular gases with low solubility that are more resistant than air-filled microbubbles to change in size when mixed with blood and that persist long enough to reach and opacify the myocardium [108].
2. The development of contrast-specific imaging modalities that take advantage of the nonlinear backscattering properties of contrast microbubbles, resulting in a considerably higher contrast-to-tissue signal than with conventional fundamental imaging [109].
3. The refined understanding of the interaction between the ultrasound beam and contrast microbubbles [110, 111], which means an improvement of endocardial border delineation, allowing improved visualization of more myocardial segments, better confidence and accuracy in the assessment of wall motion, and decreased interobserver and intraobserver variability. This allowed the design of specific contrast imaging algorithms that enable us to obtain quantitative estimates of regional MBF and myocardial blood volume [112].

In the absence of prior myocardial injury, both resting myocardial blood flow (MBF) and left ventricular function remain normal even in the presence of an epicardial coronary stenosis of up to 85% to 90% in severity (Fig. 7.4) [113]. With increases in myocar-

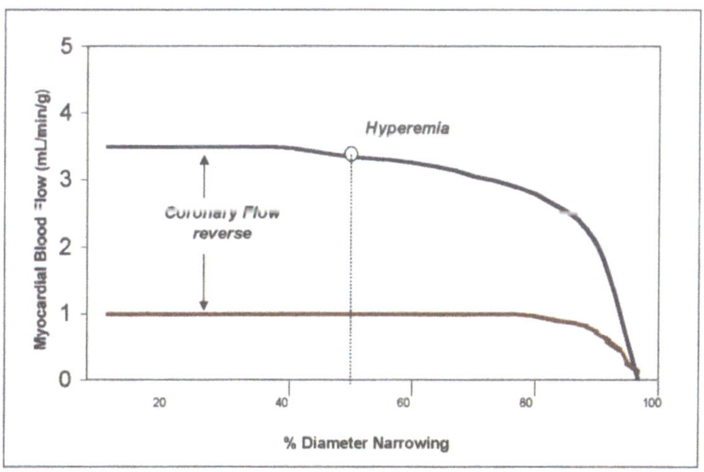

Fig. 7.4. Relationship between the percentage of coronary stenosis and MBF at rest (*dashed line*) and during hyperemia (*solid line*). Resting MBF remains constant until stenosis severity exceeds approximately 85% severity, whereas hyperemic MBF becomes attenuated in the presence of stenosis greater than about 50% severity

dial oxygen demand, MBF can usually increase four to five times above that of resting levels. Coronary arteries with stenoses that encroach 50%–85% of the luminal diameter, however, show an attenuated hyperemic response. To detect non-flow-limiting stenoses with echocardiography, therefore, adequate exercise or pharmacologic stress is used to produce supply/demand mismatch and ischemia, which results in the development of a regional wall motion abnormality. Reliance on the use of wall motion abnormalities to detect covert CAD remains a disadvantage because ischemia must be provoked, and wall motion abnormalities appear late in the ischemic cascade. With MCE, however, tissue perfusion can now also be assessed with echocardiography.

What Does Myocardial Video Intensity Represent?

When second-generation microbubbles are administered as a constant intravenous infusion, the concentration of microbubbles in the circulation will reach a steady state. Microbubble concentration in any microcirculatory unit remains constant during this period of time. Within the linear range of the microbubble concentration versus video intensity (VI) relation, areas with a lower VI will contain a lower number (mass) of microbubbles. Since concentration is equal to mass/volume, areas with a lower VI will also have a smaller blood volume (for example, areas of microvascular damage secondary to infarction.)

Because steady state VI reflects tissue blood volume, it follows that in the myocardium, the circulatory compartment (arteries, microvessels, or veins) that contains the largest proportion of the myocardial blood volume (MBV) will be most represented by steady-state myocardial VI. Therefore, steady-state myocardial VI provides an estimate of capillary blood volume.

Image Processing and Determination of Tissue Contrast Enhancement

Newer modalities such as harmonic and pulse inversion imaging have improved the signal-to-noise ratio by attempting to isolate nonlinear signals originating predominantly from microbubbles; however, nonlinear propagation of ultrasound through tissue also results in tissue harmonic signals [114, 115]. Because it is difficult to mentally track regional differences in background and to determine the subsequent change in VI produced by microbubbles, digital image processing techniques such as image alignment, averaging, video densitometry, and, finally, background-subtraction become essential.

To minimize respiratory motion and changes in location of tissue within the ultrasound sector, the patient is asked to breathe quietly during the study, and multiple images are acquired so that only high-quality and similarly positioned images within the sector are selected for digitization and video densitometric analysis. Further optimization of the alignment of digitized images can be obtained either manually or with computer cross-correlation using either custom-designed or commercially available software [116]. The tissue VI signal from aligned baseline (precontrast) and contrast-enhanced images can then be determined by placing a region of interest over the image, and the values can be digitally subtracted to obtain regional background-subtracted contrast enhancement.

The human eye can only differentiate a few shades of gray [117], but it can distinguish hundreds of hues of color, so background-subtracted images can be color-coded to better demonstrate regional differences in contrast enhancement. The pixel with the greatest VI has been assigned a level of 256, and all the others have been assigned proportionally lower values. Each pixel is then relegated a color representing the degree of contrast enhancement [118]. The images in this review have been color-coded with a heated object algorithm, in which hues of red, orange, yellow, and white represent incremental amounts of contrast enhancement.

Quantification of MBF

Methods to quantify tissue blood flow using MCE have been developed to take advantage of ultrasound/microbubble interactions. As mentioned previously, ultrasound at transmit powers used clinically can rapidly and effectively destroy microbubbles, also during in vivo imaging [119]. At steady state during a continuous intravenous infusion of microbubbles, the number of microbubbles entering or leaving any microcirculatory unit is constant, and will depend on the flow rate. After destroying microbubbles within the ultrasound beam elevation, the rate of replenishment of microbubbles into the microvessels within the beam elevation will reflect microbubble velocity and, hence, RBC velocity [120].

This concept is diagrammatically represented in Fig. 7.5. The elevation (or thickness) of the ultrasound beam is represented by a myocardium with a thickness of E (Fig. 7.5A). After microbubbles are destroyed at t_0 by a pulse of ultrasound (Fig. 7.5A), new microbubbles will begin to replenish the ultrasound beam elevation. As the pulsing interval (PI) is increased (Fig. 7.5, B–E), there is more time for replenishment to occur between each destructive pulse of ultrasound and the degree of microbubble replenishment into the elevation increases. As long as the relationship between microbubble concentration and myocardial VI is linear, VI will progressively increase at longer PIs (Fig. 7.5 lower panel) [120]. The rate in rise of VI depicts MBF velocity [120].

When the PI is long enough for the entire ultrasound beam elevation to be completely replenished with microbubbles (Fig. 7.5E), the PI versus VI relationship plateaus. As discussed earlier, steady-state plateau myocardial VI represents MBV (or capillary blood volume). Because resting MBF velocity within the capillaries is very low (≤1 mm/s), and the ultrasound beam elevation measures approximately 5 mm in thickness, a PI of approximately 5 s is usually required for the entire ultrasound elevation to completely replenish with microbubbles. Myocardial VI at a PI of greater than 5 s,

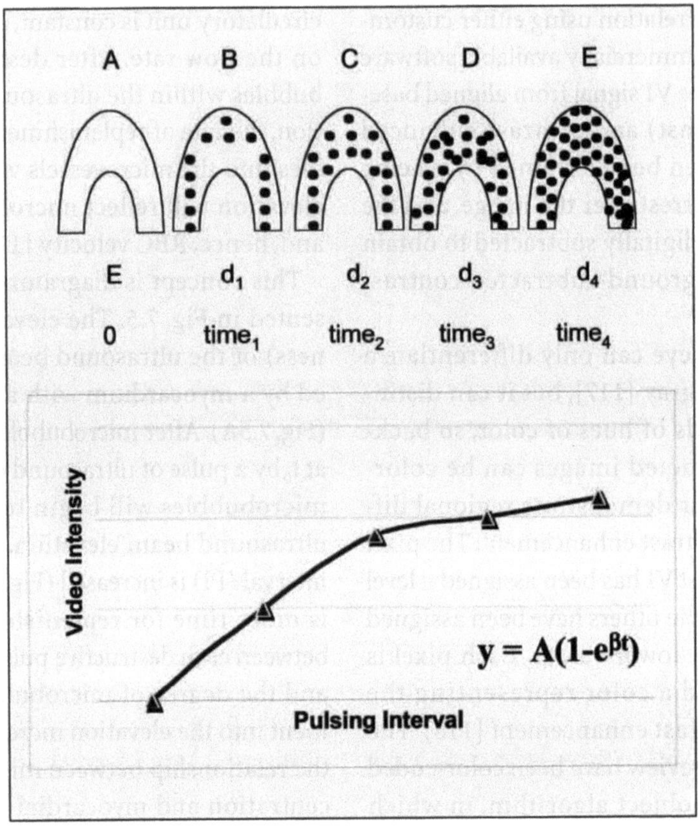

Fig. 7.5. Replenishment of myocardial microcirculation within ultrasound beam elevation (*E*) at different PIs (*t1* to *t4*) after destructive pulse of ultrasound during continuous infusion of microbubbles (*top panel*). Relation between PI and myocardial VI (*bottom panel*)

therefore, provides an assessment of regional MBV.

The PI versus myocardial VI relationship (Fig. 7.5, bottom) can be fitted to an exponential function: $y = A(1 - e^{-\beta t})$, where y is myocardial VI at a PI of t, A is the plateau VI representing MBV, and β is the rate constant representing the mean microbubble velocity. MCE can, therefore, determine both specific components of MBF: flow velocity (β) and MBV [120].

Thus, MCE can be used to not only provide insights into spatial patterns of normal and abnormal perfusion, but also to explore the adequacy of nutrient perfusion, and help to clarify flow–function relations.

Detection and Quantification of Stenosis Severity Using MBF Reserve

One advantage of using MCE for quantification of MBF velocity is that unlike Doppler, MCE is not angle dependent. An obvious application using the ability of MCE

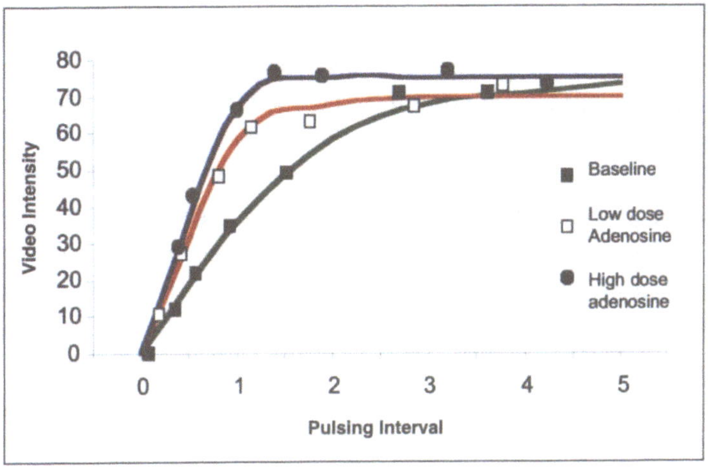

Fig. 7.6. Pulsing interval versus video intensity relationship obtained at rest (■) and during two doses of adenosine [low dose (□) or high dose (●)]

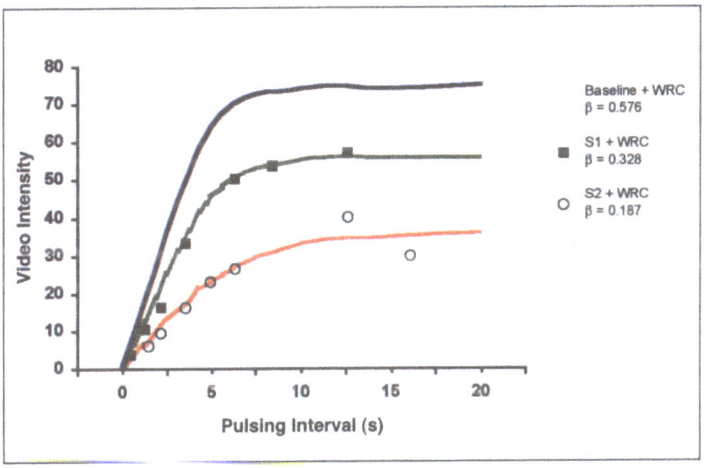

Fig. 7.7. Pulsing interval versus video intensity relationships obtained during hyperemia in the absence (_) and presence of two different non-flow-limiting stenoses (■ and ○)

to determine resting and hyperemic MBF velocity is the quantification of MBF reserve. In an animal study, different doses of adenosine (2.5 and 5.0 μg • kg^{-1} • min^{-1}) were infused directly into the coronary artery to increase MBF to different degrees. The pulsing interval versus VI curves obtained at rest (solid squares) and during the two doses of adenosine [low dose (open squares) and high dose (solid circles)] are shown in Fig. 7.6. As flow increased with adenosine, the rate of the rise of myocardial VI also progressively increased [121]. The plateau VI (or MBV) between the three stages, however, remains constant. These findings are similar to previous studies [122, 123] showing that capillary blood volume remains constant in the absence of changes in systemic hemodynamics during intracoronary adenosine. In this setting, therefore, microbubble velocity reserve is directly proportional to MBF reserve.

The abnormal flow reserve observed in the presence of physiologically significant coronary stenoses can also be determined using MCE. Figure 7.7 illustrates PI versus VI curves obtained from an animal during hyperemia in the absence and presence of two different noncritical stenoses. Decreases in peak hyperemic flow in the presence of more severe stenosis are associated with progressive decreases in microbubble velocity as depicted by the slower rate of rise in VI (solid squares and open circles) compared with that seen in the absence of a stenosis (open squares) [124].

Wei et al. have also recently shown that abnormalities of MBF velocity reserve can be quantified in patients with CAD [125]. An apical two-chamber view from a patient with a moderate stenosis in the LAD (60% by quantitative coronary angiography) was obtained at rest and during hyperemia. The images are color-coded parametric images of microbubble velocity (β), which were generated by fitting an exponential function to each pixel in the image. The value of β from each pixel was represented using a "ripening mango" algorithm in which colors progressing from dark green to light green to yellow to red represent incremental increases in β. The corresponding PI versus VI curves from the LAD (solid circles) and LCx beds (open circles) are shown (Fig. 7.8A, B). At baseline, the change in VI at different PI is similar in both the LAD and LCx beds as the stenosis was not flow-limiting at rest, and the measured microbubble velocity (β) from both beds is also similar (Fig. 7.8A). During hyperemia induced with an intravenous infusion of 140 $\mu g \cdot kg^{-1} \cdot min^{-1}$ of adenosine, however, the increase in MBF is lower in the stenosed LAD compared with the LCx bed. The color in the LAD bed therefore consists of darker hues of green (indicating lower microbubble velocities) compared with the yellow and red colors seen in the LCx bed. The measured mean microbubble velocity is also lower for the LAD compared with the LCx (Fig. 7.8B).

Patients with normal coronary arteries on angiography had significantly higher MBF velocity reserve (defined as hyperemic/resting MBF velocity) than did patients with CAD—a finding similar to that determined using intracoronary Doppler flow wire measurements. Furthermore, patients with a stenosis greater than 70% severity assessed by quantitative coronary angiography all had MBF velocity reserve of less than 1.5 as measured using MCE in our study [125]. Abnormalities of MBF reserve can therefore potentially be used to quantify noninvasively the physiologic significance of stenoses in humans.

Pharmacologic Stress

We have discussed the use of vasodilator stress to produce perfusion defects on MCE, or for the assessment of MBF velocity

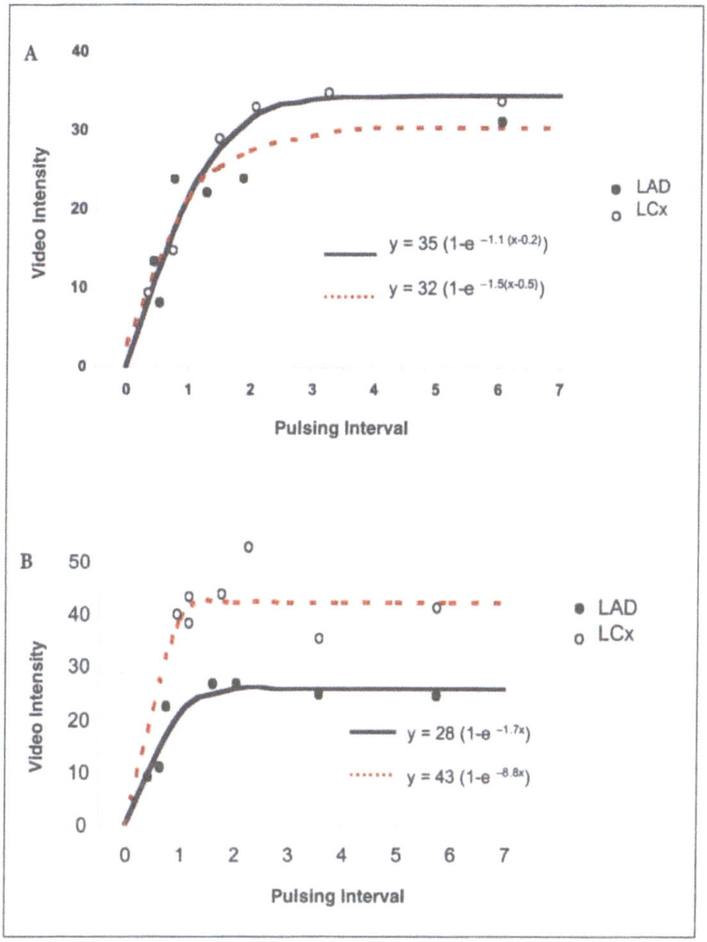

Fig. 7.8. PI versus VI curves from the LAD (■) and LCx beds (○) from a patient with moderate LAD stenosis (69% by QCA) obtained at rest (**A**) and during hyperemia (**B**)

reserve. In North America, dobutamine is more commonly used for pharmacologic stress with echocardiography compared with vasodilators like dipyridamole or adenosine. Even though dobutamine produces ischemia by increasing myocardial oxygen demand and causing a supply-demand mismatch, abnormal subendocardial blood flow reserve is also an important determinant of wall-thickening abnormalities during dobutamine stress. Figure 7.9 shows examples of the wall-thickening response at incremental doses of dobutamine in dogs with chronic coronary stenoses [126]. The animals were divided into three groups on the basis of subendocardial MBF reserve: those with a normal endocardial MBF reserve of more than 3; those with mildly reduced reserve (2 to 3); and those with a significantly impaired MBF reserve of less than 2. In the group with

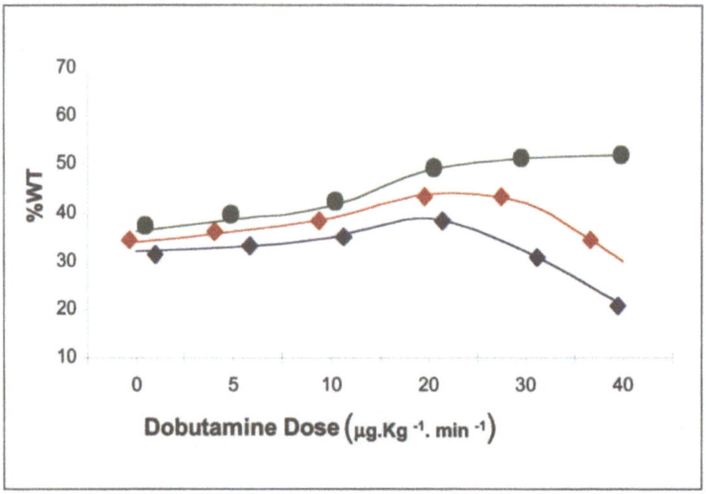

Fig. 7.9. Response of percentage of wall thicknening (%WT) at progressively higher doses of dobutamine in animals with endocardial MBF reserve of >3 (*green line*), 2 to 3 (*red line*) and < 2 (*blue line*)

normal MBF reserve, progressive increases in wall thickening are seen at higher doses of dobutamine. In the other two groups, however, a decrease in wall thickening is noted at higher doses of dobutamine, compatible with the development of ischemia from supply–demand mismatch. Not only is the degree of wall-thickening abnormality dependent on the severity of impaired subendocardial MBF reserve, but the dobutamine dose at which hypokinesis develops is also lower in the animals with lower MBF reserve. Immediately after exercise, or during dobutamine stress, a very limited time window exists for acquisition of perfusion images with MCE. It is, therefore, not possible to use high-power intermittent MCE modalities in these settings, as there is insufficient time to obtain replenishment curves from multiple windows. A number of real-time perfusion modalities have recently been developed. These techniques use an adequate transmit power to induce nonlinear oscillation of microbubbles, but it is low enough for the microbubbles to remain intact. Myocardial perfusion imaging can, therefore, be performed at high frame rates (>20 Hz), allowing simultaneous assessments of both perfusion and wall thickening.

Another advantage of these techniques is that replenishment curves can be derived rapidly over a few cardiac cycles. By transmitting a number of high-power ultrasound pulses to destroy microbubbles within tissue, and then reverting to a low-power imaging modality, replenishment of the myocardial microcirculation can be followed in real-time [127]. Similar to high-mechanical index intermittent imaging, a bed supplied by a stenosed artery will have a slower rate of rise of VI during stress than a normal bed during real-time imaging, allowing detection of stenoses [127]. Recently, clinical studies have been performed using low-power imaging during exercise [128] or dobutamine stress [129]. Good correlations were found between low-power MCE techniques for the detection of perfusion defects compared with SPECT or quantitative coronary angiography.

Because abnormal subendocardial flow is also the reason underlying the development of a supply–demand mismatch during dobutamine stress, we would also expect a slower rate of replenishment of microbubbles in a stenosed compared with a normal bed during dobutamine stress. Consequently, quantitative or qualitative assessments of regional MBF velocity can also be applied to the detection of coronary stenosis with MCE during dobutamine stress [130].

References

1. Hamaoka K, Onouchi Z, Ohmochi Y et al. Coronary arterial flow-velocity dynamics in children with angiographically normal coronary arteries. *Circulation* 1995; 92: 2.457
2. Bach RG, Kern MJ, Donohue TJ, Aguirre FU, Caracciolo EA. Comparison of phasic blood flow velocity characteristics of arterial and venous coronary artery bypass conduits. *Circulation* 1993; 88 (Suppl II): II-133
3. Gurne O, Chenu P, Polidori C, Louagie Y, Buche M, Haxhe JP et al. Functional evaluation of internal mammary artery bypass grafts in the early and late postoperative periods. *J Am Coll Cardiol* 1995; 25: 1.120
4. Ofili E0, Kern MJ, Labovitz Al et al. Analysis of coronary blood flow velocity dynamics in angiographically normal and stenosed arteries before and after endoluminal enlargement by angioplasty. *J Am Coll Cardiol* 1993; 21: 308
5. Segal J, Kern Mj, Scott NA et al. Alterations of phasic coronary artery flow velocity in humans during percutaneous coronary angioplasty. *J Am Coll Cardiol* 1992; 20: 276
6. Gould KL, Kirkeeide RL, Buchi M. Coronary flow reserve as a physiologic measure of a stenosis severity. *J Am Coll Cardiol* 1990; 15: 459
7. Klocke FJ. Measurements of coronary flow reserve: defining pathophysiology versus making decisions about patient care. *Circulation* 1987; 76: 1.183
8. Marcus ML, Wilson RF, White CW. Methods of measurement of myocardial blood flow in patients: a critical review. *Circulation* 1987; 76: 245
9. Gould KL, Lipscomb K, Hamilton GW. Physiologic basis for assessing critical coronary stenosis: instantaneous flow response and regional distribution during coronary hyperemia as measures of coronary flow reserve. *Am J Cardiol* 1974; 33: 87
10. White CW, Wright CB, Dory DB, et al. Does visual interpretation of the coronary angiogram predict the physiologic importance of a coronary stenosis? *N Engl J Med* 1984; 310: 819
11. Wilson RE, White CW. Intracoronary papaverine: an ideal coronary vasodilator for studies of the coronary circulation in conscious humans. *Circulation* 1985; 73: 444
12. Marcus M, Wright C, Dory D et al. Measurements of coronary velocity and reactive hyperemia in the coronary circulation of humans. *Circ Res* 1981; 49: 877
13. Devchak YA, Segal J, Reiner JS et al. Doppler guide wire flow-velocity indexes measured distal to coronary stenosis associated with reversible thallium perfusion defects. *Am Heart J* 1995; 129: 219
14. Kern Mj, Donohue TJ, Aguirre FV et al. Clinical outcome of deferring angioplasty in patients with normal translesional pressure-flow velocity measurements. *J Am Coll Cardiol* 1995; 25: 178
15. Pijls NHJ, de Bruync B, Peels K et al. Measurement of myocardial fractional flow reserve to assess the functional severity of coronary-artery stenosis. *N Engl J Med* 1996; 334: 1.703
16. Kern MJ, Bruyne B, Pijls NHJ. From research to clinical practice: current role of intracoronary physiologically based decision making in the cardiac catheterization laboratory. *J Am Coll Cardiol* 1997; 30: 613
17. Gould KL, Kirkeeide RL, Buchi M. Coronary flow reserve as a physiologic measure of a stenosis severity. *J Am Coll Cardiol* 1990; 15: 459
18. Wilson RE, Marcus ML, White CW. Prediction of the physiologic significance of coronary arterial lesions by quantitative lesion geometry in patients with limited coronary artery disease. *Circulation* 1987; 75: 723

19. Ardehali A, Segal J, Cheitlin MD. Coronary blood flow reserve in acute aortic regurgitation. *J Am Coll Cardiol* 1995; 25: 1.387
20. Antony I, Nitenberg A, FoultjM, Aptecar E. Coronary vasodilator reserve in untreated and treated hypertensive patients with and without left ventricular hypertrophy. *J Am Coll Cardiol* 1993; 22: 514
21. Inoue T, Sakai Y, Morooka S et al. Coronary flow reserve in patients with dilated cardiomyopathy. *Am Heart J* 1993; 125: 93
22. Akasaka T, Yoshida K, Yamamuro et al. Phasic coronary flow characteristics in patients with constrictive pericarditis: comparison with restrictive cardiomyopathy. *Circulation* 1997; 96: 1.874
23. Kern MJ, Deligonul U, Vandormael M et al. Impaired coronary vasodilatory reserve in the immediate post-coronary angioplasty period: analysis of coronary arterial velocity flow indexes and regional cardiac venous flow. *J Am Coll Cardiol* 1989;13:860
24. Strauer B. The significance of coronary reserve in clinical heart disease. *J Am Coll Cardiol* 1990; 15: 775
25. Hofmann JIE. A critical view of coronary reserve. *Circulation* 1987; 75(Suppl I): I
26. Zijlstra F, Fioretti P, Reiber J, Serruys PW. Which cine angiographically assessed anatomic variable correlates best with functional measurements of stenoses severity? A comparison of quantitative analysis of the coronary angiogram with measured coronary flow, reserve and exercise redistribution thallium-201 scintigraphy. *J Am Coll Cardiol 1988;* 12: 686
27. Demer LL, Gould KL, Goldstein RA et al. Assessment of coronary artery disease severity by positron emission tomography. Comparison with quantitative arteriography in 193 patients. *Circulation* 1989; 79: 825
28. Weyman AE, Feigenbaum H, Dillon JC, Johnston KW, Eggleton RC. Noninvasive visualization of the left main coronary artey by cross-sectional echocardiography. *Circulation* 1976; 54: 169
29. Capannari TE, Daniels SR, Meyer RA, Schwartz DC Kaplan S. Sensitivity, specificity, and predicti value of twodimensional echocardiography detec ting coronary artery aneurysms in patients with Kawasaki's disease. *J Am Coll Cardiol* 1986; 7:355
30. Yoshikawa J, Yanagihara K, Okawi T et al. Cross-sectional echocardiographic diagnosis of coronary artery aneurysms in patients with the mucocutaneous lymph node syndrome. *Circulation* 1979; 59: 133
31. Satomi G, Nakamura K, Narai S, Takao A. Systematic visualization of coronary arteries by two-dimensional echocardiography in children and infants: evaluation in Kawasaki's disease and arteriovenous fistulas. *Am Heart J* 1984; 107: 497
32. Hiraishi S, Yashiro K, Kusano S. Noninvasive vizualization of coronary arterial aneurysm in infants and young children with mucocutaneous lymph node syndrome with two dimensional echocardiography. *Am J Cardiol* 1979; 43: 1.225
33. Fisher EA, Sepehri B, Lendrum B, Luken J, Levitskyf. Two-dimensional echocardiography visualization of the left coronary artery in anomalous origin of the left coronary artery from the pulmonary artery. *Circulation* 1981; 63: 698
34. Rogers EW, Feigenbaum HM, Weyman AE, Godley RW, Johnson KW, Eggleton RC. Possible detection of atherosclerotic coronary calcification by two-dimensional echocardiography. *Circulation* 1980; 1046
35. Miyatake K, Yamagishi M, Izumi SA et al. Doppler echocardiographic approach to the blood flow of the left anterior descending coronary artery. *J Gin Ultrasound* 1988; 16: 471
36. Presti CF, Feigenbaum H, Armstrong WQF, Ryan T, Dillon JC. Digital two-dimensional echocardiographic imaging of the proximal left anterior descending coronary artery. *Am J Cardiol* 1987; 60: 1.254
37. Chen CC, Morganroth J, Ogawa S, Mardelli TJ. Detecting left main coronary artery disease by apical, cross-sectional echocardiography. *Circulation* 1980; 62: 288
38. Rink LD, Feigenbaum H, Godley RW, et al. Echocardiographic detection of left main coronary artery obstruction. *Circulation* 1982; 65: 719
39. Friedman MJ, Shan DJ, Goldman S et al. High predictive accuracy for detection of left main coronary artery disease by antilog signal processing of two-dimensional echocardiographic images. *Am Heart J* 1982; 103(2): 194-201
40. Block PI, Popp RL. Detecting and excluding significant left main coronary artery narrowing by echocardiography. *Am J Cardiol* 1985; 55: 937
41. Chandraratna PAN, Aronow WS, Murdock K, Milholland H. Left main coronary arterial patency assessed with cross-sectional echocardiography. *Am J Cardiol* 1980; 46: 91
42. Ryan T, Armstrong WF, Feigenbaum H. Prospective evaluation of the left main coronary artery using digital two-dimensional echocardiography. *J Am Coll Cardiol* 1986; 7: 807
43. Fusejima K. Noninvasive measurement of coronary artery blood flow using combined two-dimensional and Doppler echocardiography. *J Am Coll Cardiol* 1987;10:1.024
44. Douglas PS, Fiolkoski J, Berko B, Reichek N. Echocardiographic visualization of coronary artery anatomy in the adult. *J Am Coll Cardiol* 1988; 11: 5.565
45. Rogers EW, Feigenbaum H, Weyman AE, Godley RW,

Willis ER, Vakili ST. Evaluation of coronary artery anatomy in vitro by cross-sectional echocardiography. *Am J Cardiol* 1979; 43: 386

46. Ogawa S, Chen CC, Hubbard FE et al. A new approach to visualize the left main coronary artery using apical cross-sectional echocardiography. *Am J Cardiol* 1980; 45: 301
47. Ross JJ Jr, Mintz GS, Chandrasekaran K. Transthoracic two-dimensional high frequency (7.5 MHz) ultrasonic visualization of the distal left anterior descending coronary artery. *J Am Coll Cardiol* 1990; 15: 373
48. Sawada SG, Ryan T, Segar D et al. Distinguishing ischemic cardiomyopathy from nonischemic dilated cardiomyopathy with coronary echocardiography. *J Am Coll Cardiol 1992;* 19:1.223
49. Faletra F, Cipriani M, Corno R, Formentini A, Danzi GB, Pezzano A. Transthoracic high-frequency echocardiographic detection of atherosclerotic lesion in the descending portion of the left coronary artery. *J Am Soc Echocardiogr* 1993; 6:290-8
50. Faletra F, Cipriani M, De Chiara F et al. Imaging the left anterior descending coronary artery by high-frequency transthoracic echocardiography in heart transplant patients. *Am J Cardiol* 1995; 75: 855-8
51. Verez Z, Katz M, Rath S. Two-dimensional echocardiographic analysis of proximal left main coronary artery in humans. *Am Heart J* 1986; 112: 972
52. Voci P, Testa G, Plaustro G, Marino B, Campa PP. Study of the coronary flow with high resolution transthoracic echocardiography and nondirectional Doppler. *Cardiologia* 1997; 42: 849-53
53. Crowley JJ, Dardas PS, Harcombe AA, Shapiro LM. Transthoracic Doppler echocardiographic analysis of phasic coronary blood flow velocity in hypertrophic cardiomyopathy. *Heart* 1997; 77: 558
54. Hozumi T, Yoshida K, Akasaka T et al. Noninvasive assessment of coronary flow velocity and coronary flow velocity reserve in the left anterior descending coronary artery by Doppler echocardiography. *J Am Coll Cardiol* 1998; 32: 1.251
55. Kenny A, Shapiro LM. Transthoracic high-frequency two-dimensional echocardiography, Doppler and color flow mapping to determine anatomy and blood flow patterns in the distal left anterior descending coronary artery. *Am J Cardiol* 1992; 69: 1.265
56. Gramiak R, Holen J, Moss AJ, Gutierrez OH, Picone AJ, Roe SA. Left coronary arterial blood flow: noninvasive detection by Doppler US. *Radiology* 1986; 159: 657
57. Crowley JI, Shapiro LM. Transthoracic echocardiographic measurement of coronary blood flow and *reserve. J Am Soc Echocardiogr 1997; 10: 337*
58. Watanabe H, Yokoi Y, Takemoto K, et al. Assessment of the epicardial coronary flow velocity by transthoracic color Doppler echocardiography is a useful screening test for angina pectoris (abstract). *J Am Coll Cardiol* 1999; 33: 404A
59. Reeder GS, Seward JB, Tajik AJ. The role of two-dimensional echocardiography in coronary artery disease: a critical appraisal. *Mayo Clin Proc* 1982; 57: 247
60. Ronderos R, Salcedo EE, Kramer JR, Simpendorfer CC, Shirley EK. Value and limitations of two-dimensional echocardiography for the detection of left main coronary artery disease. *Cleve Clin Q* 1984; 51: 7
61. Vered Z, Katz M, Rath S et al. Two-dimensional echocardiographic analysis of proximal left main coronary artery in humans. *Am Heart J* 1986; 112: 972
62. Feigenbaum H. Transthoracic ultrasonic visualization of coronary atherosclerosis. *J Am Soc Echocardiogr* 1989; 2: 253
63. Klein LW, Weintrub WS, Agarwal JB, Seelaus PA, Katz RI, Helfant RH. Prognostic significance of severe narrowing of the proximal portion of the left anterior descending coronary artery. *Am J Cardiol* 1986; 58: 42
64. Currie PJ. Transesophageal echocardiography: new window to the heart. *Circulation* 1989; 80: 215
65. Erbel R. Transesophageal echocardiography: new window to coronary arteries and coronary blood flow. *Circulation* 1991; 83: 339
66. Taams MA, Gussenhoven El, Cornel JH et al. Detection of left coronary stenosis by transesophageal echocardiography. *Eur Heart J* 1988; 9: 1.162
67. Zwicky P, Daniel WG, Mügger A, Lichtlen PR. Imaging of coronary arteries by color-coded transesophageal Doppler echocardiography. *Am J Cardiol* 1988; 62: 639
68. Yamagishi M, Miyatake K, Beppu S et al. Assessment of coronary blood flow by transesophageal two-dimensional pulsed Doppler echocardiography. *Am J Cardiol* 1988; 62: 641
69. Pearce FB, Sheikh KH, de Bruijn NP, Kisslo J. Imaging of the coronary arteries by transesophageal echocardiography. *J Am Soc Echocardiogr* 1989; 2: 276
70. Yamagishi M, Miyatake K, Beppu S, Tanaka N, Nimura Y. Visualization of coronary blood flow by color Doppler imaging with transesophageal approach. *Chest* 1989; 96: 972
71. Yoshida K, Yoshikawa J, Hozumi T et al. Detection of left main coronary artery stenosis by transesophageal color Doppler and two-dimensional echocardiography. *Circulation* 1990; 81: 1.271
72. Reichert SLA, Visser CA, Koolen JJ et al. Transesophageal examination of the left coronary artery

with a 7.5 MHz annular array two-dimensional color flow Doppler transducer. *J Am Soc Echocardiogr* 1990; 3: 118

73. Scherem SS, Tunick PA, Slater J, Kronzon I. Transesophageal echocardiography in the diagnosis of ostial coronary artery stenosis. *J Am Soc Echocardiogr* 1990; 3: 367
74. Iliceto S, Marangelli V, Memmola C et al. Transesophageal doppler echocardiography evaluation of coronary blood flow velocity in baseline conditions and during dipyridamole-induced coronary vasodilation. *Circulation* 1991; 83: 61
75. Yamagishi M, Yasu T, Ohara K, Kuro M, Miyatake K. Detection of coronary blood flow associated with left main coronary artery stenosis by transesophageal Doppler color flow echocardiography. *J Am Coll Cardiol* 1991; 17:87
76. Samdarshi TE, Nanda NC, Gatewood RP Jr et al. Usefulness and limitations of transesophageal echocardiography in the assessment of proximal coronary artery stenosis. *J Am Coll Cardiol* 1992; 19: 572
77. Esteban E, García Fernández MA, Torrecilla EG, San Roman D, Delcán JL. Transesophageal echocardiography in the assessement of coronary artery anatomy and blood flow. *Rev Esp Cardiol* 1993; 43:46:20-7
78. Memmola C, Iliceto S, Rizzon P. Detection of proximal stenosis of left coronary artery by digital transesophageal echocardiography. Feasibility, sensitivity, and specificity. *J Am Soc Echocardiography* 1993; 6: 149
79. Memmola C, Iliceto S, Napoli VF et al. Coronary flow dynamics and reserve assessed by TEE in obstructive hypertrophic cardiomyopathy. *Am J Cardiol* 1994; 74: 1.147
80. Tardif JC, Vannan MA, Taylor K, Schwart SL, Pandian NG. Delineation of extended lengths of coronary arteries by multiplane transesophageal echocardiography. *J Am Coll Cardiol* 1994; 24: 909
81. Redberg RF, Sobol Y, Chou TM et al. Adenosine induced coronary vasodilatation during transesophageal Doppler echocardiography. Rapid and safe measurement of coronary flow reserve ratio can predict significant left anterior descending coronary stenosis. *Circulation* 1995; 92: 190
82. Vicente T, Pinar E, Pérez-Lorente F, López Candel J, Pico F, Pérez de Juan MA, Valdés M. Usefulness of transesophageal echocardiography in the diagnosis of coronary anomalies. *Rev Esp Cardiol 1996; 49: 657-62*
83. Galati A, Greco G, Goletta C, Ricci R, Serdoz R, Richichi G, Ceci V. Usefulness of dipyridamole transesophageal echocardiography in the evaluation of myocardial ischemia and coronary artery flow. *Int J Card Imaging* 1996; 12: 169
84. Cox ID, Heald SC, Murday AJ. Value of transesophageal echocardiography in surgical ligation of coronary artery fistulas. *Heart* 1996; 76: 181
85. Kasar E, Chandrianratna PA. Assessment of coronary artery aneurysms with multiplane transesophageal echocardiography. *Am Heart J* 1997; 133: 526
86. Kozakova M, Palombo C, Pratali L et al. Assessment of coronary flow reserve by transesophageal Doppler echocardiography. Direct comparison between different modalities of dipyridamole and adenosine administration. *Eur Heart J* 1997; 18: 514
87. Paraskevaidis IA, Katritsis DG, Tsiapras DP, Kyriades ZS, Korovesis ST, Kremastinos DTh. Coronary flow reserve assessment by transesophageal echocardiography identifies early restenosis of the left left anterior descending coronary artery angioplasty. *Am J Cardiol* 1997; 79: 803
88. Kozakova M, Palombo C, Pratali L, Pittella G, Galetta F, L'Abatte A. Mechanisms of coronary flow reserve impairment in human hypertension. An integrated approach by transthoracic and transesophageal echocardiography. *Hypertension* 1997; 29: 551
89. Wolford DC, Jost CM, Mache EC, Walker W, Ramanatian KB. Role of transesophageal echocardiography in the clinical management of a patient with a giant coronary artery aneurysm. *Clin Cardiol* 1997; 20: 573
90. Zehetgruber M, Mundigler G, Christ G et al. Estimation of coronary flow reserve by transesophageal coronary sinus Doppler measurements in patients with syndrome X and patients with significant left coronary artery disease. *J Am Coll Cardiol* 1995; 25: 1.039
91. Mundigler G, Zehetgruber M, Christ G, Siostzonek P. Comparison of transesophageal coronary sinus and left anterior descending coronary artery Doppler measurements for the assessment of coronary flow reserve. *Clin Cardiol 1997;* 20: 225
92. Siostrzonek P, Kranz A, Heinz G et al. Noninvasive estimation of coronary flow reserve by transesophageal Doppler measurement of coronary sinus flow. *Am J Cardiol 1993; 72:* 1.334
93. Stoddard MF, Prince CR, Morris GT. Coronary flow reserve assessment by dobutamine transesophageal Doppler echocardiography. *J Am Coll Cardiol* 1995; 25: 325
94. Gramiak R, shah PM. Echocardiography of the aortic root. *Invest Radiol* 1968; 3: 356
95. Mulvagh SL, Foley DA, Aeschbacher BC, Klarich KK, Seward JB .Second harmonic imaging of an intravenously administered echocardiographic contrast agent: Visualization of coronary arteries and measurement of coronary blood flow. *J Am Coll Cardiol* 1996;27:1519

96. Caiati C, Montaldo C, Zedda N, Bina A, Iliceto S. A new non-invasive flow reserve assessment: contrast enhanced transthoracic second harmonic *Circulation* 1999; 99: 771
97. Bartel T, Müller S, Baumgart D, Haude M, Erbel R. Measurement of coronary flow velocity using contrast-enhanced transthoracic Doppler: validation by intracoronary Doppler guide wire (resumen). *J Am Coll Cardiol* 1999; 33: 456A
98. Iliceto S, Caiati C, Aragona P, Verde R, Schlief R, Rizzon P. Improved Doppler signal intensity in coronary arteries after intravenous peripheral injection of a lung-crossing contrast agent (SHU 508 A). *J Am Coll Cardiol* 1994; 23: 184
99. Caiati C, Aragona P, Iliceto S, Rizzon P. Improved Doppler detection of proximal left anterior descending coronary artery stenosis after intravenous injection of a lung-crossing contrast agent: a transesophageal Doppler echocardiographic study. *J Am Coll Cardiol 1996;* 27:1.413
100. Carreras F. The functional study of the blood flow of internal mammary artery grafts via transthoracic doppler echocardiography . *Rev Esp Cardiol* 1999; 52:259-60
101. Jayaweera AR, Edwards N, Glasheen WP, et al. In-vivo myocardial kinetics of air-filled albumin microbubbles during myocardial contrast echocardiography: comparison with radiolabeled red blood cells. *Circ Res.* 1994;74:1157–1165
102. Ismail S, Jayaweera AR, Camarano G, et al. Relation between air-filled albumin microbubble and red blood cell rheology in the human myocardium: influence of echocardiographic systems and chest wall attenuation. *Circulation.* 1996;94:445–451
103. Wei K, Jayaweera AR, Firoozan S, et al. Quantification of myocardial blood flow with ultrasound induced destruction of microbubbles administered as a constant venous infusion. *Circulation.* 1998;97:473–483
104. Schelbert HR, Phelps ME, Hoffman EJ, Huang SC, Selin CE, Kuhl DE. Regional myocardial perfusion assessed with N-13 labeled ammonia and positron emission computerized axial tomography. *Am J Cardiol* 1979;43:209- 218
105. Bergmann SR, Herrero P, Markham J, Walsh MN. Noninvasive quantitation of myocardial blood flow in human subjects with oxygen-15-labeled water and positron emission tomography. *J Am Coll Cardiol* 1989;14:639–652
106. Bol A, Melin JA, Vanoverschelde J-L, Baudhuin T et al. Direct comparison of N-13 ammonia and O-15 water estimates of perfusion for quantification of regional myocardial blood flow by microspheres. *Circulation* 1993;87:512–525
107. Kaul S. Assessment of coronary microcirculation with myocardial contrast echocardiography: current and future clinical applications. *Br Heart J* 1995;73: 490–495
108. Porter TR, Xie F. Visually discernible myocardial echocardiographic contrast after intravenous injection of sonicated dextrose albumin microbubbles containing high molecular weight, less soluble gases. *J Am Coll Cardiol* 1995;25:509- 515
109. Vannan MA, Kuersten B. Imaging techniques for myocardial contrast echocardiography. *Eur J Echocardiogr* 2000;1:224–226
110. Tiemann K, Lohmeier S, Kuntz S, et al. Real-time contrast echo assessment of myocardial perfusion at low emission power: first experimental and clinical results using power pulse inversion imaging. *Echocardiography* 1999;16:799–809
111. Wei K, Skyba DM, Firschke C, Lindner JR, Jayaweera AR, Kaul S. Interaction between microbubbles and ultrasound: in vitro and in vivo observations. *J* Am *Coll Cardiol* 1997;29:1081–1088
112. Wei K, Jayaweera AR, Firoozan S, Linka A, Skyba DM, Kaul S. Quantification of myocardial blood flow with ultrasound-induced destruction of microbubbles administered as a constant infusion. *Circulation* 1998;97:473–483
113. Gould KL, Lipscomb K: Effects of coronary stenoses on coronary flow reserve and resistance. *Am J Cardiol* 1974:34: 48-55
114. Singh AK, Behari J: Ultrasound nonlinearity parameter (B/A) in biological tissues. *Indian J Exp Biol* 1994; 32:281-283
115. Thomas JD, Rubin DN: Tissue harmonic imaging: Why does it work? *J Am Soc Echocardiogr* 1998; 11:803-808
116. Jayaweera AR, Sklenar J, Kaul S: Quantification of images obtained during myocardial contrast echocardiography. *Echocardiography* 1994; 11:385-396
117. Kaul S: Myocardial contrast echocardiography. *Curr Probl Cardiol* 1997; 22:549-640
118. Villanueva FS, Glasheen WP, Sklenar J, et al: Successful and reproducible myocardial opacification during two-dimensional echocardiography from right heart injection of contrast. *Circulation* 1992; 85:1557-1564
119. Wei K, Skyba DM, Firschke C, Lindner JR, Jayaweera AR, Kaul S. Interaction between microbubbles and ultrasound: in vitro and in vivo observations. *J Am Coll Cardiol* 1997;29:1081-8
120. Wei K, Jayaweera AR, Firoozan S, Linka A, Skyba DM, Kaul S. Quantification of myocardial blood flow with ultrasound induced destruction of microbubbles administered as a constant venous infusion. *Circulation* 1998;97:473-83
121. Wei K, Jayaweera AR, Firoozan S, et al: Quantification

of myocardial blood flow with ultrasound induced destruction of microbubbles administered as a constant venous infusion. *Circulation* 1998; 97:473-483

122. Crystal GJ, Downey HF, Bashour F: Small vessel and total coronary blood volume during intracoronary adenosine. *Am J Physiol* 1981; 241:H194-H201
123. Eliasen P, Amtorp O: Effect of intracoronary adenosine upon regional blood flow, microvascular blood volume and hematocrit in canine myocardium. *Int J Microcirc* 1984; 3:3-12
124. Wei K, Jayaweera AR, Firoozan S, et al: Basis for detection of stenosis using venous administration of microbubbles during myocardial contrast echocardiography: Bolus or continuous infusion? *J Am Coll Cardiol* 1998; 32:252-260
125. Bin JP, Pelberg RA, Wei K, Le DE, Goodman NC, Kaul S. Dobutamine versus dipyridamole for inducing reversible perfusion defects in chronic multivessel coronary artery stenosis. *J Am Coll Cardiol* 2002; 40:167-74
126. Wei K, Ragosta M, Thorpe J, et al: Non-invasive quantification of coronary blood flow reserve in humans using myocardial contrast echocardiography. *Circulation* 2001; 103:2560-2565
127. Leong-Poi H, Le E, Rim SJ, Sakuma T, Kaul S, Wei K. Quantification of myocardial perfusion and determination of coronary stenosis severity during hyperemia using real-time myocardial contrast echocardiography. *J Am Soc Echocardiogr* 2001;14: 1173-82
128. Shimoni S, Zoghbi WA, Xie F, Kricsfeld D, Iskander S, Gobar L, et al. Real-time assessment of myocardial perfusion and wall motion during bicycle and treadmill exercise echocardiography: comparison with single photon emission computed tomography. *J Am Coll Cardiol* 2001;37:741-7
129. Porter TR, Xie F, Silver M, Kricsfeld D, Oleary E. Real-time perfusion imaging with low mechanical index pulse inversion Doppler imaging. *J Am Coll Cardiol* 2001;37:748-53
130. Leong-Poi H, Rim SJ, Le E, Fisher NG, Wei K, Kaul S. Perfusion versus function: the ischemic cascade in demand ischemia. *Circulation* 2002;105:987-92

Chapter 8

Myocardial Contrast Echocardiography in the Assessment of Patients with Chronic Coronary Artery Disease

Leopoldo Pérez de Isla • Miguel Angel García Fernández • José Luis Zamorano

Introduction

Echocardiography has been established as a very important tool for imaging the heart and the great vessels. It is readily available to cardiologists and is neither expensive nor time consuming. Similar data can be obtained using other techniques, but none of them is able to provide all the structural, functional and haemodynamic information that echocardiography does. The development of new contrast agents and new devices and methods for assessing myocardial perfusion has led to an emerging field of applications and indications for patients suffering from chronic ischaemic heart disease. Myocardial contrast echocardiography is now moving from the experimental laboratory to daily clinical practice for the evaluation of ischaemic heart disease, since the assessment of myocardial perfusion with this technique may provide important information at low additional cost.

Echocardiography Contrast Agents

Echocardiography contrast agents are excellent tracers of red blood cell kinetics [1, 2]. The development of new microbubbles, used as echocardiographic contrast agents, and new imaging modalities allows the assessment of myocardial perfusion by echocardiography. Second-generation microbubbles are composed of high-molecular-weight gases that are very difficult to diffuse. After intravenous injection of an ultrasound contrast agent, the microbubbles are passively driven by the blood flow and remain within the vascular space until they dissolve [3]. Because of dilution and dissolution, there is a continuous decrease in the number of microbubbles from the site of injection to the left heart [4]. After passing the left ventricular cavity, the microbubbles reach the myocardial circulation [5]. Thus, these agents produce left ventricular cavity opacification and a proportion of them enter the coronary circulation.

Myocardial contrast echocardiography provides images of the coronary microcirculation. The microbubbles remain in the vascular space only and do not enter the extravascular space. This is an important difference with tracers used with other imaging methods used to evaluate myocardial perfusion, which are either taken up by the myocytes or able to reach the extravascular space [6,7].

When intravenous infusion of ultrasound contrast by bolus injections is performed, only visual, qualitative judgment of myocardial perfusion is feasible. Continuous infusion of contrast agents is necessary for quantitative assessment of myocardial perfusion [8]. Also, the adjustment of echo settings is easier when a continuos infusion of echo contrast is done [3].

More extensive information about contrast agents is given in other chapters of this book.

Imaging Modalities

Although a detailed description of different imaging modalities is given in another chapter of this book, we will summarize their basic principles focusing on the understanding of the assessment of chronic coronary artery disease. Fundamental echo imaging is not a good tool with which to visualize contrast in the myocardial vessels, because the backscatter from the tissue hides the weak signals originating from the microbubbles. New developments in ultrasound imaging techniques have provided intramyocardial coronary vessel-specific imaging, which improves the separation of the signals generated by the microbubbles from those generated by the myocardial tissue. Several imaging modalities are available for use with myocardial contrast echocardiography. The main difference between

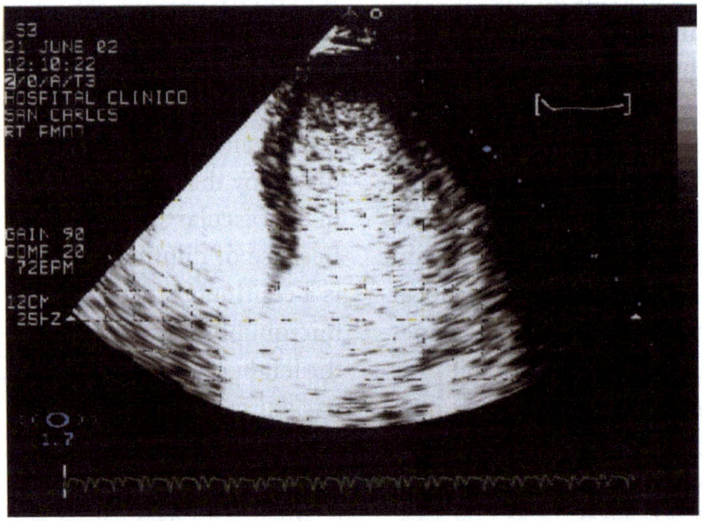

Fig. 8.1. Apical perfusion defect assessed by means of a Real Time technique (Power Modulation) after infusion of intravenous SonoVue®

these methods is the acoustic power level needed to perform the study so as to detect the microbubbles in the myocardium.

High power in the transducer is needed for harmonic imaging, ultra-harmonic imaging and harmonic power Doppler imaging (Fig. 8.1). High power produces a rapid destruction of the microbubbles. Microbubbles burst and emit a powerful signal that is collected by the transducer. The solution to the problem that microbubble destruction represents is solved by limiting the time that the heart is exposed to the ultrasound. In this way so-called triggered imaging was developed, which consists in the interruption of the transmission of the ultrasound after imaging for acquisition of one or more frames [9]. This interruption allows replenishment of the myocardium with microbubbles. Afterwards, another short period of ultrasound exposure results in myocardial contrast enhancement and almost simultaneous destruction of the microbubbles.

New techniques have been developed in order to achieve continuous display of myocardial perfusion, based on a very low emission power [10, 11]. These techniques are called real-time perfusion imaging modalities and the parameter we usually modify to obtain them is the so-called "mechanical index". This index is directly proportional to the output power of the ultrasound system and inversely proportional to the transducer frequency.

The detection of microbubbles is possible because of modifications to the pulses that are emitted. In "normal" imaging the pulses have the same polarity and amplitude. With real-time perfusion imaging, either the polarity and the amplitude are alternated. By comparing different pulses the sig-

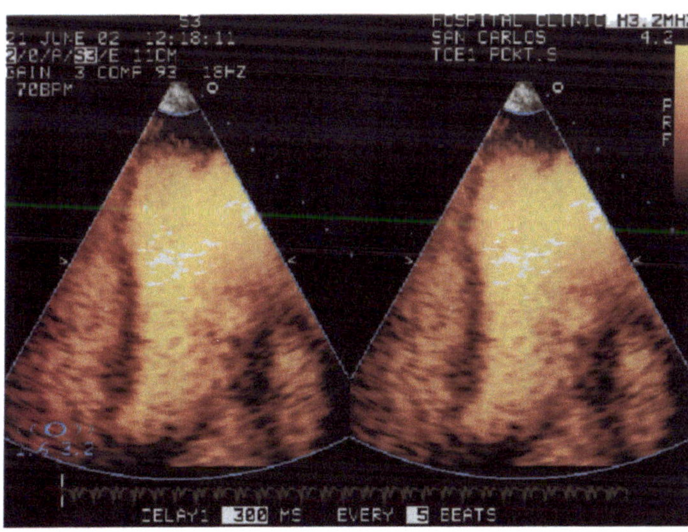

Fig. 8.2. The same case as Fig 8 1 but using Power Doppler. Note that the location and extension of the defect is similar when using different techniques

nals of the microbubbles can be detected. The signals from the tissue are very weak at low emission power, and the tissue becomes invisible. Thus, myocardial contrast signals can be analysed without background subtraction. Three myocardial contrast echocardiography methods use these technologies: coherent contrast imaging, pulse inversion and power modulation (Fig. 8.2).

Real-time imaging requires microbubbles that emit harmonics at low acoustic power. This imaging modality has many advantages: microbubbles resonate but do not burst, very few tissue harmonic signals are produced and several cycles can be obtained quickly, allowing bubble visualization even in low-flow states. Real-time tissue imaging is a new technique that uses low-power outputs to visualize echocardiographic contrast in real-time, permitting simultaneous integration of perfusion and wall thickening information.

Coronary Microcirculation

The volume of blood in the coronary circulation is 12 ml/100 g of myocardium [12]. This blood is distributed in the arterial, capillary and venous compartments in near equal proportions. A major proportion of the arterial and venous blood volume resides in epicardial vessels. Thus, almost all the myocardial blood volume present in the microcirculation is in the capillary circulation [12] (Fig. 8.3). Therefore, the capillaries are the predominant vessels in the myocardium and, moreover, during ventricular systole, when blood is milked out from arterioles and veins, what we mostly see is capillary blood volume.

Of note is that during resting conditions some capillaries allow blood red cell flow and other capillaries do not; during myocardial stress, oxygen demand is increased and a larger number of capillaries allow red cell flow.

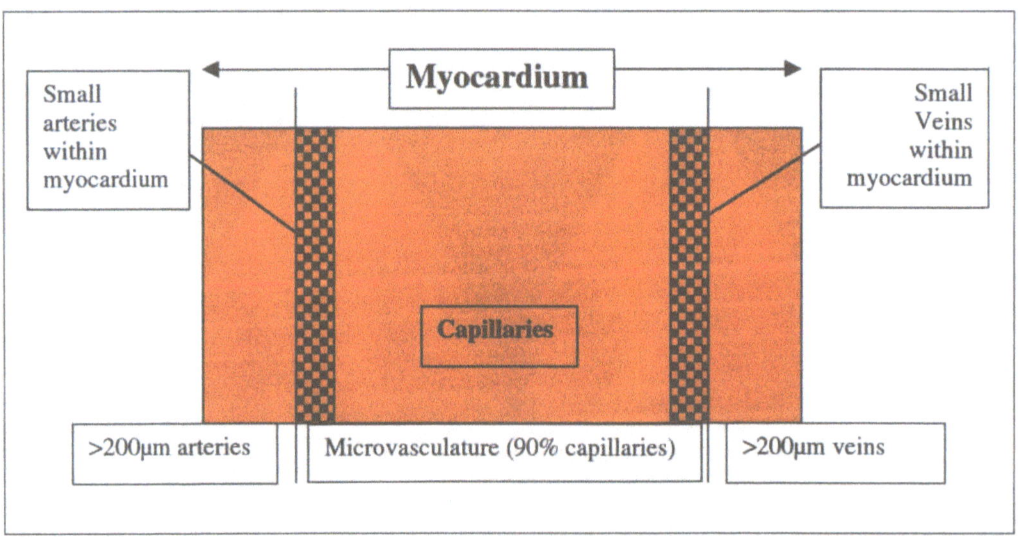

Fig. 8.3. Schematic distribution of myocardial blood volume. See details in text

This process is called "capillary recruitment".

Resting myocardial blood flow volume remains normal even in the presence of a coronary artery stenosis of up to 85%–90% in severity. Coronary arteries with a stenosis of 50%–85% of the coronary luminal diameter show a decreased hyperaemic response when myocardial oxygen demand is increased by exercise or pharmacologic stress. Myocardial blood volume decreases in the stenosed myocardial bed during hyperaemia and the degree to which it decreases is proportional to the stenosis severity. This is how perfusion defects appear.

Assessment of Myocardial Perfusion

Evaluation of myocardial perfusion is performed by examining the changes in signal intensities of the myocardium that occurred after intravenous injections of contrast. The video intensity in a specific area of myocardium is proportional to the number of microbubbles that are present in a certain moment in a specific region of myocardium [13]. Basically, there are two ways to analyse myocardial perfusion: the qualitative method and quantitative method.

Qualitative methods are based on the subjective assessment of myocardial perfusion in different regions of left ventricular myocardium. A three-degrees scale is normally used to perform this analysis. Segments with no microbubble signal are termed "no perfusion segment", segments with microbubble signal present but not normal in intensity are termed "patchy segments" and segments with a normal intensity microbubble signal are termed "normal perfusion segments". The great advantage of the qualitative assessment is its feasibility to be performed "on-line" during image acquisition. Its great disadvantage is that the human eye is not able to distinguish between the vast grey-scale that the images are shown [14]. To improve this defect, some modalities based on the colurization of signal to help the human eye to distinguish among different signal intensities have been developed [15].

Quantitative methods have been developed to avoid the subjectivity of qualitative assessment. After storing the myocardial perfusion images either on videotapes or in a digital format, they are processed and analysed "off-line" to measure video intensity. Signal quantification is performed for all the cardiac cycles stored in a region of interest previously determined. Its most important advantages are that this type of assessment allows an objective and numerical way of evaluating and comparing our results, and in this way we can differentiate among a large scale of signal intensities. Its most important disadvantages are: (1) it is necessary to perform the analysis "off-line", which is time consuming, and, (2) standard video intensity measures are not very reliable when microbubble concentration is too high, because of the nonlinear portion of the ultrasound signal–microbubble concentration curve that is reached at smaller microbubble concentration when log compression and post-processing are used [13]. To avoid this inconvenience, if we measure the signal prior to these manipulations, the relationship becomes nonlinear at much higher concentrations. This measurement is called "acoustic intensity" and is different to video intensity [16]. (Fig. 8.4).

There are two main parameters to be determined when evaluating myocardial perfusion in a quantitative basis, and both of them are the principal determinants of myocardial blood flow: myocardial flow velocity and myocardial blood volume. Myocardial blood flow is proportional to the product of myocardial blood volume and myocardial blood flow velocity.

Contrast agents may be administered as a bolus injection or as continuous perfusion. During continuous intravenous infusion of microbubbles, the amount of microbubbles entering and leaving the coronary microcirculation is constant and depends on the flow rate: by destroying them, the rate of replenishment of microbubbles into the myocardium may be assessed. Thus, the microbubble velocity can be determined. On other hand, the steady-state myocardial video intensity represents myocardial blood volume.

When using real-time methods, we can continuously measure myocardial video intensity after microbubble destruction. This destruction is achieved by a short but high-powered pulse of ultrasounds. Afterwards, video intensity is measured until the steady-state is reached. This low-power imaging technology facilitates recording of contrast replenishment, because the acquisition of the data is performed in real-time and is much shorter as compared with high-power triggered imaging. With triggered methods, using a timer or triggering ultrasound transmission to the electrocardiogram, new microbubbles are allowed to replenish the

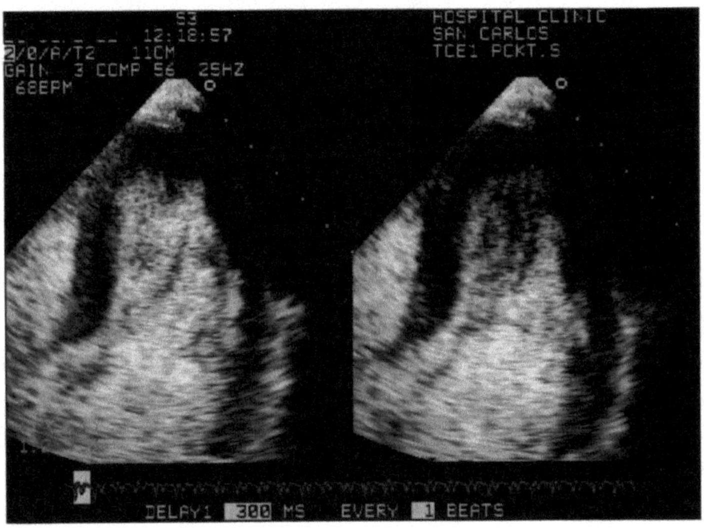

Fig. 8.4. Apical perfusion defect using ultra-harmonic technique. The perfusion defect at the apex can be seen. When comparing both images, there is perfusion signal in the myocardium (coded in *white colour*) in the left one that partially disappears in the right one (note this change at interventricular septum level, for instance). Nevertheless, there is an apical defect present in both images. It constitutes a reliable sign of absence of perfusion and, therefore, a sign that constitutes a reliable marker of lack of future functional recovery

microcirculation between destructive pulses of ultrasounds. Triggered images are acquired at different triggering intervals on the ultrasound system. For reliable measurements, acquisition of the same cross-sections is necessary, which is often difficult to achieve in sick patients. Nevertheless, some continuous low-power emission imaging methods have been developed to continuously monitor cardiac imaging between high-power ultrasound pulses. Time (measured on a continuous basis when using real-time methods or time at which ultrasound pulses were delivered if using triggered methods) versus video intensity is fitted to an exponential function: $y= A(1-e^{-\_t})$, "y" being the video intensity, "A" the video intensity plateau, "_" the microbubbles mean velocity and "t" the time [8, 17-20].

Most clinical studies have been performed using simple visual scoring. There are no comparable studies evaluating new quantitative analysis tools for assessment of perfusion, which theoretically should improve results.

Evaluation of Coronary Stenosis Using Stress Tests

Resting myocardial blood flow volume remains normal even in the presence of coronary artery stenosis of up to 85%–90% in severity [21]. Nevertheless, coronary arteries stenosis of 50%–85% of the coronary luminal diameter shows a decreased hyperaemic response when myocardial oxygen demand is increased by exercise or pharmacologic stress. Different methods have been used to detect significant coronary stenosis. For reliable myocardial contrast studies, expertise is required regarding the handling of the ultrasound contrast agents and the use of ultrasound equipment.

As in stress echocardiography and in nuclear imaging, different stress modalities may be used for myocardial contrast echocardiography. It was shown that adenosine stress was superior to dobutamine in detecting ischaemic myocardium in animals [22]. Nevertheless, to our knowledge, no clinical studies have been performed comparing different stress protocols for myocardial contrast echocardiography in humans. Exercise stress is probably the most frequent stress protocol for assessment of inducible abnormalities in left ventricular wall motion, but it has rarely been used for myocardial contrast echocardiography due to its inherent technical limitations. When triggered imaging is performed, many imaging acquisition problems appear due to patients with exaggerated respiratory and thoracic motion, wall motion artefacts may be accentuated following an increase in heart rate and inotropic state, and repeated adjustments of the trigger point may be necessary. Vasodilator stress results in a lower peak heart rate as compared with exercise or dobutamine, and facilitates acquisition of triggered myocardial contrast echocardiography images [3].

Evaluation of Myocardial Blood Flow Reserve

By administering adenosine, myocardial blood flow is progressively increased. In this setting, myocardial blood flow velocity reserve is proportional to microbubble velocity reserve as assessed by intracoronary Doppler flow wire [23]. Thus, myocardial blood flow reserve may be determined using myocardial contrast echocardiography. Decreases in peak hyperaemic flow in the presence of significant stenosis are associated with decreases in microbubble velocity compared with those seen in the absence of stenosis. Patients with a coronary stenosis of more than 70% have a myocardial blood flow reserve of less than 1.5. In conclusion, abnormalities of coronary blood flow reserve can be used to evaluate the physiological significance of stenosis.

Evaluation of Myocardial Blood Volume

Although myocardial blood flow is the best parameter for quantifying myocardial perfusion, most studies addressed differences in myocardial blood volume between single myocardial areas, rather than differences in myocardial blood flow. The presence of myocardial perfusion defects is the hallmark of coronary artery disease and its presence and magnitude have been strongly related with life expectancy and symptomatic prognosis.

Evaluation of myocardial blood volume is performed by examining the changes in signal video intensity of the myocardium that occur after intravenous injections of contrast [24,25]. Because reduction in myocardial blood flow is associated with a reduction in myocardial blood volume, estimation of myocardial blood volume can provide information regarding the severity of coronary stenosis. In the vascular bed supplied by a stenosed coronary artery, myocardial blood volume is decreased when hyperaemia occurs. A decrease in capillary density is believed to be responsible for reduced myocardial blood volume, which probably reflects the need to maintain a constant capillary hydrostatic pressure. This process is called "capillary de-recruitment".

It is possible to qualitatively visualize and quantify the amount of myocardium that is at risk due to moderate or severe coronary stenosis. Visual judgment of myocardial contrast echocardiography has been used in many studies to evaluate changes in myocardial blood volume. Quantitative analysis has been performed by measuring the regional video intensity. The time course of a bolus injection provides more information than analysing single frames. The result of computed curve-fitting has been shown to correlate well with the perfusion rate of blood to the myocardium.

Although there are many differences between radionuclide traces and myocardial contrast agents, many studies validating myocardial contrast echocardiography compared it with radionuclide imaging. Kaul demonstrated that the location of reversible and irreversible perfusion defects with myocardial contrast echocardiography is similar to that provided by single-photon emission tomography [26]. Its sensitivity and specificity in detecting segments with abnormal perfusion is 92% and 84%, respectively. The results of this approach were demonstrated in another study conducted by Heinle [27]. He found that left circumflex coronary artery territory was a frequent source of false-positive results.

Two recent papers have reported results that confirm these findings. In the first study, 100 consecutive patients with intermediate-to-high probability of coronary artery disease were evaluated using bicycle or treadmill for stress induction, real-time imaging and a bolus injection of a contrast agent [28]. That study included various imaging modalities for assessment of ischaemic heart disease. Compared with quantitative angiography, the sensitivities of myocardial contrast echocardiography, single-photon emission computed tomography and echocardiographic wall motion analyses were similar (76%). These results were confirmed by another study, which used real-time perfusion imaging too [29]. It was performed on 117 patients during dobutamine stress echocardiography by using bolus injections of echocardiographic contrast. On this occasion, myocardial contrast echocardiography was more sensitive than wall motion analysis. Overall agreement between quantitative coronary angiography and myocardial contrast echocardiography imaging on a territorial basis was 83%, as compared with 72% for wall motion. Contrast defects were detected in 17 territories subtended by arteries with significant stenosis, which had normal wall motion at stress. These results must be confirmed in larger and multicentre studies.

Evaluation of the Transmural Distribution of Myocardial Blood Flow

One of the more important advantages of myocardial contrast echocardiography over other diagnostic tools for detection of coronary artery disease is its excellent spatial resolution. In the above-mentioned studies, it was found that perfusion was more often impaired in the subendocardial than in the subepicardial layers. This feature provides a very accurate method for evaluating the distribution of myocardial blood flow, which can be used to quantify stenosis severity during stress tests. The subendocardial endocardium is the myocardial layer with a larger oxygen demand. Subsequently, it has the highest susceptibility to ischaemia. In the presence of coronary artery disease, increases in epicardial blood flow exceed those of the endocardium, resulting in decreases in the endocardial–epicardial ratio of blood flow [29]. Assessment of transmural differences represents another method quantifying stenosis severity using myocardial contrast echocardiography.

Combining Techniques

It has been reported that the combination of wall motion analysis with myocardial contrast echocardiography had the best balance between sensitivity (86%) and specificity (88%), with the highest accuracy (86%) [28]. It is possible to perform myocardial perfusion studies during continuous infusion of contrast. Under these conditions, a visual assessment, conducted by judging the speed and pattern of contrast replenishment, is performed and afterwards a sophisticated quantitative analysis is initiated.

Combined assessment of myocardial perfusion and left ventricular systolic function is able to improve the accuracy in the detection of ischaemic myocardial areas and this may have a large impact on the management of patients with coronary artery disease. The use of myocardial contrast echocardiography and wall motion analysis appears to have a diagnostic accuracy that is at least equal to that of nuclear imaging in identifying patients with significant coronary artery disease. Besides, this dual technique may help in the evaluation of patients after coronary interventions. Thus, myocardial contrast echocardiography is an important addition to classic stress echocardiography.

Evaluation of Coronary Stenosis Without Stress

The detection of coronary artery disease in the absence of previous infarction requires the application of stress to compare the results during the peak stress with the baseline results. A method that would be able to assess coronary status at rest would be very valuable. This objective could be achieved by imaging the compensatory mechanisms that maintain normal resting myocardial blood flow in the presence of a significant coronary stenosis.

Epicardial blood flow is variable during the cardiac cycle. Flow is higher in diastole than during systole [30]. The decrease in coronary blood flow during systole results from a decrease in the microvascular dimensions caused by the changing elastance of the myocardium. The compression of myocardial veins during systole results in propulsion of blood into the coronary sinus. The same process occurs in myocardial arterioles, resulting in reflux of blood into the larger arteries. Coronary arterioles dilate to maintain normal resting myocardial blood flow when a stenosis is present. Most of these arterioles are extramyocardial but some are in the myocardium. The volume of blood in these arterioles increases with the increase in the grade of stenosis severity. Retrograde displacement of blood should increase in systole when arterioles are compressed. Thus, the ratio systolic/diastolic myocardial blood volume increases with the presence of an epicardial coronary stenosis [31]. It could be measured by myocardial contrast echocardiography and could be used to detect coronary stenosis at rest, without the need for any stress.

Summarizing, contrast echocardiography provides an interesting tool that offers the potential of a complete evaluation of patients with chronic coronary artery disease. It offers not only a diagnostic tool in the evaluation of these patients but also provides prognostic information.

References

1. Jayaweera AR, Edwards N, Glasheen WP, et al. In-vivo myocardial kinetics of air filled albumin microbubbles during myocardial contrast echocardiography: comparison with radiolabeled red blood cells. Circ Res. 1994;74:1157-1165
2. Ismail S, Jayaweera AR, Camarano G, et al. Relation between air-filled albumin microbubble and red blood cell rheology in the human myocardium: influence of echocardiographic systems and chest wall attenuation. Circulation. 1996;94:445-451
3. American Society of Echocardiography Task Force on Standards and Guidelines for the use of ultrasonic contrast in echocardiography. Contrast echocardiography: current and future applications. J Am Soc Echocardiogr 2000; 13: 331-42
4. Wei K, Skyba DM, Fischke C et al. Interaction between microbubbles and ultrasound: in vitro and in vivo observations. J Am Coll Cardiol 1997; 29: 1081-8
5. Kaul S. Myocardial contrast echocardiography, 15 years of research and development. Circulation 1997; 96: 3745-60
6. Skyba DM, Camarano G, Goodman NC, et al: Hemodynamic characteristics, myocardial kinetics, and microvascular rheology of FS-069, a second-generation echocardiographic contrast agent capable of producing myocardial opacification from a venous injection. J Am Coll Cardiol 28:1292-1300, 1996
7. Keller MW, Segal SS, Kaul S, Duling B: The behavior of sonicated albumin microbubbles within the microcirculation: A basis for their use during myocardial contrast echocardiography. Circ Res 65:458-467, 1989
8. Wei K, Jayaweera AR, Firoozan S et al. Basis for detection of stenosis using venous administration of microbubbles during myocardial contrast echocardiography: bolus or continuous infusion? J Am Coll Cardiol 1998; 32: 252-60
9. Colon PJ, Richards DR, Moreno CA et al. Benefits of reducing the cardiac cycle-triggering frequency of ultrasound imaging to increase myocardial opacification with FS069 during fundamental and second harmonic imaging. J Am Soc Echocardiogr 1997; 10: 602-7
10. Tiemann K, Lohmeier S, Kuntz S, et al. Real-time contrast echo assessment of myocardial perfusion at low emission power: first experimental and clinical results using power pulse inversion imaging. Echocardiography 1999;12:266-71.
11. Hope Simpson D, Chin CT, Burns PN. Pulse inversion Doppler: a new method for detecting nonlinear echoes from microbubble contrast agents. IEEE Trans UFFC 1999;46:372-82
12. Kassab GS, Lin DH, Fung YB. Morphometry of pig coronary venous system. Am J Physiol 267:H2100-2113, 1994
13. Skyba DM, Jayaweera AR, Goodman NC, et al. Quantification of myocardial perfusion with myocardial contrast echocardiography during left atrial injection of contrast. Implications for venous injection. Circulation 90:1513-1521, 1994
14. Kaul S. Myocardial contrast echocardiography.Curr Probl Cardiol 22:549-640, 1997
15. Villanueva FS, Glasheen WP, Skienar J, et al: Successful and reproducible myocardial opacification during two-dimensional echocardiography from right heart injection of contrast. Circulation 86:1557-1564, 1992
16. Le E, Bin JP, Coggins MP, et al: Increase in myocardial oxygen consumption increases myocardial blood volume: A study using myocardial contrast echocardiography. Circulation 1001-450, 1999 (abstr)
17. Wei K, Jayaweera AR, Firoozan S, et al: Quantification of myocardial blood flow with ultrasound induced destruction of microbubbles administered as a constant venous infusion. Circulation 97:473-483, 1998
18. Wei K, Le E, Bin JP, Coggins M et al. Quantification of renal blood flow with contrast enhanced ultrasound. J Am Coll Cardiol 2001;37:1135-40
19. Schlosser T, Pohl C, Veltmann C et al. Feasibility of the flash replenishment concept in renal tissue: which parameters affect the assessment of the contrast replenishment? Ultrasound Med Biol 2001;27:937-44
20. Köster J, Schlosser T, Pohl C et al. Blood flow assessment by ultrasound-induced destruction of echocontrast agents using harmonic power Doppler imaging: which parameters determine contrast replenishment curves? Echocardiography 2001; 18: 1-8
21. Gould KL, Lipscomb K. Effects of coronary stenosis on coronary flow reserve and resistance. Am J Cardiol;34:48-55, 1974
22. Lafitte S, Matsugata H, Peters B, et al. Comparative value of dobutamine and adenosine stress in the detection of coronary stenosis with myocardial contrast echocardiography. Circulation 2001;103:2724-30
23. Wei K, Ragosta M, Thorpe J et al. Non-invasive quantification of coronary blood flow reserve in humans using myocardial contrast echocardiography. Circulation 2001; 103:2560-2565
24. Jarhult J, Mellander S. Autoregulation of capillary hydrostatic pressure in skeletal muscle during regional arterial hypo- and hypertension. Acta Phsyiol Scand 1974; 91:32-41
25. Jayaweera AR, Wei K, Coggins M, et al: The role of capillaries in determining coronary blood flow

reserve. New insights using myocardial contrast echocardiography. Am J Physiol 1999; 6:1-12363-2372
26. Kaul S, Senior R, Dittrich H et al. Detection of coronary artery disease with myocardial contrast echocardiography: comparison with 99m Te-sestamibi single-photon emission computed tomography. Circulation 1997; 96: 785 92
27. Heinle SK, Noblin J, Goree-Best P et al. Assessment of myocardial perfusion by harmonic power Doppler imaging at rest and during adenosine stress. Circulation 2000; 102: 55-62
28. Shimoni S, Zoghbi WA, Xie F et al. Real-time assessment of myocardial perfusion and wall motion during bicycle and treadmill exercise echocardiography: Comparison with single photon emission computed tomography. J Am Coll Cardiol 2001; 37: 741-7
29. Porter TR, Xie F, Silver M et al. Real-time perfusion imaging with low mechanical index pulse inversion Doppler Imaging. J Am Coll Cardiol 2001; 37: 748-53
30. Folts JD, Gallagher K, Rowe GG. Hemodynamic effects of controlled degrees of coronary stenosis in short term and log term studies in dogs. J Thorac CV Surg 1977; 73:722-727
31. Wei K, Coggins M, Bin J-P, et al. Phasic changes in video intensity can be used to detect coronary stenois at rest without need for stress. J Am Coll Cardiol 1999 (suppl A); 33:450 A

Chapter 9

Myocardial Viability: Comparison with Other Imaging Techniques

Roxy Senior

Myocardial viability may be defined as myocardium with preserved metabolic, cellular and membrane function which allows the myocardium to maintain its contractile function. Thus, the mere presence of contractile function suggests that the myocardium is viable. However, the clinical scenario where assessment of myocardial viability is an issue is when there is regional or global left ventricular dysfunction in the context of coronary artery disease. There are two broad scenarios of coronary artery disease where this can occur. The first scenario is when the reduction of contractile function with preserved metabolic, cellular and membrane function may occur when myocardial blood flow is chronically reduced ("hibernating myocardium") or when the myocardial blood flow is normal at rest but there is repetitive demand-induced ischaemia in presence of non-flow-limiting coronary artery stenosis at rest ("stunned, myocardium") [2]. The second scenario is in the setting of acute myocardial infarction (AMI) where following a period of prolonged occlusion the infarct-related artery is partially or completely open either spontaneously or by reperfusion (stunned myocardium) [3]. It is clear from the pathophysiologic description that the single most important determinant of myocardial viability is myocardial blood flow.

Myocardial Contrast Echocardiography

Myocardial contrast echocardiography (MCE) is a technique that utilises microbubbles during echocardiography [4]. These microbubbles remain entirely within the intravascular space and their presence within any myocardial region denotes the status of microvascular perfusion within that region [5, 6].

The blood present in the entire coronary circulation (arteries, arterioles, capillaries, venules and veins) is approximately 12 ml/100 g of cardiac muscle [7]. Approximately one-third of this blood is present within the myocardium itself which is termed myocardial blood volume [8]. The predominant (90%) component of the myocardial blood volume is the capillaries [8]. The myocardial signal assessed visually as contrast intensity reflects the concentration of microbubbles within the myocardium, and during continuous infusion of microbubbles, the signal intensity

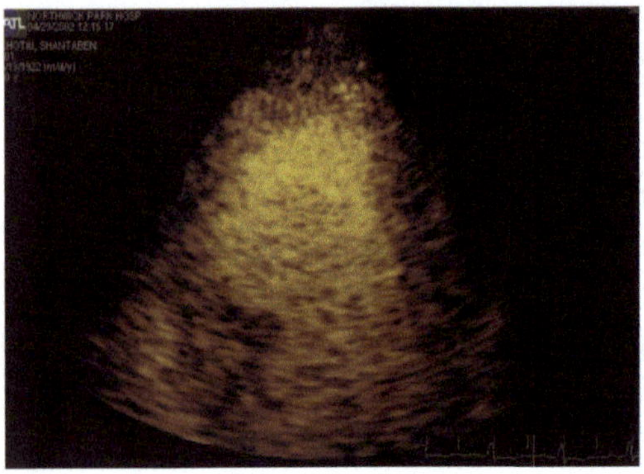

Fig. 9.1. The microbubble signal intensity after the myocardium is fully replenished with microbubbles represents myocardial capillary blood volume

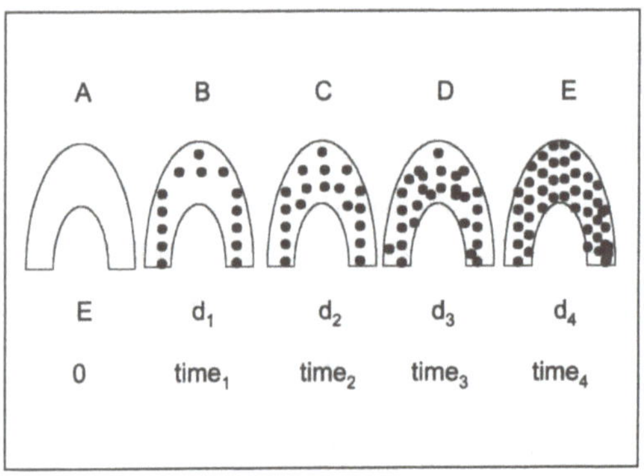

Fig. 9.2. The elevation (thickness) of the ultrasound at t_0, then replenishment of the beam elevation (d_1 through d_4, B–E) will depend on the velocity of microbubbles and the ultrasound pulsing interval (Reproduced from [10], with permission)

when the entire myocardium is fully replenished largely denotes capillary blood volume [9-11] (Fig. 9.1). Any alteration of signal in this situation must, therefore, occur principally due to change in capillary blood volume. Furthermore, it has been shown that, following destruction of microbubbles in the myocardium during high-power imaging, the replenishment of the myocardium takes approximately 5 s at rest [10] (Fig. 9.2). A decrease in myocardial blood flow results in prolongation of replenishment time which is proportional to the degree of myocardial blood flow (Fig. 9.3) [10]. Myocardial perfusion is defined as tissue blood flow at the capillary level. The two components of tissue blood flow are capillary blood volume and microbubble velocity, i.e. rate of microbubble replenishment following destruction of microbubbles. The product of these two components denotes myocardial blood flow at the tissue level [11]. Thus, MCE can detect not only capillary blood volume but, by virtue of its temporal resolution, can also assess myocardial blood flow. The technique by which myocardial blood flow may be assessed has been described in this book. Briefly, a series of high-energy ultrasound pulses are delivered to destroy microbubbles in the myocardium. Ultrasound imaging is then continued either intermittently (during high-power imaging) [10, 11] or continuously (low-power imaging) [12] to observe contrast intensity and microbubble velocity. The product of peak contrast intensity and microbubble velocity gives the measure of myocardial blood flow [10] (Fig. 9.4).

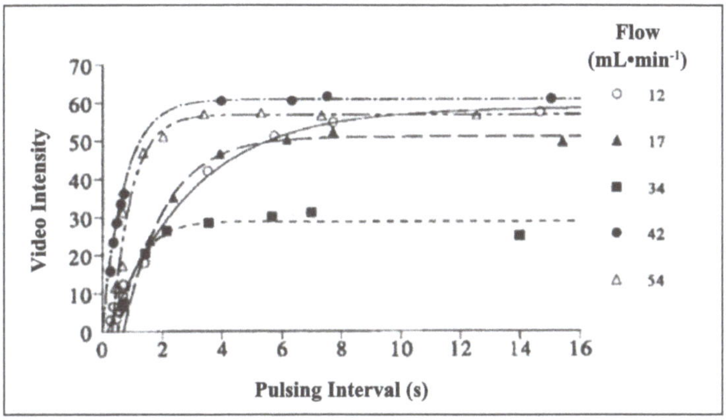

Fig. 9.3. Relationship between pulsing interval (x axis) and video intensity (y axis) at five different flow rates (Reproduced from [10], with permission)

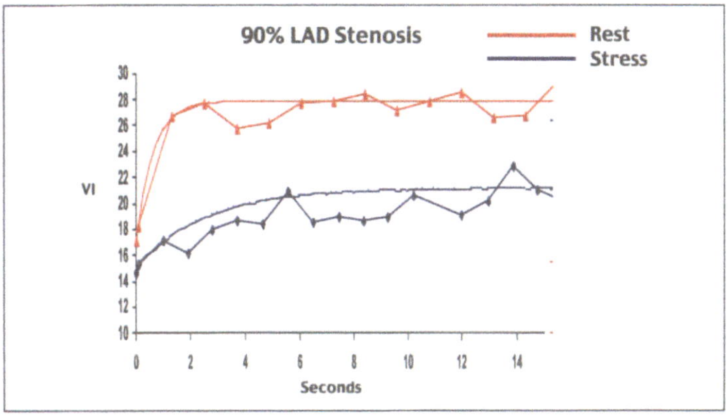

Fig. 9.4. Video intensity against time to myocardial replenishment. The product of plateau video intensity and rate of replenishment gives the measure of myocardial blood flow

Pathophysiological Basis of MCE for Detection of Myocardial Viability

The underlying basis for assessing myocardial viability with MCE is that myocardial contrast enhancement depends on an intact microcirculation. Kloner et al. noted that with AMI during occlusion of the coronary artery for more than 180 min, the degree of myocyte loss paralleled the degree of loss of microvascularisation [13] (Fig. 9.5). In a study by Ragosta et al., contrast intensity was assessed in the infarct-related region in 105 patients with recent AMI [14] by MCE during cardiac catheterisation. They noted that patients with patent infarct-related artery and good contrast intensity demonstrated improvement in contractile function compared to those patients with poor contrast score 1 month after follow-up. Janardhanan et al. similarly showed that the extent and severity of contrast defects after AMI

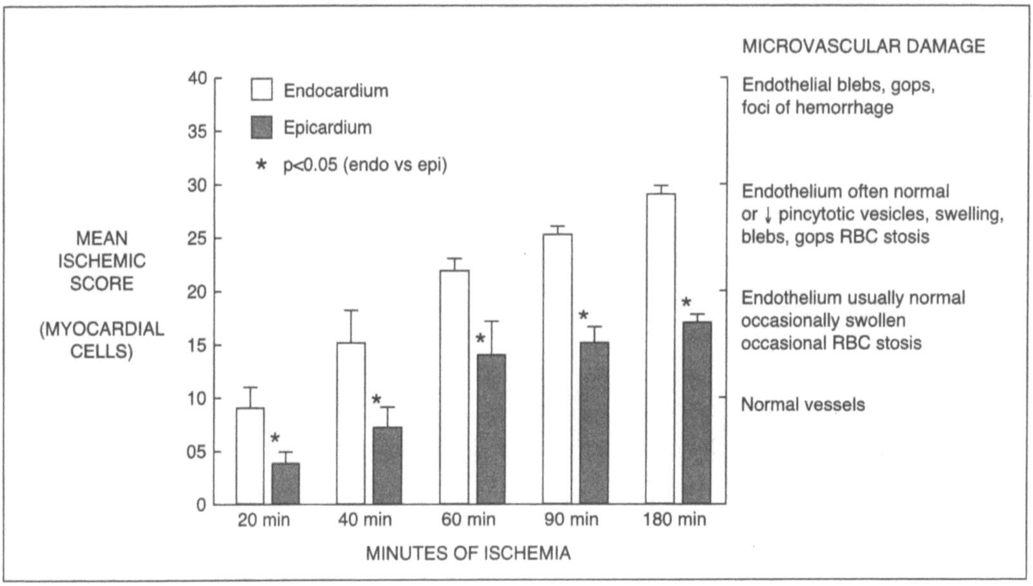

Fig. 9.5. Relationship between duration of coronary occlusion and myocyte loss and capillary derangement (Reproduced from [13], with permission)

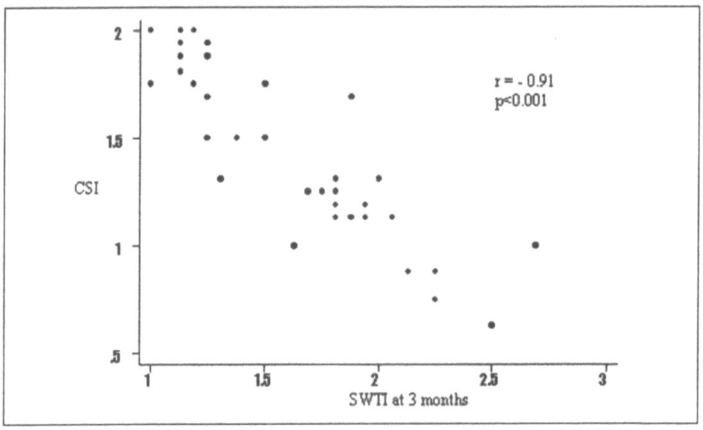

Fig. 9.6. Correlation between contrast score index (*CSI*) at baseline and systolic wall thickness index (*SWTI*) at 3 months

showed a strong inverse correlation with recovery of function at 3 months after revascularisation (Fig. 9.6) [15]. Ito and colleagues performed MCE 15 min after reperfusion was established in patients with AMI presenting within 6 h of onset of chest pain. They noted that in the 25% of their patient cohort with no myocardial opacification, despite a patent infarct-related artery, regional and global function were worse 1 month later compared with those showing opacification of the infarct bed [16]. These studies established the value of intact microvasculature after AMI as assessed by MCE to predict myocardial viability.

Detection of Myocardial Viability After AMI

The extent of myocardial necrosis after AMI is directly related to (1) total duration of coronary occlusion, (2) the extent of myocardium subtended by the occluded artery and, (3) the quality of collateral circulation. Thus, in the absence of collateral blood flow, when a coronary artery is suddenly occluded, perfusion within the infarct zone is minimal and results in myocardial necrosis which commences at the endocardium and progresses transmurally over time, so that it is transmural by 6 h (Fig. 9.7) [17]. However, in the presence of collateral-derived residual blood flow even as low as 30% (0.30 ml/min/g) of normal myocardial viability could be maintained within the occluded infarct bed [18]. Thus, following AMI the progression of myocardial necrosis may be halted if the IRA opens either spontaneously or after reperfusion therapy, if there is sufficient collateral circulation supplying the jeopardised region despite the occluded artery. Myocardial blood flow may be normal or reduced (patent but presence of severe flow-limiting stenosis at rest in the infarct-related artery, partial microembolisation of distal vessels despite patent infarct-related artery and presence of collateral blood flow) in the myocardium, which is predominantly viable in the infarct-related myocardium with largely preserved myocardial viability [19-21].

Thus, it follows, that in situations where myocardial blood flow is reduced but enough to maintain microvascular integrity, one should allow enough time for contrast microbubbles to transit to the capillaries after the initial phase of microbubble destruction. In a study of 98 patients after AMI by Swinburn et al., it was clearly shown that contrast intensity assessed early after microbubble destruction was a poor predictor of microvascular integrity compared to contrast intensity assessment late after microbubble destruction [22]. This was also shown by Coggins et al. and Laffitte et al.,

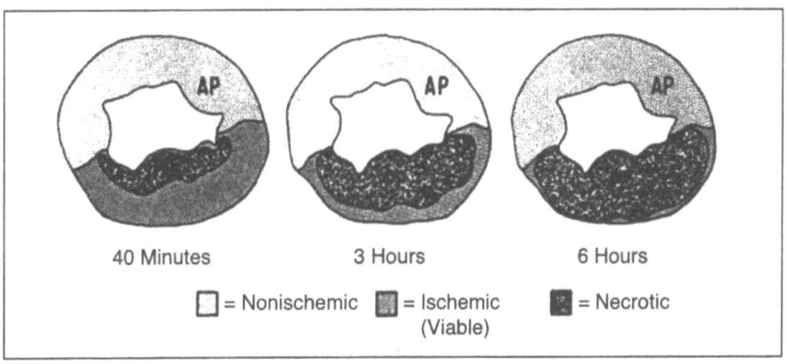

Fig. 9.7. Relationship between duration of coronary occlusion and transmural extent of myocardial infarction (Reproduced from [17], with permission)

who noted that due to variability in myocardial blood flow in the infarct-related region, assessment of contrast intensity should be continued up to 15 cardiac cycles following the destructive phase for optimum assessment of microvascular integrity (Table 9.1) [23, 24]. Figure 9.8 shows an example of two patients with AMI with and without contrast opacification in akinetic segments at 15 cardiac cycles after destruction imaging. The former recovered function whilst the latter remained akinetic [15].

Table 9.1. Perfusion defect size (PDS) at various time points after coronary occlusion and following destructive phase (modified from [23])

	Time after coronary occlusion			
	30 min	2 h	4 h	6 h
PDS at PI of 5 cardiac cycles (2.6±0.4 s)	25.8±9.0	25.4±8.4	25.3±8.3	27.8±7.6
PDS at PI of 10 cardiac cycles (5.3±0.48 s)	21.7±10.1	20.1±8.6*	21.5±9.7	24.3±9.0
PDS at PI of 20 cardiac cycles (10.6±1.5 s)	18.5±9.2*	16.8±9.1*	18.5±8.9*	20.3±9.6*
PDS at PI of 30 cardiac cycles (15.2±2.4 s)	17.7±9.5*	19.9±8.5*	17.6±9.3*	16.4±8.3*

% of LV short-axis slice
* $p<0.5$ vs PI=5 cardiac cycles

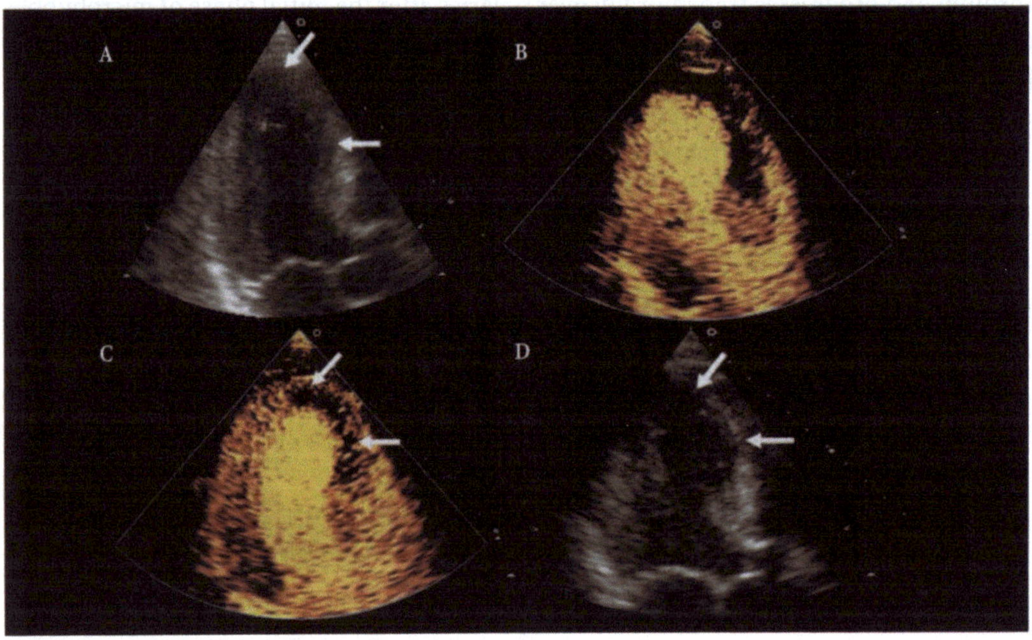

Fig. 9.8. End systolic frames of the apical three-chamber view showing (**A**) akinetic mid anterior septum and apex (*arrows*); (**B**) immediate post high mechanical index destruction frame on MCE; (**C**) lack of contrast opacification of the dysynergic segments even at 15 cardiac cycles (*arrows*); (**D**) lack of functional recovery at 12 weeks despite revascularisation (*arrows*)

Whilst assessment of microvascular integrity performed as mentioned above is a reliable indicator of myocardial viability, it may not be able to discriminate normal from minor tissue damage. In a study by Coggins et al., the authors assessed final infarct size during AMI with MCE [23]. They performed quantitative analysis using peak contrast intensity, rate of microbubble replenishment (β) myocardial and MCE derived myocardial blood flow. They found that the most significant parameter which predicted mild versus moderate reduction of myocardial blood flow assessed by radiolabelled microspheres was rate of microbubble replenishment and myocardial blood flow derived from the product of peak contrast intensity and β value (Table 9.2) [23]. In another study by Janardhanan et al., the authors also showed that microbubble velocity was the strongest predictor of contractile reserve in patients after AMI [25]. This is not surprising because β has a stronger relationship with MBF than peak contrast intensity.

Contrast intensity due to thresholding effect and sometimes indistinguishable background noise may fail to detect differences between normal and mildly reduced microvascular volume in small infarction. Since myocardial blood flow is invariably reduced even in minor infarction, microbubble velocity will be reduced and is more easily detectable. Furthermore, even as early as 1 week after AMI, a state of myocardial "hibernation" may ensue due to repetitive silent ischaemia as a result of persistence of critical flow-limiting infarct-related artery stenosis. This may result in down regulation of resting myocardial blood flow and persistent myocardial dysfunction. Thus, despite similar microvascular volume, high myocardial blood flow may maintain a higher degree of myocardial viability.

Timing of Performing MCE in Relation to Accuracy in Predicting Myocardial Viability

Restoration of epicardial coronary flow in the infarct-related region early after AMI may result in coronary hyperaemia which lasts for 3-6 h [26]. Coronary hyperaemia results in underestimation of myocardial necrosis and hence overestimation of myocardial viability. However, reactive hyperaemia disappears about 3-6 h after

Table 9.2. MCE parameters versus radiolabelled microsphere-derived myocardial blood flow (MBF) [23]

Variable % of normal	Mild reduction in MBF (>50% of normal)	Moderate reduction in MBF (25%–50% of normal)	Severe reduction in MBF (<25% of normal)
A	79±42*	88±35*	49±49*†
β	54±23**	32±12*†	25±20*†
A x β	38±21*	26±13*†	9±7*‡

* $p<0.05$ vs normal bed

† $p<0.05$ vs regions with mild reduction in MBF

‡ $p<0.05$ vs regions with moderate reduction in MBF

primary coronary intervention. The degree of coronary hyperaemia is invariably related to the extent of myocardial necrosis and directly related to the degree of patency of the infarct-related artery [27]. Following this phase, however, microvascular stunning may persist for up to 48 h [28-29]. Thus, MCE defects seen may be due to microvascular stunning which is recoverable. A study by Brochet et al. clearly showed that approximately 30% of MCE defects observed at 24 h improved at 7 days after AMI [30]. Others have also shown a similar phenomenon [27-29, 31]. However, assessment of microvascularisation approximately 3–5 days after AMI may produce optimum accuracy.

Accuracy of MCE in Predicting Myocardial Viability after AMI

Several studies using both intracoronary and intravenous MCE have demonstrated high sensitivity (75%–90%) but poorer specificity (50%–60%) in identifying recovery of contractile function after AMI. Most of these studies consisted of patients studied early after reperfusion and assessed resting function. The combination of reactive hyperaemia, dynamic nature of changes in the microcirculation early after AMI and the fact that myocardial infarction involving more than 20% of the subendocardium can render the myocardium akinetic despite significant epicardial and mid-myocardial viability [32] tend to apparently make MCE less specific for detection of myocardial viability. Technical factors like inability to distinguish microbubble signature from the underlying tissue are also important in contributing to the low specificity of MCE.

Recent studies, using background subtraction techniques, either on-line (low-power or high-power imaging, power Doppler and ultraharmonics) or off-line, assessing patients 3–5 days after AMI and assessment of contractile reserve considerably improved the specificity (80%–90%) and positive predictive value (85%–90%) of MCE [33, 34].

MCE and Chronic Coronary Artery Disease

There are only limited studies where MCE was used to predict myocardial viability in patients with left ventricular dysfunction due to chronic coronary artery disease. DeFillipi et al., Nagueh et al. and Camaraho et al. used intracoronary MCE in this group of patients. Both studies again showed high sensitivity (85%–90%) but low specificity (50%–50%) for predicting recovery of function following revascularisation [35-37]. In a recent study by Shimoni et al., 20 patients in a similar group of patients were evaluated using a continuous infusion of Optison with intermittent pulse inversion harmonics and incremental triggering [38]. The authors observed that MCE peak contrast intensity correlated with microvascular density and capillary area (biopsy of myocardium). They observed considerable overlap in microvascular density in patients with and without recovery of function following revascularisation. While peak contrast intensity showed a similar overlap in these two groups of patients, the β value (rate of microbubble replenishment) and MCE-derived myocardial blood flow were significantly lower in patients with no recovery of function compared to those with recovery of function. In light of several mechanisms proposed to account for depressed resting function in myocardial hibernation, it is conceivable that the higher blood flow measured by MCE parameters in segments with similar degrees of cellularity, fibroses and microvessel density maintained a higher level of myocardial viability.

Comparison of MCE with Other Imaging Techniques

Techniques such as positron emission tomography and single photon imaging have been used to assess myocardial viability because of its ability to either demonstrate ongoing metabolic activity in dysfunctional myocardial cells (positron emission tomography) [39] or indicate intact cell membrane (thallium-201) [40, 41] or mitochondrial function (Tc-99m sestamibi) [42-43]. Contractile reserve which is a marker of myocardial viability may be assessed by low-dose dobutamine echocardiography or cardiac magnetic resonance imaging [44-48]. Lately, gadolinium-based contrast agents with cardiovascular magnetic resonance (CMR) are used to assess late hyperenhancement of the myocardium, which reflects myocardial necrosis [49, 50]. Gadolinium DTPA is an extracellular tracer which in essence measures the interstitial space associated with myocyte loss.

Comparison with Dobutamine Echocardiography

The majority of the studies done so far used dobutamine echocardiography to compare with MCE. Numerous studies have indicated the value of dobutamine echocardiography in identifying viable myocardium [44-46]. The major determinants of contractile response during dobutamine in dysfunctional myocardium are coronary flow reserve and the extent of myocardial necrosis. Thus, despite the presence of significant viable myocardium, limited coronary flow reserve (critical flow-limiting coronary artery stenosis and/or poor collateral circulation in presence of occluded artery) may result in demand-induced ischaemia even during low-dose dobutamine and prevent contractile response [51]. Coronary artery studies in the post-thrombolytic era have clearly shown the existence of a critical residual stenosis of the infarct-related artery in a significant number of patients. Furthermore, the contractile response diminishes with an increased extent of myocardial necrosis [52]. Thus, dobutamine echocardiography has a potential to underestimate myocardial viability after AMI. In a study by Agati et al. 2 weeks after AMI, dobutamine echocardiography showed a lower sensitivity (85%) and negative predictor value (93%) compared to MCE (100% and 100%, respectively) [53]. In 24 patients after AMI, Iliceto et al. compared MCE with low-dose dobutamine echocardiography. Also in this study, MCE was more sensitive than dobutamine echocardiography in detecting myocardial viability [54]. It may be inferred that while dobutamine response suggests significant myocardial viability, absence of dobutamine response does not necessarily imply absence of viability. However, presence of homogeneous contrast opacification of these dobutamine non-responsive segments is likely to suggest significant myocardial viability and therefore is likely to translate to recovery of function during follow-up. In a study by Senior et al., the sensitivity and negative predictive value of dobutamine echocardiography for the prediction of recovery of dysynergic segments during follow-up improved significantly from 59% to 79% and from 88% to 95% when contrast opacification was observed in the dobutamine non-response segments [55]. Indeed, dobutamine and myocardial contrast echocardiography data showed that combination of dobutamine and contrast echocardiography provided the best independent predictor for the recovery of function. This was also shown in an experimental study by Meza et al. [56].

Comparison with Radionuclide Imaging

Radionuclide imaging has been used extensively to assess myocardial viability after AMI and in chronic coronary artery disease [40-43]. However, there are very few studies comparing radionuclide techniques and MCE to assess myocardial viability. Recent studies conducted with MCE in post-AMI patients demonstrated a good concordance with radionuclide myocardial perfusion imaging for the detection of myocardial perfusion [57]. Using power Doppler imaging techniques in a study of 15 post-AMI patients, agreement for presence or absence of myocardial perfusion was excellent. That study was followed by a larger study of 100 patients, in whom the concordances using harmonic B-mode and power Doppler imaging were 80% and 82%, respectively [58] (Fig. 9.9).

Nagueh et al. also performed a thallium-201 redistribution study in patients with left ventricular dysfunction and chronic coro-

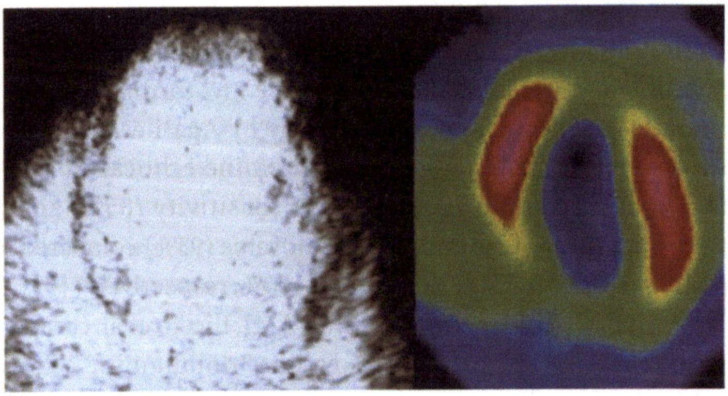

Fig. 9.9. Myocardial contrast echocardiography (*left*) showing reduced opacification (perfusion) in distal septum and apex with SonoVue. Corresponding images on ^{99m}Tc-sestamibi scan (*right*) showing identical perfusion defect. These suggest non-viable myocardium [58]

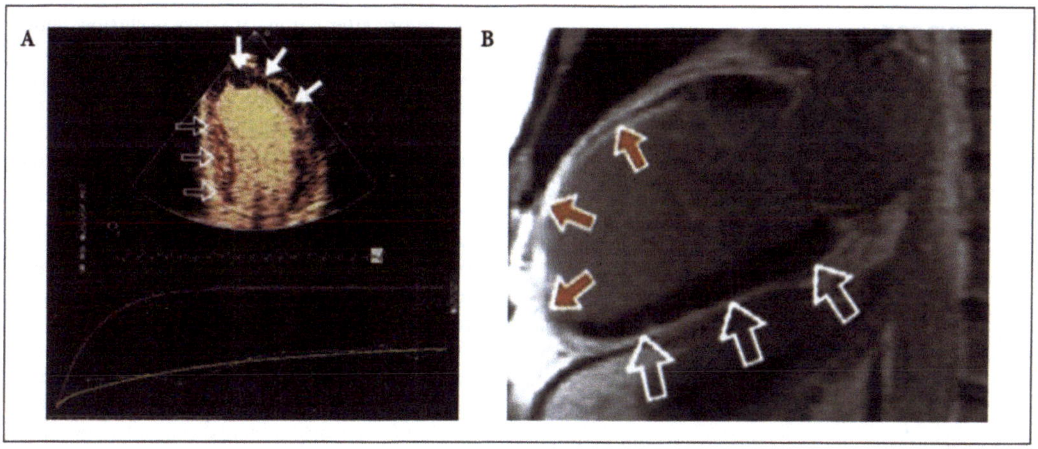

Fig. 9.10. Example of a patient who sustained an anterior myocardial infarction. **A** *Top*: Apical two chamber view on MCE with absence of contrast opacification (*solid arrows*) at the apex and anterior wall, which were akinetic. The normal, remote segments (*outlined arrows*) show normal contrast intensity. **A** *Bottom*: Replenishment curves in the akinetic segment (*yellow*) demonstrates very low microbubble velocity and myocardial blood flow remote, normal segment (*red*). **B** The corresponding image on CMR demonstrates TEI>75% in the akinetic segments compared to normal remote segment

nary artery disease. Both MCE and thallium-201 were similar in predicting recovery of function after revascularisation [36]. However, the technique and understanding of MCE has improved considerably since then. It is likely that with the improved technique, sensitivity and specificity will be higher than radionuclide techniques. The major limitations of radionuclide imaging for reliable detection of myocardial viability are tracer kinetics and partial volume effect.

Comparison with Cardiovascular MRI

Gadolinium-enhanced MRI has been shown to accurately detect the transmural extent of myocardial infarction. In the only study to date comparing MCE with infarct transmurality using contrast-enhanced MRI following AMI, Janardhanan et al. clearly showed that correlates of myocardial perfusion assessed by MCE clearly classifies the transmural extent of myocardial infarction with a high degree of accuracy [25] (Fig. 9.10).

Conclusion

Myocardial contrast echocardiography has evolved over the years so that it can now be applied clinically for evaluation of myocardial viability. The advancement of the quantitation technique has now made it possible for MCE to be used reliably for the assessment of myocardial viability.

References

1. Rahimtoola SH. A perspective on the three large multicenter randomised clinical trials of coronary bypass surgery for chronic stable angina. *Circulation* 1985; 72: V123-35
2. Vanoverschelde JL, Wijns W, Depre C et al. Mechanisms of chronic regional post-ischaemic dysfunction in humans: new insights from the study of noninfarcted collateral-dependent myocardium. *Circulation* 1993; 87: 1513-32
3. Baronial E, Loner RA. The stunned myocardium: prolonged, postischemic ventricular dysfunction. *Circulation* 1982; 66: 1146-9
4. Kaul S, Force T. Assessment of myocardial perfusion with contrast two dimensional echocardiography. In Weyman AE (ed): Principles and Practice of Echocardiography. 2nd ed. Philadelphia: Lea and Febiger 1993: 687-730
5. Kaul S. Clinical applications of myocardial contrast echocardiography. *Am J Cardiol* 1992; 69-46H-55H
6. Kaul S, Jayaweera AR. Myocardial contrast echocardiography has the potential for the assessment of coronary microvascular reserve. *J Am Coll Cardiol* 1993; 21: 356-358
7. Kassab GS, Lin DH, Fung YB. Morphometry of pig coronary venous system. *Am J Physiol* 1994; 267 (6 Pt 2): H2100-13
8. Kaul S, Jayaweera AR. Coronary and myocardial blood volumes: noninvasive tools to assess the coronary microcirculation? *Circulation* 1997; 96: 719-724
9. Linka AZ, Sklenar J, Wei K, Jayaweera AR, Skyba DM, Kaul S. Spatial distribution of microbubble velocity and concentration within the myocardium: insight into transmural distribution of myocardial blood flow and volume. *Circulation* 1998; 98: 1912-1920
10. Wei K, Jayaweera AR, Firoozan S, Linka A, Skyba DM, Kaul S. Quantification of myocardial blood flow with ultrasound-induced destruction of microbubbles administered as a continuous infusion. *Circulation* 1998; 97: 473-483
11. Wei K, Linka A, Jayaweera AR, Firoozan S Goodman NC, Kaul S. Basis of stenosis detection by myocardial contrast echocardiography during venous administration of microbubbles: bolus or continuous infusion? *J Am Coll Cardiol* 1998; 32: 252-260
12. Tiemann K, Lohmeier S, Kuntz S, Köster J, Pohl C, Burns PN, Porter TR, Nanda NC, Lüderitz B, Becher HL. Real-time contrast echo assessment of myocardial perfusion at low emission power: first experimental and clinical results using power pulse inversion imaging. *Echocardiography* 1999; 16: 799-809
13. Kloner RA, Rude RE, Carlson N, et al. Ultrastructural evidence of microvascular damage and myocardial cell injury after coronary artery occlusion: which comes first? *Circulation* 1980; 62: 945-952
14. Ragosta M, Camarano G, Kaul S, Powers ER, Sarembock IJ, Gimple LW. Microvascular integrity indicates myocellular viability in patients with recent myocardial infarction. New insights using myocardial contrast echocardiography. *Circulation* 1994; 89: 2562-9
15. Janardhanan R, Swinburn J, Greaves K, Senior R. Usefulness of Myocardial Contrast Echocardiography using low power continous imaging early after acute myocardial infarction to predict late functional left ventricular recovery. *Am J Cardiol* 2003
16. Ito H, Tomooka T, Sakai N. Yu H, Higashina Y, Fujii K, Masuyama T, Kitabatake A, Minamino T. Lack of myocardial perfusion immediately after successful thrombolysis. A predictor of poor recovery of left ventricular function in anterior myocardial infarction. *Circulation* 1992; 85: 1699-1705
17. Reimer KA, Jennings RB. The "wavefront phenomenon" of myocardial ischemic cell death. II. Transmural progression of necrosis within the framework of ischemic bed size (myocadium at risk) and collateral flow. *Lab Invest* 1979; 40: 633-44
18. Jugdutt BI, Hutchins GM, Bulkley BM, Becker LC. Myocardial infarction in the conscious dog: three-dimensional mapping of infarct, collateral flow and region at risk. *Circulation* 1979; 60: 1141-50
19. Johnson WB, Malone SA, Bantely GA, Anselone CG, Bristow JD. No reflow and extent of infarction during maximal vasodilatation in the porcine heart. *Circulation* 1988; 78: 462-472
20. Vanhecke J, Flaeng W, Borgers M, Jan I, Van de Werf F, De Geest H. Evidence for decreased coronary flow reserve in viable postischemic myocardium. *Circ Res* 1990; 67: 1201-1210
21. The TIMI Study Group. Comparison of invasive and conservative strategies after treatment with intravenous tissue plasminogen activator in acute myocardial infarction: results of the Thrombolysis in Myocardial Infarction (TIMI) phase II trial. *N Engl J Med* 1989; 320: 618-627
22. Swinburn JMA, Lahiri A, Senior R. Intravenous myocardial contrast echocardiography predicts recovery of dysynergic myocardium early after acute myocardial infarction. *J Am Coll Cardiol* 2001; 38: 19-25
23. Coggins MP, Sklenar J, Le DE, et al. Noninvasive Prediction of Ultimate Infarct Size at the Time of Acute Coronary Occlusion Based on the Extent and Magnitude of Collateral-Derived Myocardial Blood Flow. *Circulation* 2001; 104: 2471-2477
24. Lafitte S, Higashiyama A, Masugata H, Peters B, Strachan M, Kwan OL, DeMaria AN. Contrast echocar-

diography can assess risk area and infarct size during coronary occlusion and reperfusion: experimental validation. *J Am Coll Cardiol* 2002; 39: 1546-54
25. Janardhanan R, Moon JCC, Pennell DJ, Senior R. Prediction of the extent of myocardial necrosis and contractile reserve after reperfusion therapy following acute myocardial infarction: comparison between myocardial contrast echocardiography and contrast enhanced cardiovascular magnetic resonance. *J Am Coll Cardiol*, 2003; 41(6): 4394
26. Kaul S, Villaneuva FS. Is the determination of myocardial perfusion necessary to evaluate the success of reperfusion when the infarct related artery is open? *Circulation* 1992; 85: 1942-1944
27. Villanueva FS, Glasheen WP, Sklenar J, Kaul S. Characterization of spatial patterns of flow within the reperfused myocardium using myocardial contrast echocardiography: implications in determining the extent of myocardial salvage *Circulation* 1993; 88: 2596-2606
28. Agati L, Voci P, Vilotta F et al. Influence of residual perfusion within the infarct zone on the natural history of left ventricular dysfunction after acute myocardial infarction: a myocardial contrast echocardiographic study. *J Am Coll Cardiol* 1994; 24: 336-42
29. Ito H, Iwakura K, Masuyama T, Hori M, Higashino Y, Fujii K, Minamino T. Temporal changes in myocardial perfusion patterns in patients with reperfused anterior wall myocardial infarction. Their relation to myocardial viability. *Circulation* 1995; 91: 656-62
30. Brochet E, Czitrom B, Darila-Cohen D, et al. Early changes in myocardial perfusion patterns after myocardial infarction: relation with contractile reserve and functional recovery. *J Am Coll Cardiol* 1998; 32: 2011-7
31. Czitrom D, Karila-Cohen D, Brochet E, et al. Acute assessment of microvascular perfusion patterns by myocardial contrast echocardiography during myocardial infarction: relation to timing and extent of functional recovery. *Heart* 1999; 81: 12-16
32. Myers JH, Stirling MC, Choy M, et al. Direct measurement of inner and outer wall thickening dynamics with epicardial echocardiography. *Circulation* 1986; 74: 164-72
33. Swinburn J, Senior R. Real-time contrast echocardiography - a new bedside technique to predict contractile reserve early after acute myocardial infarction. *Eur J Echocardiogr* 2002; 3: 95-99
34. Main ML, Magalski A, Chee NK, Coen MM, Skolnick DG, Good TH. Full-motion pulse inversion power Doppler contrast echocardiography differentiates stunning from necrosis and predicts recovery of left ventricular function after acute myocardial infarction. *J Am Coll Cardiol* 2001; 38: 1390-4
35. deFilippi CR, Willett DL, Irani WN et al. Comparison of myocardial contrast echocardiography and low-dose dobutamine stress echocardiography in predicting recovery of left ventricular function after coronary revascularization in chronic ischemic heart disease. *Circulation* 1995; 92: 2863-2868
36. Nagueh SF, Vaduganathan P, Ali N, et al. Identification of hibernating myocardium: comparative accuracy of myocardial contrast echocardiography, rest-redistribution thallium-201 tomography and dobutamine echocardiography. *J Am Coll Cardiol* 1997; 29: 985-993
37. Camarano G, Ragosta M, Gimple LW et al. Identification of viable myocardium with contrast echocardiography in patients with poor left ventricular systolic function caused by recent or remote myocardial infarction. *Am J Cardiol* 1995; 75: 219-219
38. Shimoni S, Frangogiannis NG, Aggeli CJ, et al. Microvascular structural correlates of myocardial contrast echocardiography in patients with coronary artery disease and left ventricular dysfunction: implications for the assessment of myocardial hibernation. *Circulation* 2002;106:950-6
39. Di Carli MF, Davidson M, Little R et al. Value of metabolic imaging with positron emission tomography for evaluating prognosis in patients with coronary artery disease and left ventricular dysfunction. *Am J Cardiol* 1994; 73: 527-33
40. Bonow RP, Dilsizian V, Cuocol A, Bacharach SL. Identification of viable myocardium in patients with chronic coronary artery disease and left ventricular dysfunction. Comparison of thallium scintigraphy with reinjection and PET imaging with ^{18}F-fluorodeoxyglucose. *Circulation* 1991; 83: 26-37
41. Kitsiou AN, Srinivasan G, Quyyumi AA, Summers RM, Bacharach SL, Dilsizian V. Stress-induced reversible and mild-to-moderate irreversible thallium defects. Are they equally accurate for predicting recovery of regional left ventricular function after revascularization? *Circulation* 1998; 98: 501 508
42. Udelson J, Coleman P, Metherall J et al. Predicting recovery of severe regional ventricular dysfunction comparison of resting scintigraphy with ^{201}T1 and ^{99m}Tc-sestamibi. *Circulation* 1994; 89: 2552-2661
43. Bisi G, Sciagra R, Santoro GM, Rossi V, Fazzini PF. Technetium-99m sestamibi imaging with nitrate infusion to detect viable hibernating myocardium and predict post revascularisation recovery. *J Nucl Med* 1995; 46: 1994-2000
44. Senior R. Kaul S and Lahiri A. Myocardial viability on echocardiography predicts long term survival after revascularisation in patients with ischaemic congestive heart failure. *J Am Coll Cardiol* 1999; 33: 1848-1854
45. Senior R, Lahiri A. Dobutamine echocardiography

predicts functional outcome after revascularisation in patients with dysfunctional myocardium irrespective of the perfusion pattern on resting thallium-201 imaging. *Heart* 1999; 82: 668-673
46. Afridi I, Grayvurn PA, Panza JA et al. Myocardial viability during dobutamine echocardiography predicts survival in patients with coronary artery disease and severe left ventricular dysfunction. *J Am Coll Cardiol* 1998; 32: 921-926
47. Dendale PA, Franken PR, Waldman GF et al. Low-dosage dobutamine magnetic resonance imaging as an alternative to echocardiography in the detection of viable myocardium after acute myocardial infarction. *Am Heart J* 1995; 130: 134-140
48. Baer FM, Voth E, LaRosee et al. Comparison of dobutamine transesophageal echocardiography and dobutamine magnetic resonance imaging for detection of residual myocardial viability. *Am J Cardiol* 1996; 78: 415-419
49. Kim RJ, Fieno DS, Parrish TB et al. Relationship of MRI delayed contrast enhancement to irreversible injury, infarct, age, and contractile function. *Circulation* 1999; 100: 1992-2002
50. Kim RJ, Wu E, Rafael A. The use of contrast-enhanced magnetic resonance imaging to identify reversible myocardial dysfunction. *N Engl J Med* 2000; 43: 1445-53
51. Sklenar J, Camarano G, Ismail S, Goodman N, Kaul S. The effect of coronary stenosis on contractile reserve after acute myocardial infarction: implications in using dobutamine echocardiography for assessing extent of myocardial salvage after reperfusion. [Abstract]. *Circulation* 1994; 90 (suppl): 1-1172
52. Kaul S. Dobutamine echocardiography for determining myocardial viability after reperfusion: experimental and clinical observations. *Eur Heart J* 1995; 16: 17-23
53. Agati L, Voci P, Luongo R et al. Combined use of dobutamine echocardiography and myocardial contrast echocardiography to predict recovery of regional dysfunction after coronary revascularization in patients with recent myocardial infarction. *Eur Heart J* 1997; 18: 771-9
54. Iliceto S, Galiuto L, Marchese A et al. Analysis of microvascular integrity contractile reserve, and myocardial viability after acute myocardial infarction by dobutamine echocardiography and myocardial contrast echocardiography. Am J Cardiol 1996; 77: 441-5
55. Senior R, Swinburn JM. Incremental value of myocardial contrast echocardiography for the prediction of recovery of function in dobutamine non-responsive myocardium early after acute myocardial infarction. *Am J Cardiol* 2003; 91(4): 397-402
56. Meza MF, Kates MA, Barbee RW, Revall S, Perry B, Murgo JP, Cheirif J. Combination of dobutamine and myocardial contrast echocardiography to differentiate postischaemic from infracted myocardium. *J Am Coll Cardiol* 1997; 29: 974-84
57. Senior R, Kaul S, Soman P, Lahiri A. Power Doppler harmonic imaging: a feasibility study of a new technique for the assessment of myocardial perfusion. *Am Heart J* 2000; 139: 245-51
58. Krishnamani R and Senior R. Evaluation of myocardial viability after myocardial infarction. *European Heart J* 2002; 4 Supp C: C35-C38

Chapter 10
Myocardial Contrast Echocardiography and Inflammatory Response

José Azevedo • José Luis Zamorano • Miguel Angel García Fernández

In recent years, myocardial contrast echocardiography (MCE) has undergone many advances through remarkable developments in echocardiographic contrast agents pharmacodynamics and ultrasound technology [1-7]. The use of MCE has nowadays clear clinical indications, such as cardiac cavities opacification, improved endocardial border definition and quantification of myocardial perfusion. Recently, major progress has been made in MCE application for myocardial perfusion, especially under acute ischaemia and postischaemic conditions [1-3].

The new second-generation MCE agents are suitable for transpulmonary circulation, reaching the left side cardiac cavities and systemic circulation. MCE agents have a physiological behaviour in the circulation very similar to red blood cells [6, 7]. These MCE agents are safe and metabolically inactive. However, the dynamic change in size and electrostatic forces may alter its interaction with the surrounding circulating cells and endothelial wall, both in the arterial and venous vascular territories [4-7]. This is particularly true for the coronary microcirculation and capillaries. As the size of the coronary vessel diameter is gradually reduced by progressive atherosclerotic processes or acute thrombosis, these phenomena achieve a greater pathophysiological importance. During acute coronary syndromes and myocardial ischaemia, an inflammatory response can be observed with a wide range of intensity which is directly related to the degree of instability of the coronary artery atherosclerotic plaque [8-11]. The activities of the leucocyte or monocyte type of circulating inflammatory cells are the main factors responsible for the onset of instability of these coronary atherosclerotic lesions [9, 11].

Inflammation is a dynamic process that involves different types of molecules and cells inside the vascular, extravascular and interstitial space. A first group of cell adhesion molecules, called selectins (E-, P- and L-selectins), intervene in this initial stage, immobilising the circulating leucocyte to the endothelial wall, especially under low-flow conditions. The endothelial cell membrane of the venules can express E- and P-selectins, while L-selectins are exposed in the surface membrane of the activated leucocytes [12, 14]. The leucocytes then suffer a process of capture and rolling along the endothelial wall surface always according to the blood flow direction. Interaction between activated leucocytes and the endothelial wall takes place through the effect of intercellular adhesion (ICAM-1) and vascular cell adhesion (VCAM-1) molecules [9, 10]. Through the action of several selectins, activated leucocytes are more exposed to local cytokines and extravascular chemoattractant factors. Several sequential steps occur from margination, activation and adhesion, and finally aggregation and transmigration. Leucocytes become more activated, and are attracted and migrate to the extravascular space [4, 11, 14]. The interaction between leucocytes, monocytes, platelets and the surrounding circulating elements and antigens becomes more complex as the lumen of the microcirculation vessels and capillaries is gradually reduced [15, 16].

The capillary vascular territory is very sensitive to dynamic changes in size, diameter, capacitance and volume. Inflammation and micro-thrombosis can reduce the size of the lumen of small capillaries, leading to an abrupt cessation of coronary blood flow [4]. Also, the phenomena of thrombus fragmentation, distal migration and embolisation can produce a significant reduction of coronary capillary bed capacitance. This phenomenon of distal coronary embolisation from the critical stenotic lesion becomes even more important during coronary interventions, such as direct atherectomy and balloon angioplasty. Percutaneous coronary interventions are methods that are used to seal the vulnerable atherosclerotic plaque in culprit and unstable lesions. In fact, after coronary interventions, many different phenomena may occur, some of them as unexpected complications of these invasive methods. The culprit or other atherosclerotic plaques can remain unstable or rupture. A single atherosclerotic lesion reducing the blood flow to a critical level can lead to multiple occlusions located at the distal small coronary vessels and capillaries. This unsuccessful coronary interventions can be described by MCE study as a no-reflow phenomenon, because of distal migration and embolisation of a significant portion of the culprit lesion or other atherosclerotic plaques. Usually, in these cases, we can observe a slight increase in serum levels of C-reactive protein and troponine I biomarkers, revealing that a recent small vessel occlusion and myocardial necrosis have occurred. In these cases of unsuccessful coronary intervention, the MCE study frequently shows multiple areas without contrast filling or a dominant patchy pattern.

Coronary collateral circulation can be open through the recruitment of capillaries, a phenomenon that may occur during acute coronary syndromes including acute myocardial infarction (AMI). These events may take place during acute coronary syndromes such as non-ST elevation AMI, where the inflammatory process is more intense. In this particular type of acute coronary syndrome, the degree of coronary artery disease is more severe and diffuse throughout the capillary territory. The inflammatory makers, such as C-reactive protein, may reach higher values, indicating that the myocardial inflammatory reaction after ischaemia is more intense. From our experience with MCE in acute coronary syndromes, in this particular type of non-ST elevation AMI with increased C-reactive protein levels, there is a greater reduction of MCE distribution within the left ventricular myocardium. Another difference is the presence of a dominant MCE patchy pattern in this particular type of ischaemic myocardial pathology. The MCE video intensity difference between perfused and non-perfused myocardial areas is not so crisp, indicating that a diffuse process is taking place and collateral vessels may have already developed. A better delineation between perfused and non-perfused myocardial areas can be found in non-ST elevation AMI, comparing endocardial layers versus meso-epicardial regions, as was previously demonstrated by other authors [17, 18].

In contrast, in ST elevation AMI associated with a great epicardial vessel abrupt occlusion usually secondary to acute coronary artery thrombosis, the collateral circulation does not have enough time to develop during the acute ischaemic process. In these AMI cases the delimitation of the perfused versus non-perfused myocardial areas by MCE is more clear. Also, the difference in MCE video intensity between the perfused and non-perfused myocardial areas is higher.

Interaction with MCE microbubbles and leucocytes sets the basis for imaging of the inflammatory process. The dynamics of MCE microbubbles suffer a significant change due to microcirculation occlusion and ischaemic myocardium. Endothelial wall oedema, coronary capillary occlusion, local microthrombosis, extracellular matrix exposure, followed by the entry of albumin and lipid debris into the circulation create the conditions for a strong interaction with MCE microbubbles. The MCE microbubbles become trapped in this network and can be subjected to phagocytosis [14, 19, 20]. Ischaemia potentiates the inflammatory cell mechanisms and cytokine concentration. During ischaemia and reperfusion injury, MCE microbubbles can be attached to leucocytes, through albumin and other surface receptors [9]. The degree of MCE microbubble persistence and retention within the coronary microcirculation is directly related to the number of activated resident leucocytes, a marker of the extent of the inflammatory process secondary to myocardial ischaemia.

The binding mechanisms of leucocytes to MCE microbubbles are different depending on the composition of their shell. MCE microbubbles rich in albumin will bind to endothelial cell ICAM-1 and leucocytes through β2 integrin Mac-1 [9, 10]. On the other hand, lipid-rich MCE microbubbles interact with leucocytes through complement molecules [12, 13]. The change of microbubble shell composition and environment can modify the inflammatory cell reponse. Also, the MCE microbubble shell composition can be modified, incorporating specific antibodies to cytokines that can be expressed in the injured endothelial wall.

The composition of the MCE microbubble

shell modulates the inflammatory response by the leucocytes. The enrichment of the microbubble shell with amino acids, small proteins and phospholipids, such as serine or phosphatidylserine, will increase the complement binding and consequently leucocyte reactivity [13]. The degree of interaction between the MCE microbubbles and leucocytes can be changed and potentiated through the modification in the relative composition of their protein–lipid shell. Usually, the concentration of complement deposits over the MCE microbubble shell will also increase its antigenic power and cellular reactivity [13].

Specific ligands or monoclonal antibodies of cell adhesion molecules such as ICAM and VICAM-1, which are overexpressed in the inflamed and denuded endothelial surface, will increase the retention of leucocytes inside the microcirculation [10-12]. The selection of ligands to specific molecules depends on their specificity as markers of inflammation, the raise in serum concentrations as a consequence of inflammation compared with its normal basal values. The timing and amplitude of the serum level increase in the inflammatory acute phase molecules can potentially detect inflammation in early stages of this process. Molecules with different patterns of inflammatory response can be selectively targeted using specific ligands on the surface of MCE microbubbles.

The persistence of MCE microbubbles in the microcirculation after phagocytosis by monocytes and leucocytes led to new strategies in promoting its retention in specific areas. The degree of leucocyte retention could be a marker of the intensity and extension of the inflammatory process. Specific and non-specific receptors that bind to albumin or lipid components of the microbubble shell can be targeted and become antigenic for circulating and especially resident leucocytes [12]. These receptors exposed in the surface of the microbubble shell become the target of specific and labelled antibodies. Another option is to use a chemical spacer or ligand to these surface receptors that will increase the antigenic power of these molecules. The circulating time of these MCE microbubbles can be reduced and they can become trapped within the microcirculation and capillaries by resident or inflammatory cells of specific areas involved in the pathologic process, thereby increasing the time of retention. These surface antigens bound to labelled antibodies can be viewed and identified by different imaging techniques [16-18]. The interaction between MCE microbubbles and leucocytes set the basis for non-invasive imaging of the inflammatory process [16-20].

Myocardial inflammation is a consequence of several cardiac pathologies including the post-ischaemic myocardial cell lesion. During this inflammatory process, an abnormal interaction between circulating activated leucocytes and ischaemic and dysfunctioning myocardium takes place, leading to additional and further cell injury. In these pathological conditions, several steps occur, including leucocyte activation and recruitment and myocardial monocyte and inflammatory cell infiltration. Several molecules can be produced and delivered into the microcirculation and cellular and tissue metabolic systems activated including, monocyte chemoattractant protein-1, matrix metalloproteinase-increased activity expression, tissue renin angiotension system upregulation. All these phenomena may lead to severe coronary microcirculation occlusions resulting in the disorganisation and degeneration of cardiac myocytes. During the early period of the acute myocardial injury phase, several mediators can be involved in this inflammatory process. The receptor expression at the surface of the inflammatory cells creates an interactive antigenic net. Surface cell membrane antigens define not only the cell type, population and activation, but also its metabolic status. Other cell functions are also related with the surface interactive antigenic net, such as cell adhesion, transmembrane migration, cell line recruitment and traffic.

Among these molecules, the role of pro-inflammatory cytokines and membrane cell molecules is important, such as interleukin-1 beta, nitric oxide synthase-2 (NOS2), tumour necrosis factor-alpha (TNF-alpha), CD11b and CD43 [21]. Quantitative MCE can be used to localise and determine the non-ischaemic, ischaemic and necrotic areas, as well as the risk areas and regions supplied by collateral coronary blood flow. The experimental laboratory work done by the group of Lindner and colleagues raised the possibility of targeting circulating and adherent leucocytes with MCE, and of analysing the severity of the post-ischaemic myocardial tissue inflammation [18]. In this study, quantitative MCE data were compared with radionuclide imaging using tissue myeloperoxidase activity tracers, and a good correlation between theses two methods was obtained (r=0.81).

However, during the time course of the acute ischaemic myocardial injury, the inflammatory and cell mediators change and acquire a different role and degree of metabolic importance. Moreover, additional inflammatory and coagulation pathways can be activated. These metabolic changes are associated with the disorganisation of the microcirculatory coronary vasculature, trapping circulating and inflammatory cells within its dense network.

Lindner and colleagues also studied the persistence of MCE microbubbles within coronary microcirculation after ischaemia/reperfusion myocardial injury. They used fluorescein-labelled albumin microbubbles as an MCE agent and visualised them in the cremaster muscle microcirculation by intravital microscopy, under ischaemia/reperfusion and after the injection of TNF-alpha. In this experimental model, they studied the behaviour of MCE agents as a marker of myocardial inflammation after ischaemia/reperfusion injury. MCE microbubbles were found attached to activated leucocytes adherent to the venular endothelial wall. The degree of MCE microbubble adherence and persistence increased by TNF-alpha, was independent of the microbubble shell size and composition, and was directly related to the density of activated leucocytes on the vessel wall. Other factors could promote the inhibition of these phenomena, acting as mediators such as heat, fibrinogen, complement, leucocyte selectin and β2-integrin

Mac-1 [19]. In another paper published in the literature, the same authors showed that the MCE albumin microbubble persistence was closely associated with the degree of microvascular endothelial glycocalix damage and cell membrane integrity [9].

MCE can also allow non-invasive imaging of the inflammatory process through the detection of phagocytosed microbubles. Microbubbles can be targeted to intercelullar molecule-I bound to activated coronary endothelial cells, or to the Mac-1 and β2 integrin binding to denatured proteins that mediate leucocyte cell-substrate adhesion.

Cell adhesion molecules located at the surface of the monocyte cell membrane can also be related to the degree of inflammation. The concentration and surface density of these cell adhesion molecules in the leucocytes and monocytes increase their binding capacity to MCE microbubbles. Other binding molecules and ligands can establish the link between circulating phagocytes and MCE microbubbles. With increased inflammatory response, MCE microbubbles can be trapped within the microcirculation, leading to the closure of capillary flow and increased time of residence of these circulating particles.

Later, rapid hypertrophy of the non-ischaemic myocardium takes place in 4 weeks, reduced pro-collagen gene expression and collagen accumulation in the necrotic areas, while interstitial fibrosis progresses up to 20 weeks. The molecular factors related with these cellular and metabolic phenomena remain unknown.

In great arterial vessels such as the carotid arteries, the same principles and MCE strategies can be applied. Specific monoclonal antibodies against ICAM-1 have been developed and incorporated in the MCE microbbubles. Selective monoclonal antibodies can bind directly to the endothelial surface of carotid atherosclerotic plaques rich in these molecules [22]. The degree of inflammation within the atherosclerotic plaque is directly related to its instability and vulnerability, a characteristic that can be monitored using modified MCE microbubbles [22].

Other authors have also suggested new emerging applications for MCE, such as targeted delivery of genetic and pharmaceutical products as direct microbubble therapeutic vehicles or materials [17, 23-30]. In the near future, the development of new diagnostic and imaging methods in the field of immunocytochemistry, histochemistry and molecular biology techniques can be very helpful in the characterisation of the inflammatory process of acute myocardial ischaemia [23-30]. MCE microbubbles have proved to be a useful tool for the non-invasive assessment of myocardial inflammation. The future will reveal their role as therapeutic agents in a variety of pathological processes including myocardial ischaemia, reperfusion injury and inflammation.

References

1. Klibanov AL. Targeted delivery of gas-filled microspheres, contrast agents for ultrasound imaging. Adv. Drug Deliv Rev 1999; 37: 139-157
2. Alkan-Onyuksel H, Demos S, Lanza G, Vonesh M, Klegerman M, Kane B, Kuszak J, McPherson D. Development of inherently echogenic liposomes as ultrasonic contrast agents. J Pharm Sci 1996; 85: 486-490
3. Demos SM, Alkan-Onyuksel H, Kane BJ, Ramani K, Nagaraj A, Greene R, Klegerman M, McPherson D. In vivo targeting of acoustically reflective liposomes for intravascular and transvalvular ultrasonic enhancement. J Am Coll Cardiol 1999; 33: 867-875
4. Springer TA. Adhesion receptors of the immune system. Nature 1990; 346: 425-434
5. Ley K. Molecular mechanisms of leucocyte recruitment in the inflammatory process. Cardiovasc Res 1996; 32: 733-742
6. Skyba DM, Camarano G, Goodman NC, Price RJ, Skalat TC, Kaul S. Hemodynamics characteristics, myocardial kinetics and microvascular rheology of FS-069, a second generation echocardiographic contrast agent capable of producing myocardial opacification from a venous injection. J Am Coll Cardiol 1996; 28: 1292-1300
7. Lindner JR, Song J, Jayaweera AR, Sklenar J, Kaul S. Microvascular rheology of Definity microbubbles after intra-arterial and intravenous administration. J Am Soc Echocardiogr 2002; 15: 396-403
8. Keller MW, Spotnitz WD, Mathew TL, Glasheen WP, Watson DD, Kaul S. Intraoperative assessment of regional myocardial perfusion using quantitative myocardial contrast echocardiography. J Am Coll Cardiol 1990; 16: 1267-1279
9. Lindner JR, Ismail S, Spotnitz WD, Skyba DM, Jayaweera AR, Kaul S. Albumin microbubble persistence during myocardial contrast echocardiography is associated with microvascular endothelial glycocalix damage. Circulation 1998; 98: 2187-2197
10. Villanueva FS, Jankowski RJ, Klibanov S, Pina ML, Alber SM, Watkins SC, Brandenburger GH, Wagner WR. Microbubbles targeted to intercelullar molecule-I bind to activated coronary endothelial cells. Circulation 1998; 98: 1-5
11. Lindner JR, Dayton PA, Coggins MP, LeyK, Song J, Ferrara K, Kaul S. Non-invasive imaging of inflammation by ultrasound detection of phagocytosed microbubles. Circulation 2000; 102: 531/538
12. Davies GE. The Mac-1 and p159,95 β2 integrins binding denatured proteins to mediate leucocyte cell-substrate adhesion. Exp Cell Res 1992; 200: 242-252
13. Comis A, Esterbrook-Smith SB. Inhibition of serum complement haemolytic activity by lipid vesicles containing phosphatidylserine. FEBS Lett 1986; 197: 321-327
14. Lindner JR, Song J, Christiansen J, Klibanov AL, Xu F, Ley K. Ultrasound assessment of injury and inflammation using microbubbles targeted to P-selectin. Circulation 2001; 104: 2107-2112
15. Christiansen JP, Song J, Matsunaga T, Lindner JR. Microbubbles targeted to the platelet IIb/IIIa integrin adhere to microvascular thrombi in vivo (abstract). Circulation 2001; 102305
16. Lanza GM, Wallace KD, Scott MJ, Cacheris WP, Abendschein DR, Christy DH, Sharkey AM, Miller JG, Gaffney PJ, Wickline SA. A novel site-targeted ultrasonic contrast agent with broad biomedical application. Circulation 1997; 95: 3334-3340
17. Gunda M, Mulvagh SL. Recent advances in myocardial contrast echocardiography. Current opinion in cardiology 2001 July; 16(4): 231-9
18. Christiansen JP, Poi L, Klibanov AL, Kaul S, Lindner JR. Non invasive imaging of myocardial reperfusion injury using leucocyte-targeted contrast echocardiography. Circulation 2002; Apr 16: 105(15) : 1764-7
19. Lindner JR, Coggins MP, Kaul S, Klibanov AL, Brandenburger GH, Key K. Microbubble persistence in the microcirculation during ischemia/reperfusion and inflammation is caused by integrin- and complement-mediated adherence to activated leucocytes. Circulation 2000 Feb 15; 101(6): 668-75
20. Dayton PA, Chomas JE, Lum A, Lindner JR, Simon SI, Ferrara KW. Optical and acoustical dynamics of microbubble contrast agents inside neutrophils. Biophys J 2001; 80: 1547-1556. The road from concept to reality. Echocardiography 2001; 18: 339-347
21. J. Monge, J. Cortez, M.H. Custódio, L. Bronze, M. Vieira, J. Azevedo, A. Aleixo, M.G. Morais. Contrast echocardiography and its relationship with the intensity of the inflammatory response in the acute phase of myocardial infarction. Eur Heart J 2002; Vol 14, Abstr. Suppl.-Pag 715 (abstract)
22. Hiser W, Porter T, Li S, Deligonul U, Rice J, Kilzer K, Radio S. Inhibition of carotid artery neointimal formation after balloon injury using ultrasound targeted deposition of antisense to c-myc protooncogene bound to intravenously delivered perfluorocarbon microbubbles (abstract). J Am Soc Echocardiogr 1998; 11: 498
23. Newman CM, Lawrie A, Brisken AF, Cumberland DC. Ultrasound gene therapy: on 24. Bao S, Thrall BD, Miller DL. Transfection of a reposter plasmid into cultured cells by sonoporation in vitro. Ultrasound Med Biol 1997; 23: 943-959
25. Shohet RV, Chen S, Zhou YT, Wang Z, Meidell RS, Unger RH, Grayburn PA. Echocardiographic destruc-

tion of albumin microbubble directs gene delivery to the myocardium. Circulation 2000; 101: 2554-2556
26. Chen S, Shohet RV, Frenkel P, Mayer S, Unger RH, Grayburn PA. Successful expression of plasmid DNA in rat myocardium by ultrasound-targeted microbubble destruction. J Am Coll Cardiol 2001; 37: 407A
27. Christiansen JP, French BA, Matsumura M, Klibanov Lindner JR. Transfection of plasmid DNA in muscle tissue with ultrasound and cationic microbubble vesicles (abstract). J Am Soc Echocardiogr 2001; 14: 426
28. Skyba Dm, Price RJ, Linka AJ, Skalak TC, Kaul S. Direct in vivo visualisation of intravascular destruction of microbubbles by ultrasound and its local effects on tissue. Circulation; 98: 290-293
29. Porter TR, Iversen PL, Li S, Xie F. Interaction of diagnostic ultrasound with synthetic oligonucleotide-labeled perfluorocarbon-exposed sonicated dextrose albumin microbubbles. J Ultrasound Med 1996; 15: 577-584
30. Lindner JR. Evolving applications for contrast ultrasound Am J Cardiol 2002; 90: 72J-80J

Chapter 11

Myocardial Perfusion Imaging During Stress Using Contrast Echocardiography

Mark J. Monaghan

Introduction

Evaluation of reversible ischaemia and understanding the physiological significance of known coronary lesions are one of the most important applications of functional cardiac testing. Several investigation modalities compete for this important role in the management of patients with known or suspected coronary artery disease. Included in this diagnostic armamentarium are stress electrocardiography, stress sestamibi, stress cardiac magnetic resonance imaging (stress CMR) and more recently, stress myocardial contrast echo (stress MCE). Myocardial perfusion abnormalities during stress are important predictors of clinical outcome and appear to be superior to the angiographic evaluation of the coronary anatomy alone [1-3].

The classical ischaemic cascade, as illustrated in Fig. 11.1, demonstrates that one of the first indicators of an imbalance between myocardial oxygen demand and supply is a reduction in myocardial perfusion. MCE has the ability to demonstrate both myocardial blood volume and velocity on a regional basis. The combination of these two parameters has been shown to represent myocardial blood flow [4-7] and we can assume that this is directly proportional to myocardial perfusion. Therefore, stress MCE has the potential to facilitate evaluation of stress-induced changes in myocardial perfusion. Since we know that these occur early in the ischaemic cascade [8], they should be more sensitive markers than chest pain, ECG changes or regional wall motion/thickening abnormalities. In addition, the excellent spatial resolution of MCE affords significant advantages over nuclear techniques. Cost, availability and patient preference also mean that stress MCE can be a more appropriate investigation than stress CMR in the evaluation of reversible ischaemia.

This chapter considers the methodology, advantages and disadvantages of stress MCE in the management of this important patient group.

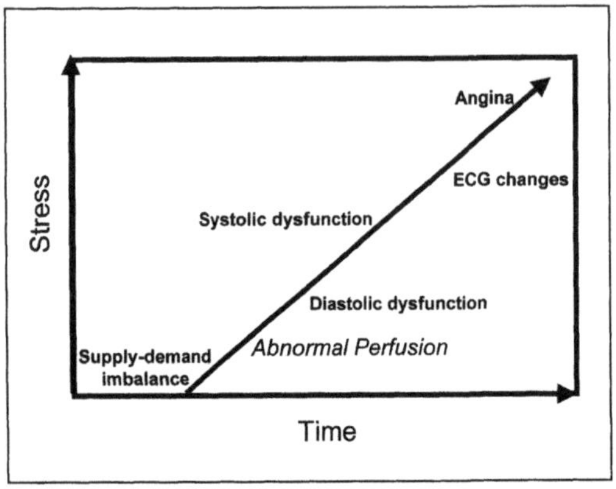

Fig. 11.1. The classical ischaemic cascade demonstrating the sequence of events that occur during stress induced ischaemia. Abnormalities in myocardial perfusion occur earlier than mechanical or ECG changes. Therefore, methods which are able to detect stress induced perfusion abnormalities should have good sensitivity for diagnosing reversible ischaemia

Principles of Stress MCE

The intensity of backscattered ultrasound (i.e. video intensity) from a unit volume of myocardium is directly proportional to the number of scattering interfaces within that volume of myocardium [4-6]. During MCE studies, those interfaces will consist of tissue structures and contrast microbubbles. Most contrast-specific imaging modalities suppress tissue signals so that the backscattered ultrasound signal intensity is mainly due, and proportional to, to the number of contrast microbubbles within the unit volume of myocardium. Since the contrast microbubbles are entirely contained within the vascular volume, the number of microbubbles, and hence backscattered signal intensity, is proportional to the blood volume within the myocardium being imaged [4, 7]. Hence, the video intensity of the contrast signal we measure or see on the screen is directly proportional to myocardial blood volume.

Ischaemia, as generated during stress in myocardial segments subtended by epicardial coronary vessels with flow-limiting lesions, results in a relative reduction in myocardial blood flow [8, 9]. Myocardial blood flow is directly proportional to the product of blood volume and velocity [9-12]. Both these parameters can be readily evaluated and appreciated during stress MCE, using a variety of techniques, as described below. The basic principle of evaluating a reduction in regional myocardial blood volume during stress-induced ischaemia is outlined in Fig. 11.2.

MCE techniques can be described as either destructive or non-destructive imaging methods [4], see also Chapter 2. The former techniques largely rely on contrast destruction to work and include harmonic imaging, harmonic power Doppler (Angio), and pulse inversion imaging. These techniques operate at a high ultrasound transmit power (mechanical index MI) and need to utilise intermittent imaging. Therefore, wall motion information is not available. Low-output (low MI) techniques have also been developed and these methods minimise contrast destruction because of low power, thereby facilitating real-time imaging of myocardial contrast, together with wall motion and thickening information. Both of these types of techniques can be utilised for stress MCE studies.

Contrast agents vary in terms of their microsphere composition. As described in Chapter 2, different shell types and differ-

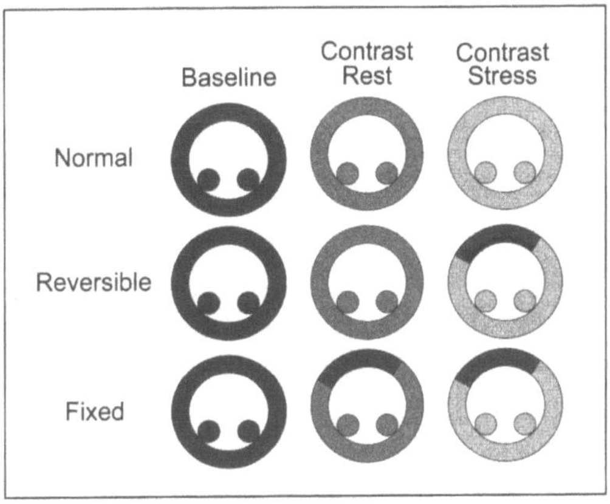

Fig. 11.2. The basic principles of qualitative evaluation of stress MCE images. Following administration of contrast, the myocardial video intensity increases, representing contrast within the myocardial blood volume. During stress, myocardial blood volume should increase and therefore the myocardial signal intensity should be greater than at rest. In myocardial segments supplied by coronary vessels with reduced flow reserve (reversible ischaemia), myocardial blood volume will decrease, resulting in a reduction in the contrast signal. This is often most evident in the sub-endocardium where ischaemia is greatest. Myocardial segments with fixed perfusion defects will show a reduced contrast effect at both rest and stress when compared to normally perfused territories

ent encapsulated gases lead to a range of acoustic properties between the various commercially available agents. Some contrast agents are more suited to destructive imaging methods because the contained gas is very soluble in blood (usually air or nitrogen), meaning that these microbubbles disappear rapidly when exposed to an ultrasound field of sufficient intensity. Contrast agents containing microbubbles with high-molecular-weight gases, which are relatively insoluble in blood, are more suited to low-MI continuous imaging methods.

Contrast agents can be administered either via a bolus injection or continuous infusion. Bolus injections have the advantages of using lower contrast volumes (less cost) and are simple to administer. However, they often result in attenuation in the image plane for a transient period and there is often only a short period, during the decay phase, when the contrast agent concentration is appropriate for analysis of myocardial blood volume.

Infusions of contrast agents are more complex to administer and usually require a larger volume of agent. However, they require less operator involvement during the stress study, it is easier to adjust the infusion rate to optimise myocardial opacification without excessive attenuation and a constant contrast concentration is more suited to quantification of myocardial blood flow.

The final variable in the methodology for stress MCE is the choice of stress agent. The choice is really between a positive inotrope such as dobutamine or arbutamine, or a coronary vasodilator such as dipyridamole or adenosine [13-15].

These two classes of drugs work in different ways and each have their own advantages and disadvantages. The inotropes work by increasing myocardial oxygen demand and this in turn causes an increase in myocardial blood flow. However, in myocardial segments supplied by vessels with poor coronary flow reserve, flow is unable to increase and, in order to maintain adequate coronary perfusion pressure, capillary de-recruitment occurs. This autoregulation mechanism means that myocardial blood volume effectively decreases in these segments and, therefore, the backscatter con-

Table 11.1. Basic methodological variables that can be combined during a Stress MCE protocol

Imaging method	Contrast agent type	Administration method	Stress agent
Non-destructive low MI	High MW gas, semi-permeable shell	Bolus	Inotrope
Destructive high MI	Low MW gas, impermeable shell	Infusion	Vasodilator

The possible range of combinations is very large. For example, destructive high MI imaging such as harmonic power Doppler could be used with a contrast containing a high-molecular-weight gas like SonoVue (Bracco), administered via a constant infusion using a positive inotropic agent such as dobutamine

trast signal intensity decreases as explained previously.

Coronary vasodilators work by using the "coronary steal" phenomenon. Myocardial blood flow increases substantially in perfusion beds supplied by coronary vessels with normal flow reserve and no flow-limiting lesions. However, a drop in perfusion pressure occurs across flow-limiting coronary lesions and blood flow is diverted towards normal perfusion territories. The reduced perfusion pressure means that capillary de-recruitment occurs in ischaemic territories. This capillary de-recruitment results in reduced myocardial blood volume and reduced re-perfusion rates following destruction. As previously explained, both of these parameters can be evaluated from the myocardial contrast signal.

The basic variables involved in stress MCE are summarised in Table 11.1. The range of possible combinations in terms of methodology is very large. So far, the ideal combination has not been found.

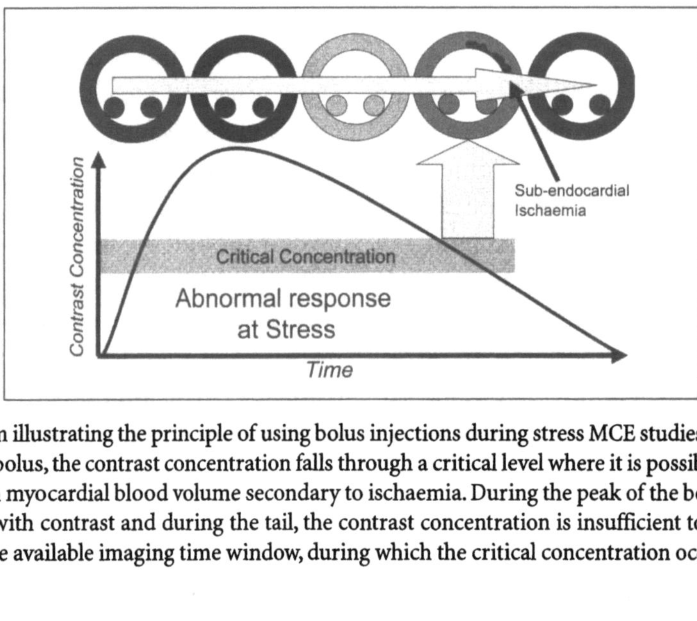

Fig. 11.3. Diagram illustrating the principle of using bolus injections during stress MCE studies. During the wash-out phase of the bolus, the contrast concentration falls through a critical level where it is possible to visualise spatial differences in myocardial blood volume secondary to ischaemia. During the peak of the bolus, the myocardium is saturated with contrast and during the tail, the contrast concentration is insufficient to cause myocardial opacification. The available imaging time window, during which the critical concentration occurs, is fairly short

Bolus Injections with Real-Time Imaging

Bolus contrast injections are probably more suited to being used in combination with real-time, non-destructive, low-MI imaging techniques. This has the advantage of allowing simultaneous evaluation of wall motion and perfusion, using contrast enhancement. These real-time low-MI imaging techniques usually provide excellent endocardial definition at adequate frame rates. Myocardial perfusion information is therefore incremental to the wall motion data and this methodology provides an excellent starting point for performing stress MCE studies [16].

As illustrated in Fig. 11.3, during the decay portion of the contrast bolus, the contrast concentration in the myocardium falls to a critical level, where it is possible to differentiate ischaemia-induced differences in myocardial blood volume. This is usually visualised initially in the sub-endocardium as a dark rim, whilst the sub-epicardium remains bright. As the contrast concentration decays further, the entire transmural extent of the myocardium becomes dark. Spatial variations in contrast enhancement during the bolus decay phase are critical aids to recognising ischaemic segments. A homogeneous, transmural decay in contrast intensity (mirrored in other segments at the same image depth) simply represents contrast decay, whereas heterogeneous opacification and especially a dark sub-endocardium, is highly suggestive of stress-induced ischaemia.

Myocardial segments that remain unopacified during the entire contrast administration usually represent infarcted and irreversibly ischaemic tissue. This is especially the case if a significant resting wall motion abnormality is present.

Although it is sometimes useful to record baseline myocardial contrast studies at rest, we know that even in the presence of an epicardial coronary stenosis of more then 80%, resting myocardial blood flow will be normal. Therefore, if resting wall motion and thickening is normal in an individual segment, one can usually assume that perfusion will be normal and a contrast study at this point may be superfluous. If myocardial contrast opacification is absent in a normally contracting segment at rest then this represents an artefact due to attenuation or inadequate gain/ultrasound penetration. During stress, we would expect changes in perfusion to be evident before wall motion abnormalities [6]. Therefore, the stress MCE images can be taken, if required, at a submaximal stage.

This technique can be utilised successfully during conventional dobutamine stress echocardiography, since at low doses, dobutamine does act as a coronary vasodilator [8] and during stress ischaemia, changes in myocardial blood volume will occur, as described previously. The fact that this methodology can be used during dobutamine stress further underlines its suitability as a starting point for performing these types of studies.

Figure 11.4a illustrates a case of a patient with an occluded LAD stent, where the distal part of the LAD is supplied by collaterals from the right coronary artery (Fig.

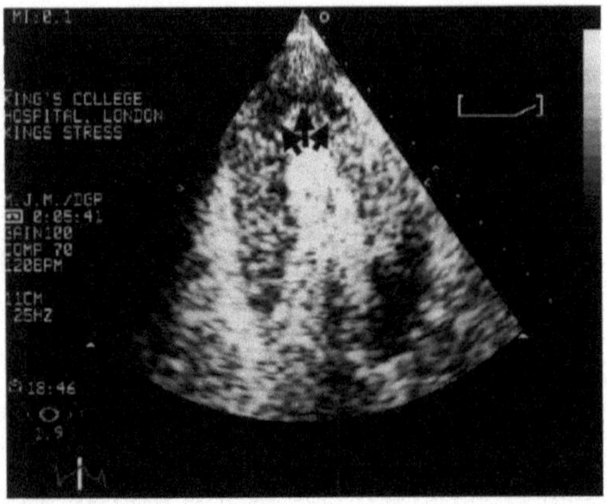

Fig. 11.4a. End-systolic apical 4 chamber image acquired during real-time low MI imaging (power modulation) at peak dobutamine stress with a contrast bolus injection. This patient had had a left anterior coronary artery stent implanted 8 weeks previously and had been referred for stress MCE because of a recurrence of his symptoms. An apical sub-endocardial perfusion defect (arrowed) is clearly seen. Reduced myocardial contrast in the basal lateral segments represents a contrast attenuation artefact

11.4b). The image shown is an apical four-chamber view taken at peak dobutamine stress (40µg/kg/min) during a contrast bolus injection. Coronary flow reserve is clearly reduced in the distal LAD territory and the myocardial contrast signal is reduced in the apical subendocardial territory. A stress-induced wall motion abnormality was also evident in the same region. The excellent spatial resolution afforded by MCE is illustrated in this case, where it is possible to see the reduction in contrast enhancement confined to the sub-endocardium.

A suggested protocol for stress MCE, using a contrast infusion, is illustrated in Fig. 11.5. Multiple bolus injections could be substituted for an infusion, with the limitations previously described.

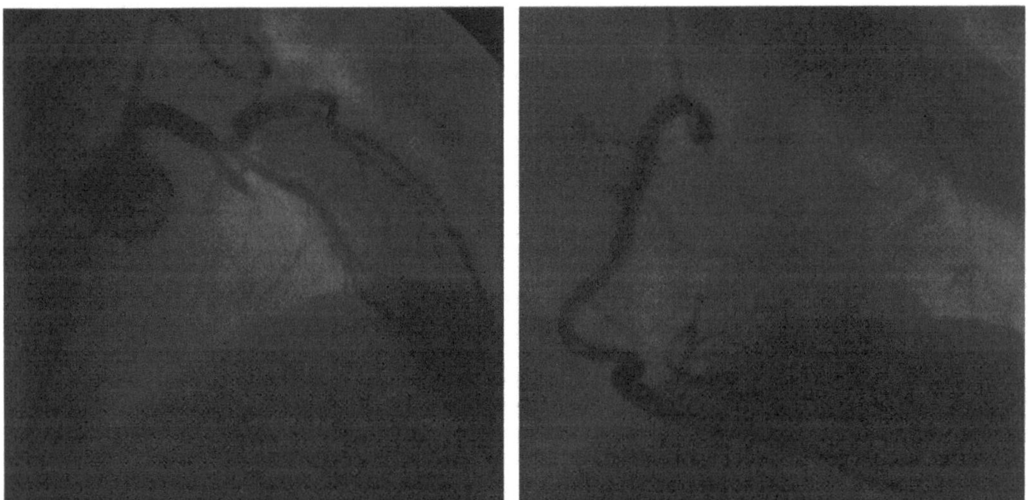

Fig. 11.4b. Coronary angiogram from the same patient shown in figure a. The left anterior descending artery is completely occluded at the location of the implanted stent. Right coronary angiography demonstrates collateral flow into the distal left anterior descending artery (beyond the stent)

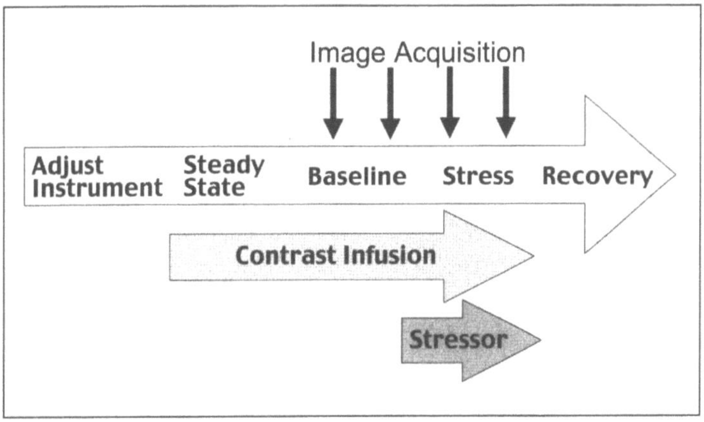

Fig. 11.5. Suggested stress MCE protocol. As described, although a contrast infusion is ideal, multiple bolus injections could be utilised. Similarly, image acquisition could be either using low MI non-destructive real-time imaging or a destructive imaging modality with intermittent imaging

Destruction, Reperfusion Real-Time Imaging

When low MI, real-time imaging is used during stress MCE it is best to employ a "negative bolus" technique in combination with a contrast infusion. The contrast infusion rate is set at a level which provides adequate myocardial opacification without contrast attenuation. Again, good endocardial definition is nearly always obtained, although if the myocardium is very bright, it can be difficult to differentiate it from the left ventricular cavity.

The low-MI imaging methodology typically uses an output MI of <0.3, and often <0.1 (depending on the contrast agent characteristics). If a few frames (usually 5-10) of high output power (MI>1.0) are fired, then contrast microspheres will be destroyed. This usually results in the myocardial contrast effect disappearing, whereas the left ventricular cavity remains bright because the contrast concentration is significantly greater in the cavity. The wash-in of contrast into the myocardium, following destruction can then be observed.

Careful adjustment of contrast infusion rate and machine settings is critical to ensure that complete contrast destruction in the myocardium occurs, without significant cavity destruction. Off-line analysis of the images allows for a region of interest to be positioned within individual myocardial segments. The contrast signal intensity can then be plotted as a reperfusion curve, as illustrated in Fig. 11.6. As previously described, the slope of the curve is proportional to blood flow velocity and the plateau to blood volume. The product of both parameters is proportional to absolute blood flow, which will be reduced in ischaemic zones. A comparison before and after stress (especially vasodilator) will permit an assessment of coronary blood flow reserve.

However, a semi-quantitative approach

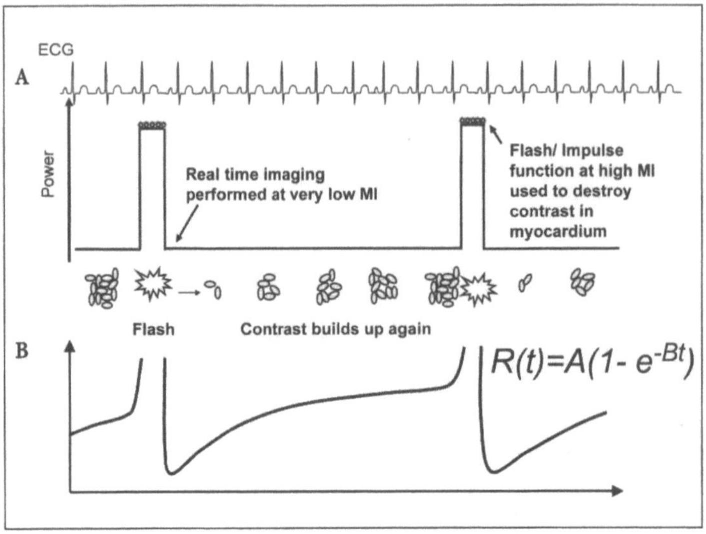

Fig. 11.6. Diagram illustrating the basic principles of low MI real-time perfusion imaging with flash/impulse contrast destruction. Following the destruction frames, contrast re-perfuses into the myocardium. **A** The plateau portion of the re-perfusion curve is proportional to myocardial blood volume. **B** The initial slope of the curve is proportional to blood flow velocity. R(t) is proportional to myocardial blood flow

can also be taken by direct observation of the number of cardiac cycles taken for an individual segment to reperfuse. Delayed reperfusion (>3-4 cycles), especially in the sub-endocardium, is highly suggestive of ischaemia. During stress, increased myocardial blood flow should mean that an individual segment will reperfuse more quickly than at rest.

There is a naturally occurring cyclic variation in the myocardial contrast effect [17, 18] and this, together with segmental motion, can make interpretation of these images in a real-time mode difficult. Therefore, it is often easier to use a triggered capture mode on the ultrasound system, so that only end-systolic or end-diastolic frames are stored. Subsequent analysis of these frames, without the confounding effects of cyclic intensity variations and wall motion, is often easier.

Again this methodology can be used with both inotropic or vasodilator stress, as previously outlined. In practice, it is most commonly utilised with vasodilator stress since it is perfusion alone rather than perfusion and wall motion data that are being analysed. An example of this technique is illustrated in Fig. 11.7.

Parametric imaging software is currently under development. This will provide colour-coded images where the colours assigned to individual myocardial segments are dependent upon the time taken for contrast to re-perfuse following flash destruction. This may provide a more readily appreciated visual display of myocardial blood flow and could be performed before and during stress.

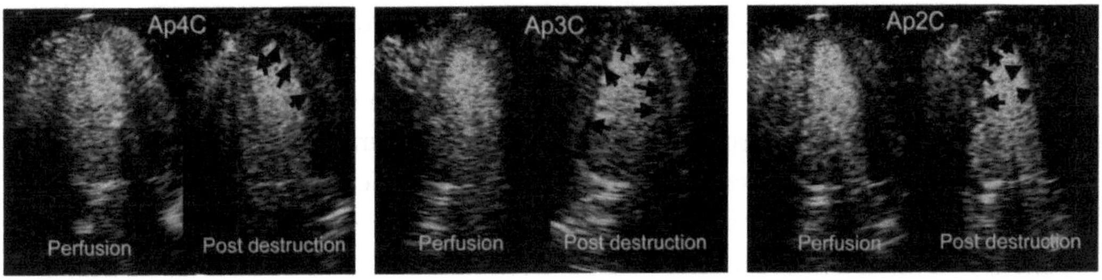

Fig. 11.7a. Dipyridamole stress contrast study using a contrast infusion and Power Modulation Low MI imaging. Apical End-systolic images acquired immediately before (perfusion) and one beat post high MI destruction frames (post destruction). Post destruction images demonstrate patchy sub-endocardial perfusion defects (arrowed) in all coronary perfusion beds

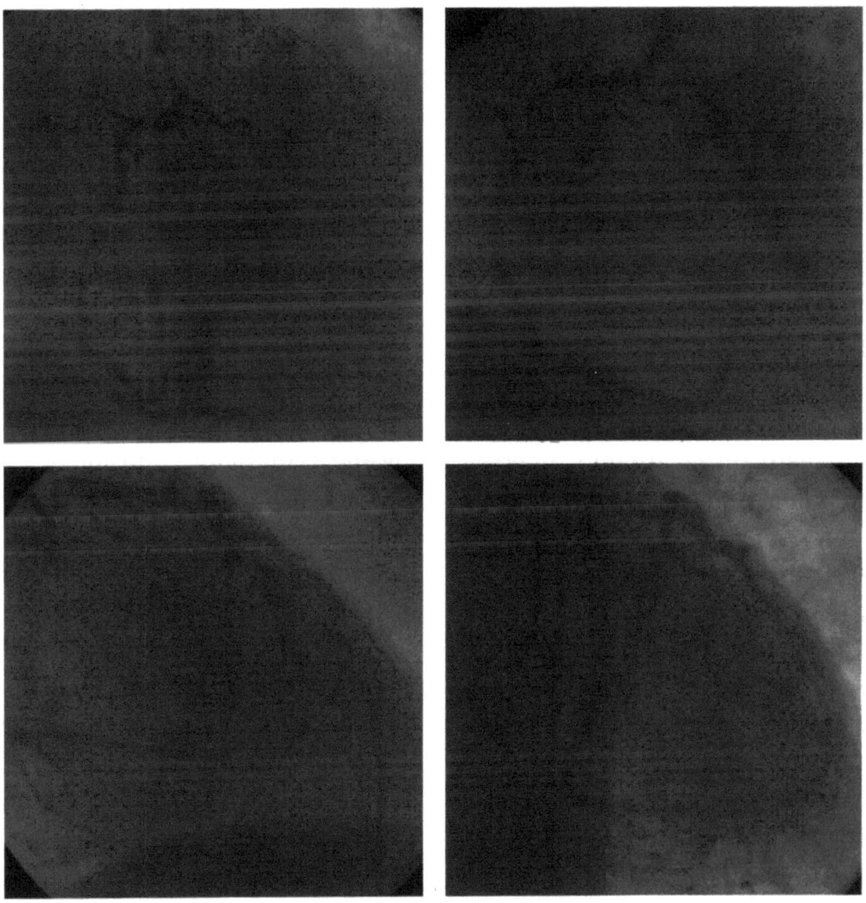

Fig. 11.7b. Coronary angiography subsequently obtained from the same patient. Significant multivessel disease is demonstrated

Destructive, Intermittent Imaging

As previously mentioned, this type of methodology may cause destruction of contrast microspheres within the myocardium (second harmonic imaging, pulse inversion imaging). In addition, the destruction and subsequent disappearance of the microspheres paradoxically enables their detection with harmonic power Doppler methodology. Due to contrast destruction, these methods are utilised with intermittent imaging and therefore no wall motion data are available.

By varying the triggering interval from one frame every cardiac cycle to up to one frame every ten cycles it is possible to obtain data on myocardial blood flow. It is important to step through an acquisition sequence where the triggering interval is varied and increased in a stepwise fashion. Software on some ultrasound systems permits the creation of a triggering sequence which simplifies and standardises image acquisition.

During long triggering intervals it can be difficult to maintain a constant scan plane, since the echocardiographer has no moving landmarks. It is possible on some ultrasound systems to utilise low-MI real-time imaging ("monitoring mode") between the high MI destructive frames and this certainly makes performing intermittent imaging much easier.

The other important issue during this type of stress MCE imaging is to decide which part of the cardiac cycle should be used for the trigger acquisition point. Although there is no absolute rule, end-systole is most commonly utilised because the myocardium is thicker, the left ventricular cavity is small and contrast attenuation is limited. Setting up the instrument controls for this type of imaging requires considerable experience in order to avoid artefacts caused by wall motion, contrast attenuation or incomplete contrast destruction.

Since myocardial blood flow increases during stress we would expect that reperfusion will ocurr with shorter trigger intervals than at baseline. For example, during vasodilator stress using either dipyridamole or adenosine, the normal coronary flow reserve response results in blood flow increasing by a factor of 4. Therefore, at rest it may take a trigger interval of four cardiac cycles for an individual segment to reperfuse, whereas under maximum coronary vasodilation, reperfusion should occur in one cycle. Thus we can compare baseline images with a trigger interval of four cycles to stress images acquired with a one-cycle interval.

An example of this technique is shown in Fig. 11.8a. This study was performed using intermittent harmonic power Doppler imaging and a continuous infusion of a contrast agent (CardioSphere, Point Biomedical), which was especially developed for destructive imaging techniques. The baseline images are acquired using a four-beat triggering interval and demonstrate relatively homogeneous perfusion in all segments. On the other hand, during dipyridamole stress, the images acquired at a one-beat interval demonstrate a reversible perfusion defect in the septal and apical lateral segments. These segments are seen to reperfuse when the triggering interval is extended to four beats. This demonstration of a perfusion

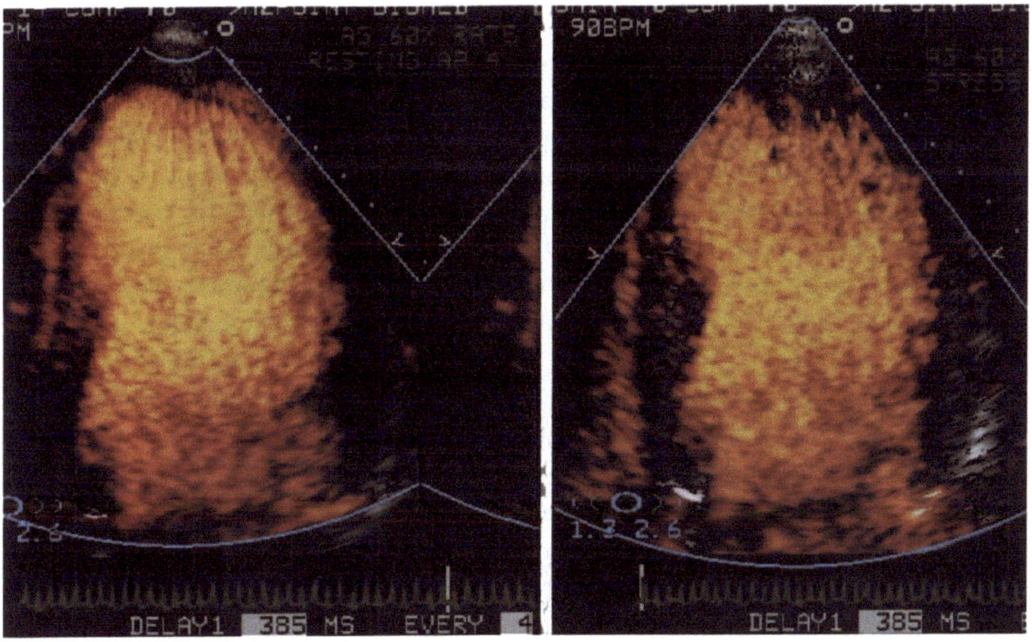

Fig. 11.8a. Apical 4 chamber Intermittent harmonic power Doppler images acquired at a 4 beat trigger interval at rest and 1 beat during dipyridamole infusion. Cardiosphere (Point Biomedical) contrast agent was utilised using a continuous infusion during this study. Fixed defects seen at rest and stress are noted in the apical and proximal septal segments. Reversible defects are noted in the more distal septal and apical lateral segments

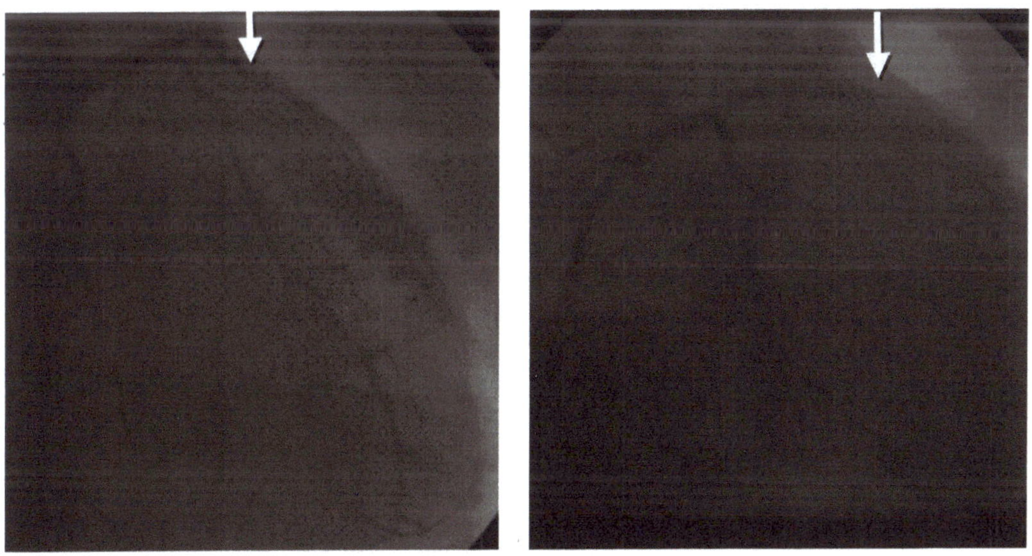

Fig. 11.8b. Left coronary angiogram from the patient whose stress MCE images are shown in figure 11.8a. An occluded left anterior descending coronary artery is seen

defect during stress at a one-beat interval, which then reperfuses with longer triggering intervals is a sensitive indicator of a reversible perfusion defect. A fixed perfusion defect (at rest and stress) is seen in the proximal septum and apex. The coronary angiogram from this patient is shown in Fig. 11.8b,c and demonstrates an occluded left anterior descending artery and severe right coronary artery disease.

Although this form of stress MCE is usually performed with vasodilator stress, it can also be utilised with inotropic stress. As previously mentioned, coronary physiology dictates that during stress-induced ischaemia, relative reductions in myocardial blood volume, secondary to capillary de-recruitment, will result in slower reperfusion into ischaemic territories. Therefore, at short triggering intervals during stress, a perfusion defect may be visualised. An example utilising dobutamine stress with intermittent harmonic power Doppler is shown in Fig. 11.9. Increased wall motion, due to the inotropic effect, may result in more wall motion artefacts when this type of stress is used. Consequently, harmonic power Doppler is more commonly used in combination with vasodilator stress.

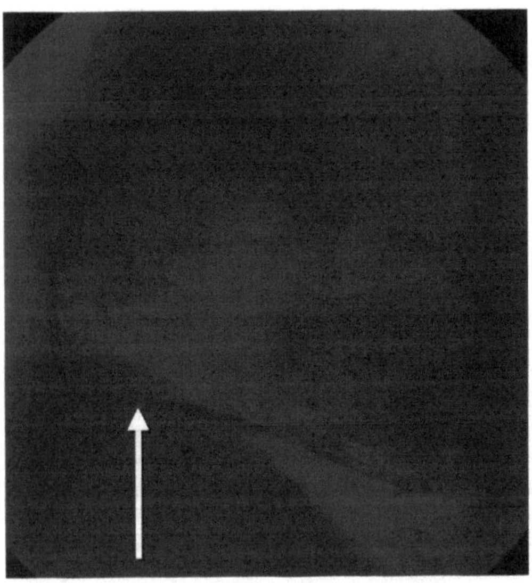

Fig. 11.8c. Right coronary angiogram from the patient whose stress MCE images are shown in figure 11.8a. Severe right coronary artery disease is seen

Although efforts to optimise stress MCE studies have so far mainly concentrated on evaluating perfusion in the left ventricular myocardium, it is possible to evaluate right ventricular myocardial perfusion [19]. However, contrast attenuation is more problematic in the right ventricle and therefore careful attention to appropriate imaging planes is required.

Limitations of Stress MCE

Although excellent research data strongly suggest that these techniques will have a major clinical role in the future, current clinical practice has been slow to adopt stress MCE as an alternative method for evaluating reversible ischaemia. There are undoubtedly many reasons for this but some of the most important ones include the lack of available training in these techniques for non-invasive cardiologists, late development of appropriate contrast-specific imaging software, lack of consensus about the appropriate combination of methodologies to perform a successful study, difficulties in obtaining reliable MCE data in the far and wide ultrasound scan planes, and artefacts caused by contrast attenuation and wall motion etc.

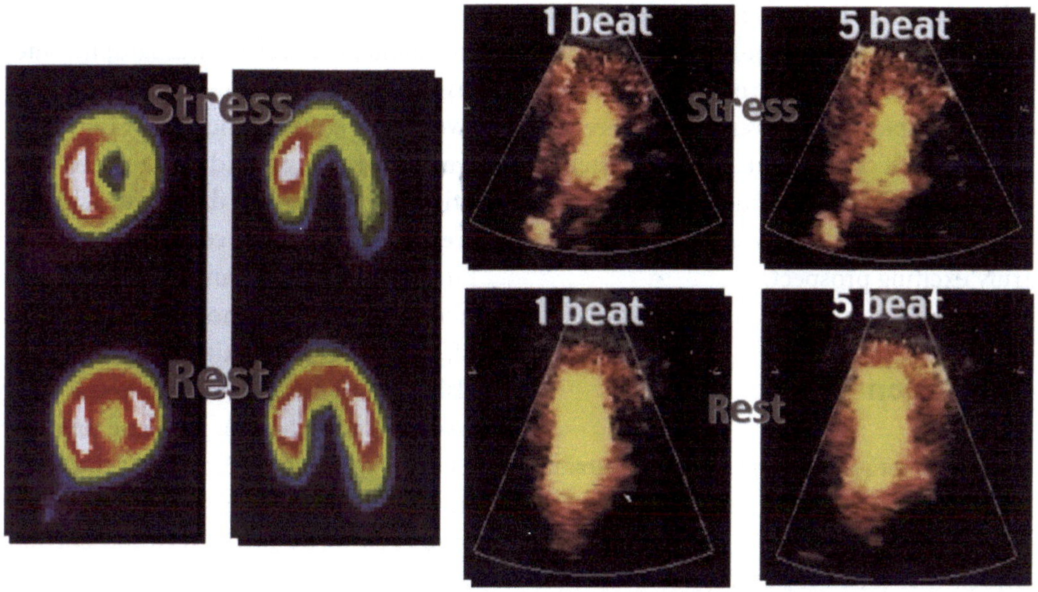

Fig. 11.9a. Simultaneously acquired resting and peak dobutamine stress Sestamibi and harmonic power Doppler images during ultrasound contrast infusion. Stress Sestamibi images demonstrate a reversible lateral wall perfusion defect. A similar defect is demonstrated in the power Doppler apical 4 chamber images. During 1 beat end-systolic triggering at rest a lateral wall perfusion defect is noted and this fills in at a 5 beat interval. However, during peak stress, the same defect is present both at 1beat and 5 beat triggering intervals, consistent with reversible ischaemia in this territory

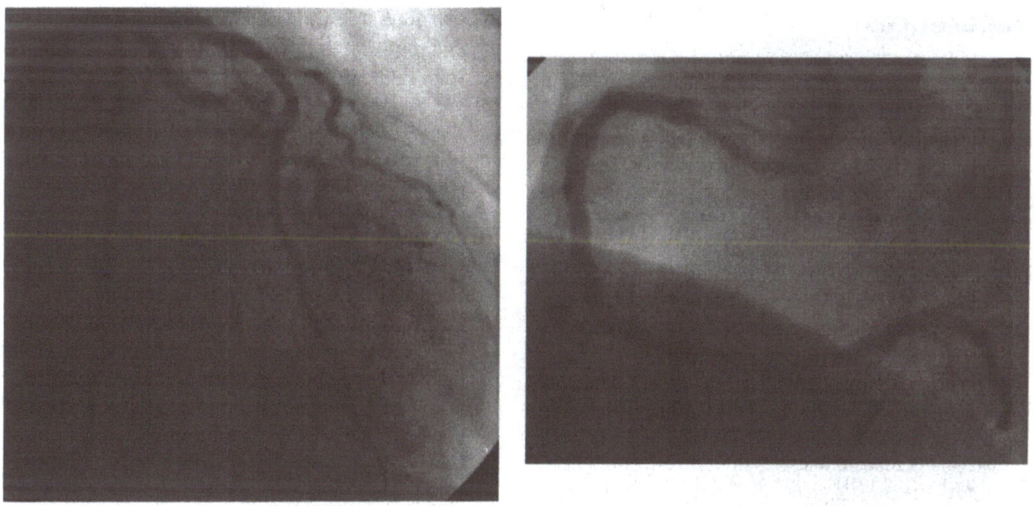

Fig. 11.9b. Coronary angiogram from the patient illustrated in figure 11.9a. It demonstrates an occluded left circumflex artery with collaterals plus diseased left anterior descending and right coronary arteries, both of which had undergone previous PTCA procedures. Postero-basal LV wall hypokinesis was also noted during peak dobutamine stress, consistent with reversible ischaemia

Despite these limitations, interest in this field remains extremely high and the remaining obstacles to progression of stress MCE are rapidly being overcome. The recent development of real-time 3D echo systems, that work effectively with contrast, creates the possiblility of 3D stress MCE, which is a truly exciting prospect.

Conclusion

One of the earliest consequences of reversible myocardial ischaemia is a relative reduction in myocardial perfusion. MCE can detect myocardial contrast parameters which are directly related to perfusion at both rest and stress. This technology therefore has the potential to increase the diagnostic sensitivity for the detection of reversible ischaemia over and above that already established for conventional stress echocardiography. Since stress MCE can be used in combination with conventional stress echocardiography techniques and can provide enhanced wall motion *plus* perfusion data, it should also increase our diagnostic confidence.

Finally, other important advantages over other competing technologies include its cost, time, excellent spatial resolution, it is a bedside technique, the ability to assess other intracardiac structures at the same time and the lack of ionising radiation. For these reasons, stress MCE is likely to become the preferred technique for functional cardiac imaging in the future.

References

1. Gibson RS, Watson DD, Craddock GB, Crampton R, Kaiser D, Denny M, Beller G: Prediction of cardiac events after uncomplicated myocardial infarction: A prospective study comparing pre-discharge exercise thallium 201 scintigraphy and coronary angiography. Circulation 1983; 68: 321-336
2. Ladenheim ML, Kotler TS, Pollock BH, Berman DS, Diamond GA: Incremental prognostic power of clinical history, exercise electrocardiography and myocardial perfusion scintigraphy in suspected coronary artery disease. Am J Cardiol 1987; 59: 270-277
3. Camarieri A, Picano E, Landi P, Michelassi C, Pingitore A, Minardi G, Gandolfo N, Seveso G, Chiarelli F, BologneseL, Chiaranda G, Sclavo H, Previtali M, Margana F, Magaia O, Bianchi F, on behalf of investigators EPIC study: Prognostic value of dipyridamole echocardiography early after myocardial infarction in elderly patients. J Am Coll Cardiol 1993; 22: 1809-1815
4. Becher H, Burns P. Handbook of contrast echocardiography. 62. 2000. Springer
5. Wei K, Skyba DM, Firschke C, Jayaweera AR, Lindner JR, Kaul S. Interactions between microbubbles and ultrasound: in-vitro and in-vivo observations. J Am Coll Cardiol 1997; 29: 1081-1088
6. Wei K, Jayaweera AR, Firoozan S, Linka A, Skyba DM, Kaul S. Quantification of myocardial blood flow with ultrasound-induced destruction of microbubbles administered as a continuous venous infusion. Circulation 1998; 97: 473-483
7. Wei K. Assessment of myocardial blood flow and volume using myocardial contrast echocardiography. Echocardiography. 19(5): 409-16, 2002 Jul
8. Leong-Poi H, Rim S, Le E, Fisher N, Wei K, Kaul S: Perfusion versus function: The ischaemic cascade in demand ischaemia. Circulation. 2002; 105: 987-992
9. Masugata H, Peters B, Lafitte S, et al. Comparison of open- and closed-chest canine model for quantification of coronary stenosis severity by myocardial contrast echocardiography. Invest Radiol 2003; 38: 44-50
10. Wei K, Jayaweera AR, Firoozan S, et al. Quantification of myocardial blood flow with ultrasound-induced destruction of microbubbles administered as a constant venous infusion. Circulation 1998; 97: 473-483

11. Masugata H, Peters B, Lafitte S, et al. Quantitative assessment of myocardial perfusion during graded coronary stenosis by real-time myocardial contrast echo refilling curves. J Am Coll Cardiol 2001; 37: 262-269
12. Galiuto L, May-Newman K, del Balzo U, Flaim S F, Iliceto S, DeMaria A. Assessment of Coronary Stenoses of Graded Severity by Myocardial Contrast Echocardiography. Journal of the American Society of Echocardiography. 15(3): 197-205, March 2002
13. Bin JP. Pelberg RA. Wei K. Le DE. Goodman NC. Kaul S. Dobutamine versus dipyridamole for inducing reversible perfusion defects in chronic multivessel coronary artery stenosis. Journal of the American College of Cardiology. 40(1): 167-74, 2002 Jul 3
14. Morcerf F. Moraes A. Carrinho M. Dohmann HJ. Study of coronary flow reserve with intravenous use of microbubbles (contrast echocardiography) and adenosine: protocol for clinical application in patients suspected of having coronary heart disease. Arquivos Brasileiros de Cardiologia. 78(3): 281-98, 2002 Mar
15. Ronderos RE. Boskis M. Chung N. Corneli DB. Escudero EM. Ha JW. Charlante C. Rim SJ. Portis M. Fabris N. Camilletti J. Mele AA. Otero F. Porter TR. Correlation between myocardial perfusion abnormalities detected with intermittent imaging using intravenous perfluorocarbon microbubbles and radioisotope imaging during high-dose dipyridamole stress echo. Clinical Cardiology. 25(3): 103-11, 2002 Mar
16. Mor-Avi V, Caiani EG, Collins KA, et al. Combined assessment of myocardial perfusion and regional left ventricular function by analysis of contrast-enhanced power modulation images. Circulation 2001; 104: 352-357
17. Wei, K. Le, E. Jayaweera, Ananda R. Bin, J. Goodman, N. Craig BS. Kaul, S. Detection of Noncritical Coronary Stenosis at Rest Without Recourse to Exercise or Pharmacological Stress. Circulation. 105(2): 218-223, January 15, 2002
18. Bekeredjian R. Hansen A. Filusch A. Dubart A. da Silva K. Hardt S. Korosoglou G. Kuecherer H. Cyclic Variation of Myocardial Signal Intensity in Real-time Myocardial Perfusion Imaging. Journal of the American Society of Echocardiography. 15(12): 1425-1431, December 2002
19. Vargas-Barron J. Pena-Duque M. Roldan FJ. Romero-Cardenas A. Espinola-Zavaleta N. Ferez-Santander S. Detection of right ventricular myocardial perfusion and contractile reserve by contrast echocardiography and low dose dobutamine in myocardial infarction after successful right coronary angioplasty. Archivos de Cardiologia de Mexico. 72(1): 49-52, 2002 Jan-Mar

Chapter 12

Myocardial Contrast Echocardiography in Acute Myocardial Infarction

Esther Pérez David • Teresa López Fernández • José Luis Zamorano
Miguel Angel García Fernández

Introduction

For the last 20 years, pharmacological or mechanical reperfusion therapy, focused on restoration of patency of the infarct-related artery, has been the cornerstone of the initial treatment of acute myocardial infarction (AMI). A large number of clinical trials have shown that complete recanalization of the occluded epicardial coronary artery significantly improves short and long-term prognosis [1-3]. It has also been shown that in order to improve prognosis it is essential to minimize the time from onset of symptoms to recanalization of infarct-related artery [4].

However, it has also been demonstrated that restoration of normal flow in the epicardial coronary artery does not automatically lead to improvement of myocardial perfusion [5, 6]. A major problem in the treatment of AMI is the potentiation of bulk fibrin emboli, which is promoted by either fibrinolytic therapy or primary angioplasty. In spite of infarct-related artery patency, microvascular damage and obstruction may persist and hamper the reflow to the postischemic bed.

Therefore, the need for imaging methods to evaluate myocardial microcirculation in this setting is increasingly recognized. Myocardial contrast echocardiography (MCE) can be extremely useful for assessing microvasculature function. This evaluation is important both during acute coronary occlusion, to define risk area, and also after reperfusion therapy, to rule out microvascular damage. It has the advantage of being a quick technique that can be performed in the coronary unit, at the patient's bedside.

In this chapter, applications of MCE in AMI will be discussed, especially focusing on reperfused myocardial infarction. Experimental models of acute ischemia have been very useful to learn about myocardial microcirculation pathophysiology. In the last few years, plenty of information regarding the clinical utility of MCE in AMI has also been published and will be reviewed.

Acute Coronary Occlusion

Experimental Models of Acute Coronary Occlusion

Functional Area at Risk

In experimental models, it has been demonstrated that 30–45 min after coronary occlusion, myocardial necrosis is initiated in the subendocardium and progresses to the epicardium over time in a wavefront pattern (Fig. 12.1). If patency of the infarct-related artery is restored shortly after occlusion, a subendocardial infarction can be demonstrated; if coronary occlusion is maintained, progressive transmural necrosis will develop as a result. In the experimental model from Reimer et al., viable and potentially salvageable subepicardial muscle persisted for at least 3 h after the onset of ischemia [7].

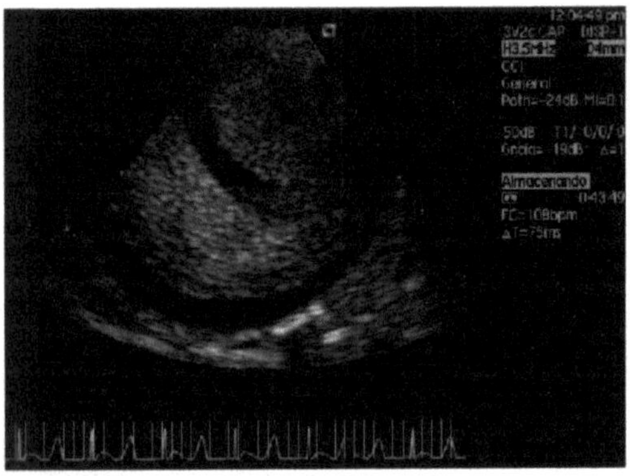

Fig. 12.1. In acute ischemia, myocardial necrosis is initiated in the subendocardium and progresses to epicardium over time in a wavefront pattern. In this MCE image, obtained after a subtotal LAD coronary occlusion, a perfusion defect can be seen that is larger in the subendocardium

Normal myocardial blood flow (MBF) is approximately 1ml/min per gram of tissue, and normal myocardial thickening is approximately 35%. When MBF diminishes, so does myocardial thickening and akinesia is observed with MBF that corresponds to 30% of normal values. However, myocytes can remain viable at as little as 25% of normal MBF if myocardial oxygen demand remains low [7]. These areas of viable myocytes are not able to maintain a normal contractile function due to their low supply of MBF, but their capabilities are still intact and contractile function may recover if oxygen delivery improves.

When prolonged coronary occlusion takes place, not only the myocytes but also the microvasculature suffers a structural damage. The most extensive microvascular damage takes place in severely necrotic areas [8]. This is the basis for the use of MCE in AMI, which allows us to study the integrity of myocardial microcirculation.

MCE is the first technique to allow "in vivo" definition of the risk area in real time on the basis of a sharp gradient in MBF between normal and underperfused myocardium [9]. In fact, the initial application of MCE was to define the regions of the myocardium perfused by coronary arteries and their branches, as well as the size of the hypoperfused region that appeared following coronary occlusion.

The risk area can be defined using MCE in two different ways. Initially, experimental models were made with intracoronary contrast injections distal to the site of occlusion. This determines a "positive risk area" which corresponds to the perfusion bed size reflected by anterograde perfusion, not including collateral flow. On the contrary, when contrast is injected proximal to the site of occlusion, the area failing to show contrast enhancement or "negative risk area" defined by MCE corresponds to the area not supplied by either anterograde flow or collateral flow through adjacent vessels and allows a "functional risk area" to be defined [9]. Depending on the extent of collateral flow, the functional risk area will invariably be smaller than the anatomical risk area.

This utility of MCE in defining risk area has been confirmed in the case of peripheral intravenous administration of contrast agents and by using novel imaging modalities meant to selectively enhance contrast signals [10].

The risk area can be more accurate for risk stratification than hemodynamic variables or left ventricular ejection fraction (LVEF). Due to compensatory mechanisms, hemodynamic variables only become abnormal when the area at risk is very large (25%–40% of the left ventricle). LVEF becomes abnormal earlier, when the area at risk is of moderate size (18%), but nevertheless is not able to differentiate among AMI size for smaller risk areas [11].

Serial MCE studies have been performed in an experimental model by Kaul et al, determining the relationship between duration of coronary occlusion and risk area/infarct size ratio [11]. As it has been demonstrated with other techniques, the duration of the occlusion is strongly correlated to the ultimate extent of the AMI size in MCE studies and also to the ratio risk area/infarct size. If there is very little or no residual collateral-derived MBF, most of the risk area undergoes necrosis within 6 h.

Relation Between Collateral-Derived Residual MBF in the Risk Area and Ultimate Infarct Size

The estimation of ultimate infarction size with MCE is not as straightforward as risk area in the presence of total coronary occlusion. Experimental studies have demonstrated that histologic infarct size is usually smaller than the risk area defined using MCE. The area of true necrosis show variable sparing of the subepicardial region (Fig. 12.2). When the endocardial and epicardial extent of AMI are compared to similar measures of the risk area, the epicardial extent of risk area overestimates the epicardial extent of the established necrosis. The duration of the occlusion is an impor-

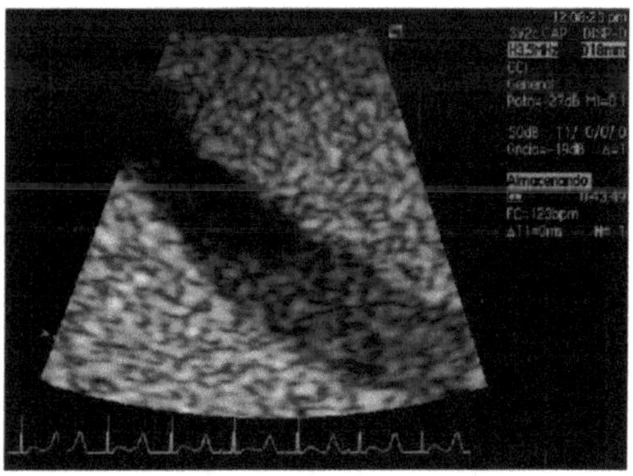

Fig. 12.2. Experimental studies have demonstrated that in acute myocardial infarction the area of true necrosis shows variable sparing of the subepicardial region. The degree of subepicardial sparing is related to the duration of the coronary occlusion and also to the degree of collateral flow to the risk area

tant factor in this discrepancy, because the transmural extent of AMI increases with the duration of coronary occlusion.

However, many experimental data have demonstrated that even for a given duration of coronary occlusion the final extent of AMI shows a great variability. This is due to the fact that not only the duration of coronary occlusion, but also other factors such as the size of the risk area and the amount of residual myocardial blood flow (MBF) within the risk area play a role in determining the final extent of AMI. The main factor that determines residual MBF in the risk area is the extent of collateral flow.

MCE is an excellent technique for evaluating collateral perfusion. Information from angiography can only be obtained for vessels larger than 100 μm in size, whereas most collaterals are much smaller. Probably for this reason a poor correlation between the angiographic collateral score and myocardial opacification from collateral vessels with MCE has been reported [12]. Spatial changes in collateral perfusion caused by altering the collateral driving pressure have been accurately measured with MCE. Kaul et al. in a canine experimental model demonstrated that manipulation of the perfusion pressure of the left anterior descending coronary artery could modify the perfusion and function of the acutely occluded left circumflex coronary [13].

This ability of MCE to identify collateral-derived MBF has long interested cardiologists, because it could allow the ultimate size of infarct shortly after coronary occlusion to be predicted. Kemper suggested using delayed low levels of myocardial opacification with MCE for detection of collateral-derived blood flow in the range that may allow myocyte survival and predict the mean transmural extent of AMI [14].

More recently, it was proposed by Coggins et al. to noninvasively determine ultimate infarct size by defining magnitude and spatial extent of collateral-dependent residual MBF within the risk area with MCE [15]. In an experimental model, intermittent harmonic imaging was used for MCE at pulsing intervals of <1 to 30 cardiac cycles. It was observed that during coronary occlusion, MCE perfusion defect size at prolonged pulsing intervals (PI >10.6±1.5 s) was smaller than measured at short pulsing intervals (PI 2.6±0.4 s) and the former correlated with infarct size in postmortem staining, whereas the latter correlated best with the risk area. The use of prolonged pulsing intervals allowed some degree of collateral-derived residual contrast refilling within the risk area and therefore was more strongly associated with ultimate infarct size. Interestingly, the extent of abnormal wall thickness markedly overestimated infarct size and correlated much better with the risk area than with ultimate infarct size. This recent study has greater clinical interest because it has been performed with venous contrast agents.

Clinical Utility of MCE in Nonreperfused AMI

Diagnostic Value of MCE in the Acute Phase of AMI Prior to Reperfusion Therapy

The concept of area at risk has been used widely in the clinical scenario [16, 17]. The value of intracoronary MCE in the delineation of an area at risk of necrosis during total coronary occlusion is well established (Figs. 12.3, 12.4) [18].

More recently, intravenous contrast agents have also been used for this purpose. A multicenter European trial performed with intravenous Sonazoid and harmonic imaging showed a high sensitivity of intravenous MCE for the detection of perfusion defects in patients with total occlusion of the infarct-related vessel, especially for anterior AMI. A group of 55 patients underwent serial perfusion studies before and after primary percutaneous transluminal coronary angioplasty (PTCA). In patients with anterior AMI, evaluation of perfusion defects was feasible on admission in 24 of 24 patients (100%) and in the remaining patients, who had an inferior AMI, diagnosis was feasible in 26 of 31 patients (84%). All patients with anterior AMI showed a perfusion defect except three patients; in these three patients, the infarct-related artery was open in the first angiography performed and showed a TIMI flow grade 3. The results of MCE in inferior AMI are not so accurate for this purpose. 13 of 23 patients did not show a perfusion defect in spite of a TIMI flow grade 0 in angiography. Although these results could be partly explained by the presence of collateral circulation, they may also be related to the existence of a smaller area at risk in inferior AMI that would be more difficult to diagnose with MCE [19].

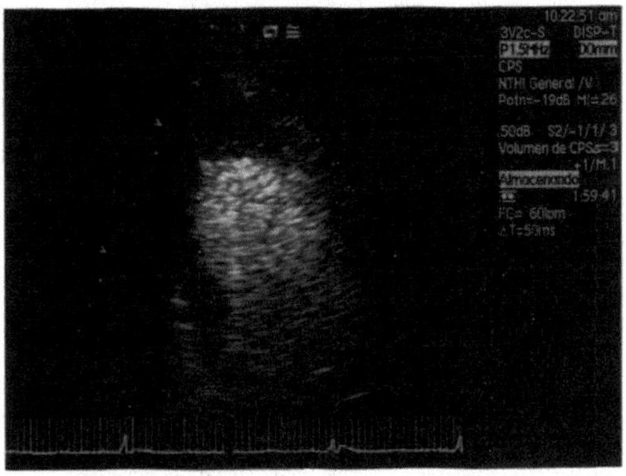

Fig. 12.3. A clear perfusion defect can be seen in this MCE study performed before angiography in this patient, admitted to the CCU for ACS. In anterior AMI, a multicenter european study demonstrated that it was possible to identify perfusion defects in 100% of the patients with a coronary occlusion

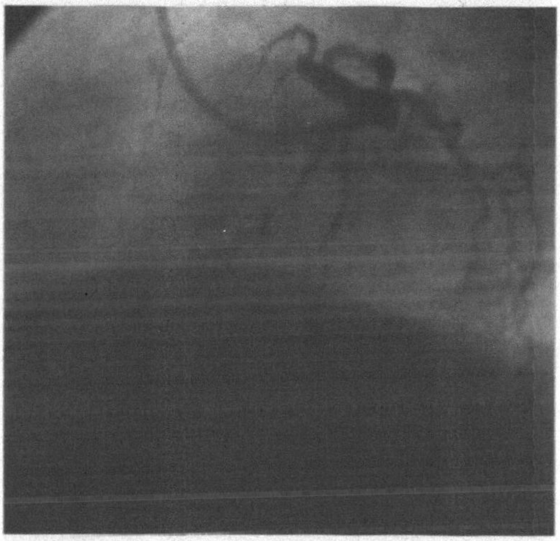

Fig. 12.4. Coronary angiography from the patient corresponding to Fig. 12.3. A proximal LAD occlusion was seen in the cath lab. The final result after primary PTCA was good

In a clinical setting, it would be more suitable to triage patients with AMI in the acute phase on the basis of the potential "worst-case scenario" ultimate infarction size than on the basis of risk area, because as we previously discussed the former can vary widely due to variability in collateral-derived residual MBF (Figs. 12.5A-C, 12.6). The size of irreversible myocardial injury can be defined with infarct-avid imaging agents

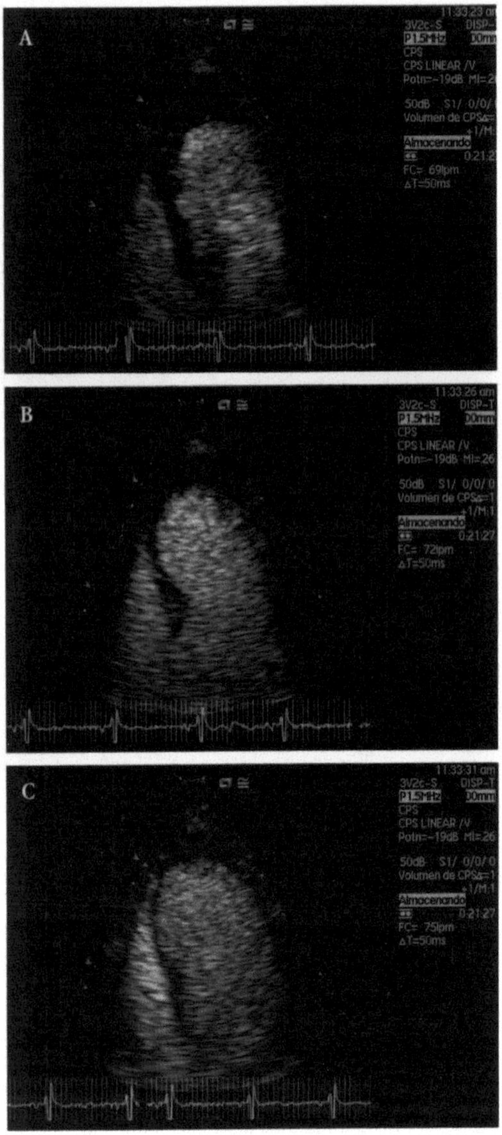

Fig. 12.5. Sequential images from a MCE study performed in a patient admitted to CCU for anterior myocardial infarction. In this case, shortly after microbubble destruction, hardly any myocardial refilling can be seen in the apical 4-chamber view (**A**). In the second image, nice refilling can be seen in the lateral wall and basal septum, but a large perfusion defect can still be seen (**B**). If a longer period of time is allowed for myocardial refilling, the extent of the perfusion defect is slowly reduced, suggesting the presence of collateral flow to the risk area (**C**)

such as Tc pirophosphate and I-labeled antimyosin antibodies. Unfortunately, these agents can be used when myocardial injury has already occurred but cannot predict infarct size at the time of occlusion. MCE could potentially play a role in this unanswered question, but clinical data evaluating MCE for this purpose are lacking.

Risk Stratification of Nonreperfused AMI After the Acute Phase with MCE

In a clinical setting, MCE is very useful for identifying collateral perfusion in presence of an occluded infarct-related artery. Sabia et al. established the percentage of perfusion bed supplied by collaterals before PTCA in 33 patients with recent MI and an occluded infarct-related artery (IRA) using MCE. For

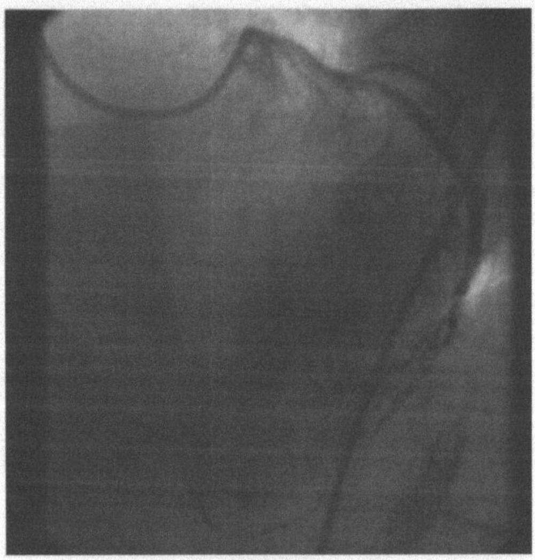

Fig. 12.6. Coronary angiography corresponding to the patient from Fig. 12.5. In this case, despite the LAD occlusion, the distal part of the vessel is refilled with collateral circulation coming from the LCx. Final infarct size will probably be smaller than expected due to the protective effect of this residual flow

this purpose, the size of the occluded bed was defined in patients after successful PTCA by injecting contrast directly into the opened IRA and expressed as a percentage of the myocardium in the short-axis view and compared to the perfusion defect observed prior to PTCA. Similar data have been obtained from patients with chronic MI [12, 20].

Evaluation of collateral-derived myocardial blood flow is important for evaluating the prognosis of patients with MI and for choosing the revascularization strategy, even after the acute phase. Myocardial tissue with residual MBF can be spared from necrosis even during persistent coronary occlusion lasting several days, although this low level of MBF may not be enough for maintaining a normal regional function. In such patients, revascularization of the IRA and improvement of anterograde coronary flow may lead to an improvement of regional function during follow-up, as demostrated by Sabia et al [21]. In this clinical study, MCE was performed to assess the percentage of the infarct bed perfused by collateral flow in 43 patients who had had an AMI 2 days to 5 weeks earlier and were referred to the catheterization laboratory for definition of their coronary anatomy. The IRA was successfully opened by angioplasty in 80% of the cases. Among the patients in whom angioplasty was successful, the 23 in whom more than 50% of the infarct bed was supplied by collateral flow had better wall motion and greater improvement in wall motion at 1 month than the 9 in whom less than 50% of the bed was supplied by collateral flow.

Interestingly, the degree of improvement in function was not influenced by the length of time between the infarction and the attempted angioplasty, demonstrating that the myocardium may remain viable for a prolonged period in many patients with acute infarction and an occluded IRA.

These findings have provided a physiological basis for the "open-artery hypothesis". The open-artery hypothesis suggests that a patent IRA confers a survival benefit greater than that expected from myocardial salvage alone, which extends beyond the time when preservation of left ventricular function is expected [22]. For this reason, MCE can play a role in the prognostic evaluation of patients with non-reperfused AMI, determining potentially viable segments and selecting patients who could benefit most from a delayed angioplasty of the IRA.

MCE in reperfused AMI: the Problem of No-reflow

No-reflow: Experimental Data

The no-reflow phenomenon was first described by Kloner et al. in 1974 [8]. This group discovered that prolonged ischemia of an epicardial coronary artery resulted in structural damage in the microvasculature that interfered with normal flow to myocytes, even when normal flow was restored in the epicardial artery. In this model, dogs were subjected to 40 or 90 min of proximal coronary artery occlusion. When the coronary occlusion was relieved after 40 min, blood flow was restored to the damaged myocardium as assessed with perfusion markers such as thioflavin S and carbon black. However, after 90 min of coronary occlusion, there was only partial restoration of blood flow to the myocardial tissue, despite the elimination of the coronary occlusion. Perfusion defects were more prominent in the subendocardium, in a similar manner to the ischemic wavefront phenomenon [7].

Anatomic no-reflow zones were examined with electron microscopy and significant capillary damage was observed. The most common findings were swollen endothelium and intraluminal endothelial protrusion and, less commonly, intraluminal plugging of platelets, fibrin and leukocytes.

No-reflow appears to be a process rather than an immediate event that occurs at the moment of reperfusion. Experimental studies have shown that the no-reflow area increases with time after reperfusion [23, 24]. During the ischemic phase, initial no-reflow zones appear to be related to endothelial damage and myocyte edema. With reperfusion, additional edema, myocyte contraction, platelets, fibrin and leucocyte plugging occur. These phenomena produce an expansion of the no-reflow zones during the first hours of reperfusion [25].

The most important factor involved in no-reflow is duration of coronary occlusion. If myocardial ischemia due to coronary occlusion has been sufficiently prolonged and severe, microvascular integrity is lost, and it is not possible to restore normal blood flow to the cardiac myocytes despite relief of the coronary occlusion. For this reason, the no-reflow area is confined to areas of infarcted tissue and indicates severe necrosis, as was demonstrated by Kemper in a canine model of coronary occlusion and reperfusion [9]. No-reflow may eventually produce inadequate healing of the cardiac scar or stop the development of future collaterals.

No-reflow has been extensively studied in experimental models with different techniques, such as nuclear imaging [26], contrast-enhanced magnetic resonance [27] and PET [28]. However, most information available about no-reflow has been obtained with MCE. No-flow to the area at risk following opening of the epicardial coronary artery [29] or a paradoxical persistence of the bubbles in the myocardium [30] are usually the manifestations of the no-reflow phenomenon.

Anatomical integrity of the microvasculature does not necessarily imply preserved function, and thus the microvessel vasodilating reserve may also be impaired [31]. A good correlation between the extent of infarction measured by triphenyltetrazolium chloride staining and the decrease in vascular conductance during maximal vasodilation with adenosine has been observed [32]. Functional impairment is not permanent in viable reperfused myocardium. Vanhaecke et al. showed in an experimental model that in viable reperfused tissue, as delineated by triphenyltetrazolium chloride staining, reflow in basal conditions is unimpaired. Endogenous coronary flow reserve is intact at the start of reperfusion, decreases by more than half after 2.5 h, and recovers completely within 1 week [33].

For many years, experimental MCE studies were performed with intracoronary injections of contrast agents. In the second half of the 1990s, Porter was the first to demonstrate that a contrast agent (PESDA, perfluoropropane-exposed sonicated dextrose albumin) administered via peripheral venous injection could visually identify myocardial perfusion abnormalities, and that finding was confirmed by other authors [34, 35]. This finding was absolutely relevant for clinical studies, as discussed in the next section.

Experimental Data: Dynamics of Myocardial Blood Flow After Reperfusion

The dynamics of microvascular flow shortly after reperfusion is spatially and temporally complex and variable. In the reperfused bed, regions of hyperemia, impaired flow reserve, low-reflow, and no- reflow can coexist.

With MCE three situations can be described within the infarcted bed:

- Severely necrotic area: this region, generally endocardial, will present anatomically damaged microcirculation and therefore no reflow with contrast echo.
- Partially necrotic area: this is an intermediate situation in which microcirculation function may be impaired even if little or no structural damage exists. Different patterns can be found, ranging from low reflow to normal or hyperemic flow with impaired flow reserve.
- Stunned area: this region will present structurally intact microcirculation, with preserved or hyperemic flow.

Cobb et al. were the first group to design an experiment to examine local effects of acute cellular injury on regional myocardial blood flow. They analyzed, after 2-h complete coronary occlusion and reperfusion, the relationship between radiolabeled microsphere-derived regional blood flow at 15 s, 15 min, 4 h and 3 days and the extent of subsequent cellular necrosis in tissue samples from the ischemic zone. Importantly, blood flow to acutely injured regions remained equal to or larger than flow to nonischemic regions 15 min after reperfusion, but at 4 h and 3 days after reperfusion, flow was significantly decreased in regions with greater than 50% infarction [36]. This was the first experimental evidence of the phenomenon of reactive hyperemia that transiently occurs after myocardial ischemia (Fig. 12.7A, B). Other studies have demonstrated that no-reflow occurs acutely on reperfusion in some areas, which are unable to reperfuse on reflow, but elsewhere a delayed fall in flow to areas that initially received adequate reperfusion is observed. Areas that showed late impairment of flow invariably demonstrated contraction band necrosis, whereas areas of immediate no-reflow showed the typical pattern of coagulation necrosis [23]. If severe necrosis exists, the ability to generate a hyperemic response is dramatically reduced.

These findings suggest that any flow tracer technique can underestimate infarct size if it is performed shortly after reperfusion. This has been confirmed in MCE examinations, performing serial studies after reperfusion. Villanueva et al. using a canine model of coronary occlusion–reperfusion, performed intracoronary contrast injections 15 min, 45 min, 2 h and 3 h after reflow, observing that at 15 min after reflow, MCE defect size underestimated infarct size by 50% [37]. It is admitted that the spatial extent of the no-reflow phenomenon esti-

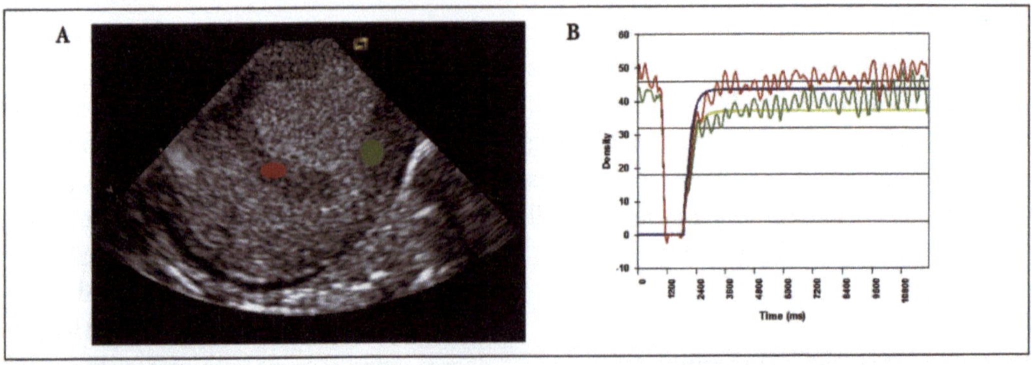

Fig. 12.7. Experimental studies have shown that blood flow to acutely injured regions remained equal to or larger than flow to nonischemic regions shortly after reperfusion. This phenomenon is known as reactive hyperemia. In this example, occlusion of proximal LAD was followed by reperfusion. Two ROIs were defined in anterior septum (ROI1, colour red) and posterior wall (ROI2, colour green) (**A**). Quantitative analysis showed that myocardial refilling slope and peak signal intensity were slightly higher in anterior septum (**B**)

mated with MCE is proportional to the spatial extent of necrosis, but infarct size is consistently underestimated [38].

It has been suggested that dipyridamole be i.v. administered to more accurately estimate infarct size shortly after reperfusion. The basis of dipyridamole use is that some regions with hyperemic flow within the ischemic bed may have some degree of functional impairment. Exogenous vasodilatation unmasks abnormalities in coronary vascular reserve specific to infarcted tissue. In the presence of dipyridamole, MCE accurately predicts the extent of infarction as early as 15 min after reperfusion [31]. Interestingly, impairment of coronary flow reserve remained relatively stable between 15 min and 3 h after reperfusion. Some concern exists, however, about the safety of administration of dipyridamole in the acute phase of myocardial infarction and this strategy is not currently used for estimation of infarct size in the clinical scenario. Another concern related to this strategy is that some groups have described microvascular stunning with reversible ischemia, comparable to myocardial stunning [39]. If this concept is accepted, vasodilators in the acute phase of AMI could also overestimate actual infarct size.

In conclusion, shortly after reperfusion, regions of no-reflow can be identified as resting perfusion defects, which correspond to areas with severe structural damage. Even though the extension of these perfusion defects is proportional to the real infarct size, perfusion defect size may fluctuate over time. Infarct size is most accurately measured in the presence of a vasodilator when MCE is performed shortly after reperfusion but an alternative strategy is assessing infarct size when hyperemic response has abated. Controversy still exists regarding when is the best moment to evaluate it, but it is generally admitted that hyperemic response has completely disappeared 48 h after AMI [40].

Clinical Data: Value of MCE for the Diagnosis of No-reflow

The real interest in no-reflow arose more than 15 years after Kloner's initial experimental models focused on that subject, when coronary angiographies began being performed to confirm the efficacy of thrombolytics. The first clinical data on no-reflow were described by Ito et al. in 1992, who investigated myocardial perfusion dynamics with MCE after thrombolysis in acute anterior myocardial infarction. MCE studies with intracoronary injections were performed before and immediately after successful reflow. Improvement in global and regional left ventricular function was greater in patients that showed significant contrast enhancement within the risk area than in the rest of patients, showing a residual contrast defect. The conclusions of this study were crucial: first, it underlined that angiographically successful reflow was not enough to confirm a successful myocardial reperfusion in AMI patients; besides, it confirmed in a homogeneous group of patients that a residual contrast defect in the risk area demonstrated immediately after reflow was a predictor of poor functional recovery [41].

Moreover, when transluminal coronary interventions became a widely used technique for reperfusion of AMI, the same finding of no-reflow was described in the catheterization laboratory immediately after patency of the infarct-related artery was restored. Clinical presentation was often sudden and dramatic: the dye stagnated in the coronary artery and the patient complained of chest pain, sometimes followed by hemodynamic compromise. These cases were easily diagnosed by angiography; however, more subtle cases of no-reflow were soon reported with normal angiographic data. Another study with MCE by Ito et al.

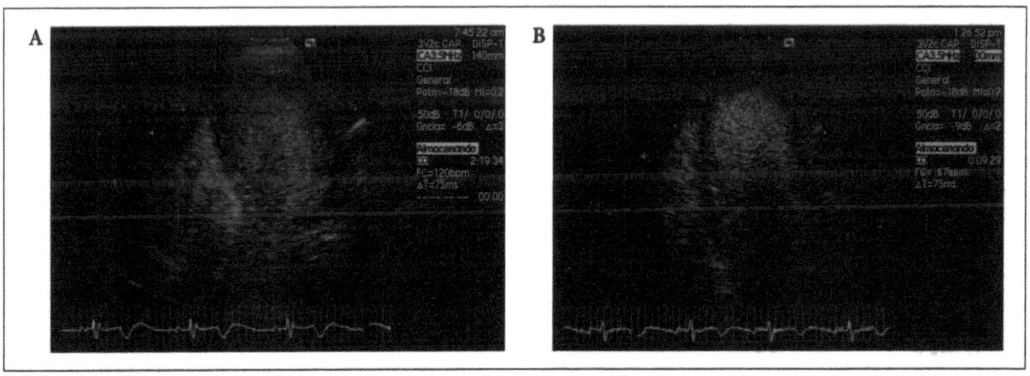

Fig. 12.8. A. MCE study corresponding to a patient admitted to the CCU for acute myocardial infarction (4 chamber apical view). A perfusion defect can be seen in the distal segments and apex; however, some residual flow can be seen in the risk area. Coronary angiography showed a severe lesion in the mid-LAD, but the coronary artery was open. **B.** After primary angioplasty, the perfusion defect is more severe, suggesting the presence of no-reflow. Primary angioplasty can contribute to microvascular damage because it can produce platelet microemboli

showed that more than 25% of patients with apparently brisk epicardial flow did not have adequate myocardial perfusion (Figs. 12.8, 12.9) [5].

This study demonstrated again that classical angiographic data were clearly insufficient to evaluate microvascular circulation. In the early 1980s, an angiographic classification of coronary blood flow patterns, thrombolysis in myocardial infarction (TIMI) was established. Grade 0 refers to no flow at all after the obstruction point. Grade 1 corresponds to material flowing beyond the area of obstruction but fails to opacify the entire artery. In grade 2, opacification of the entire artery distal to the occlusion point is observed but at a slower rate than normal, and grade 3 refers to normal coronary flow. TIMI classification was widely used but was only able to identify very severe no-reflow, which can be observed in TIMI 2 flow. Despite no obstructive lesion of the vessel, TIMI 2 flow is caused by advanced microvascular damage and is a highly specific predictor of poor outcome in patients with AMI. However, this finding has a low sensitivity in the detection of no-reflow; the final result of a TIMI 3 flow after primary angioplasty in the infarct-related artery does not preclude microvascular damage [42].

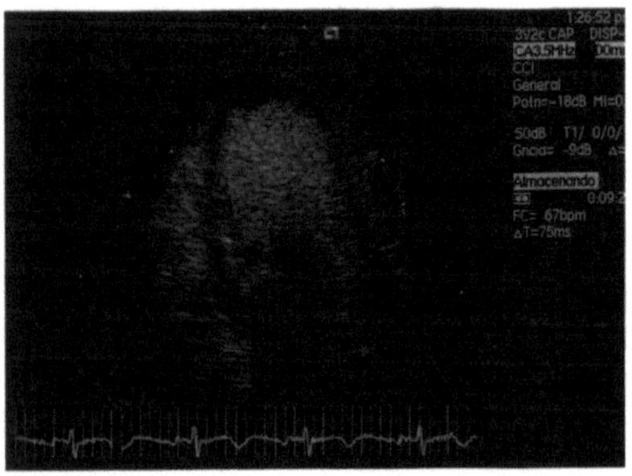

Fig. 12.9. In this case, final angiographic result was good (TIMI flow grade 3). Classical angiographic data are clearly insufficient to evaluate microvascular circulation. Ito et al have shown that more than 25% of patients with apparently brisk epicardial flow do not have adequate myocardial perfusion

This finding agrees with several studies that evaluated the ECG behavior after primary thrombolysis or coronary intervention. Persisting ST elevation after primary angioplasty (ST elevation ≥50% compared to ECG on admission) is found in more than one third of patients who undergo successful primary PTCA and has implications on clinical outcome [43, 44]. Moreover, it has been demostrated that rapid reduction in ST-segment elevation after direct coronary angioplasty or thrombolysis is associated with adequate reflow in MCE studies with intracoronary injections of contrast. On the contrary, if there is impaired microvascular perfusion in MCE, the ST elevation persists (see Fig. 12.10A-D) [45].

The pathophysiology of no-reflow observed in patients is partly different from experimental models of acute ischemia based on ligation of a coronary artery. In patients with AMI, reperfusion therapy plays an important role in the production of no-reflow. Either thrombolytic therapy or catheter-based reperfusion therapy promote the release of blood clots and platelet plugs in the microcirculation, which produce microemboli [46]. Moreover, with the increased use of stenting in catheter-based reperfusion of AMI, the problem of ather-

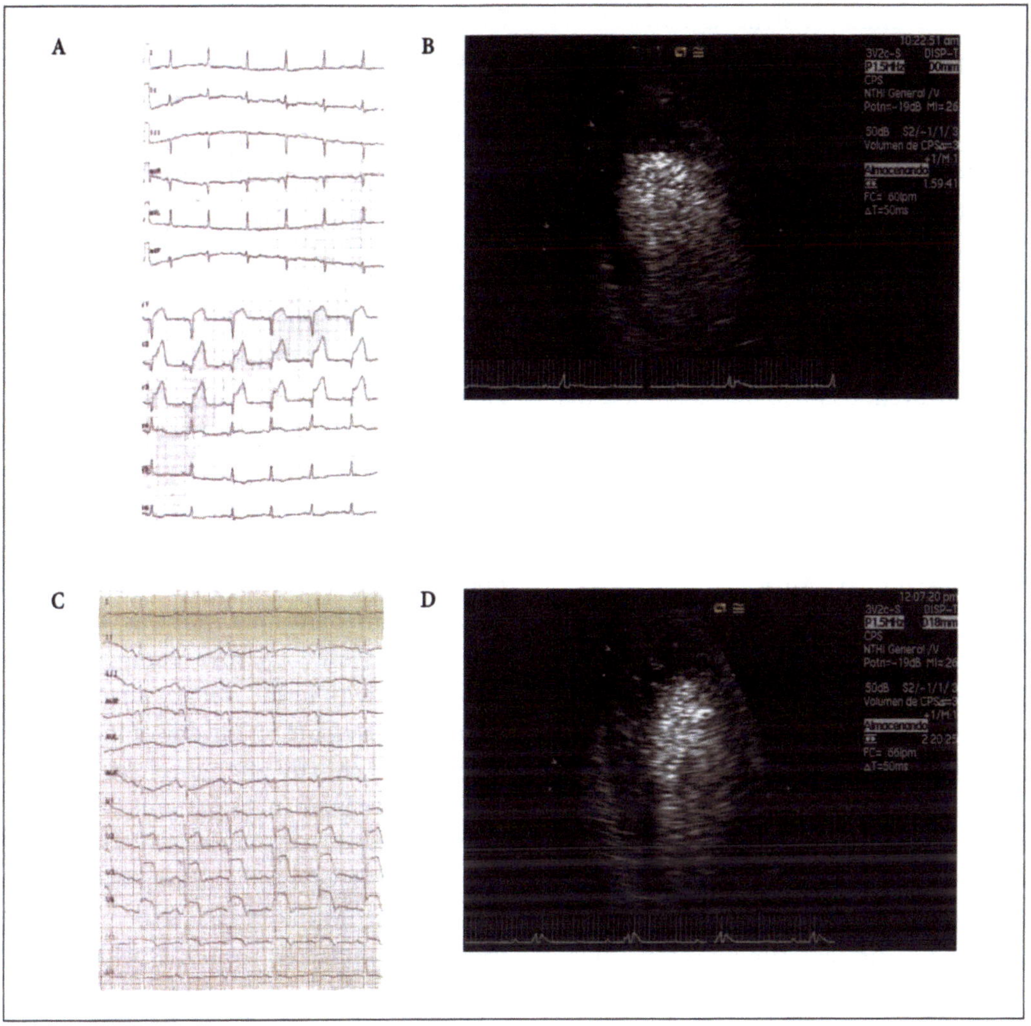

Fig. 12.10. In this patient admitted to CCU for anterior acute myocardial infarction, ST-segment elevation in the precordial leads and a clear perfusion defect can be seen before angiography (**A-B**) Despite a good angiographic result after primary PTCA, ST-segment elevation persists (**C**) and a smaller perfusion defect is still present in the MCE study (**D**)

osclerotic debris microemboli is exacerbated [6].

Although initial studies were made with intracoronary contrast injections, more recent studies have been published administering intravenous contrast in reperfused AMI, thus allowing noninvasive MCE studies [47,48]. The impact of this change in contrast administration (from intracoronary to intravenous) on the results of MCE is not fully understood yet. Probably, the no-reflow phenomenon has to be redefined for the use of an intravenous contrast agent, because nonphysiological high-pressure perfusion, which is present for intracoronary injections, is avoided for intravenous injection. It has been pointed out by some authors that more perfusion defects are observed after patency has been restored compared to previous intracoronary studies, but this finding remains controversial [19, 49]. Moreover, the meaning of this finding is not straightforward. Intravenous MCE may show a different detection rate in intermediate-or low-perfusion areas, but on the other hand it could be more reliable, because it is performed in more physiological conditions than intracoronary MCE.

Clinical Data: Dynamic Changes in Myocardial Blood Flow After Reperfusion in AMI

As discussed in previous paragraphs, several groups have shown in experimental models that a contrast defect may not be seen or may underestimate infarct size if MCE is performed immediately after reperfusion due to transient reactive hyperemia. However, the clinical scenario may present somewhat more significant differences compared to experimental models, especially if thrombolytic therapy is used as reperfusion therapy. The problem is that these differences are generally unpredictable. If a significant stenosis still exists at the time of reperfusion, it might limit hyperemia and allow a more accurate definition of infarct size shortly after reperfusion, but this is generally not the case, especially after primary PTCA. It is more frequent to see a nonsignificant residual stenosis; in this situation, variable degrees of reactive hyperemia can be found.

On the other hand, the occurrence of "microvascular stunning" (i.e., transient microvascular dysfunction due to ischemic injury) has also been demonstrated in experimental models and could also happen in AMI in humans. In conclusion, ischemic microvascular damage may be reversible or progressive after coronary reflow [39].

Temporal trends in MCE reflow patterns were studied in humans and, in a similar manner as shown in experimental models, temporal variability after AMI was observed. Ito et al. assessed microvascular function using MCE with intracoronary injections of sonicated ioxaglate on the day of infarction (before and shortly after coronary reflow) and 4 weeks later in 45 patients with successfully reperfused anterior AMI [50]. MCE images were analyzed determining corrected contrast intensity (baseline contrast intensity subtracted from the peak values in gray scale) in the risk area and in the normal posterior wall, and calculating the ratio of these (PI ratio). A general trend towards improvement in microvascular flow to the infarct bed at 28 days was noted, but the degree of improvement as assessed with the change in the PI ratio varied among patients. In patients with no-reflow, the spatial extent of the area of MCE no-reflow was reduced in the convalescent stage and the PI ratio increased in the late stage of infarction, suggesting that no-reflow could be partially reversible. PI ratio was still lower in the area of MCE no-reflow than in the area with MCE reflow, indicating that the microvasculature was less dense in the infarct region not only in the acute phase but also in the convalescent stage. As demonstrated in other studies, those patients that showed persistent no-reflow had the poorest systolic function recovery at follow-up evaluation.

Interestingly, correlation between PI ratio at day 1 and late-stage regional wall motion was rather poor, whereas it was much better when PI ratio was evaluated at day 28. Another interesting finding of this study is that a few patients with MCE reflow showed new areas of no-reflow in the late stage that had not been identified in the acute phase. These results are in agreement with previous experimental reports that recommended avoiding performing MCE during the period of reactive hyperemia that occurs shortly after reperfusion. Another study performed in anterior AMI successfully treated with primary PTCA with MCE shortly after reflow and 1 month later showed an association between persistent defects on MCE and intramyocardial hemorrhage on magnetic resonance imaging, a phenomenon which reflects severe microvascular injury [51].

More recently, dynamic changes in microvascular perfusion have also been assessed with intravenously injected contrast agents, obtaining similar results. Kamp et al. performed a serial evaluation of perfusion defects with intravenous Sonazoid and harmonic imaging in 59 patients with a first AMI episode, immediately before primary PTCA, 1 h and 12–24 h after PTCA. The extent of the perfusion defect at 12–24h was a predictor of systolic functional recovery at 4 weeks follow-up [19].

Another aspect of dynamic changes in MCE that is not fully understood is the progressive recovery of myocardial perfusion in the area of no reflow in the days following AMI, as was pointed out by Ito [50]. Brochet et al. demostrated that patients with reperfused AMI who showed an improvement of contrast score from day 1 (shortly after reflow) to day 9 more frequently exhibited contractile reserve at dobutamine echocardiography than patients with sustained no-reflow. These patients also showed significant improvement in wall motion at follow-up [52]. It is generally accepted that the reversible portion of no-reflow area is always outside the necrotic area. In contrast to reactive hyperemia this phenomenon of improvement of perfusion within the no-reflow area is progressive. It has been related to transient microvascular obstruction [46].

Value of MCE for Prediction of Systolic Functional Recovery in Reperfused AMI

As discussed in the previous section, microcirculation damage and no-reflow only appear in areas of necrotic myocardium. The basis for using MCE to evaluate myocardial viability is that regions with microvascular damage (corresponding to severe necrosis and therefore probably nonviable) will appear as contrast perfusion defects. MCE after reperfusion could be more exact than regional systolic function for this purpose. Several days after reflow, systolic function of the whole risk area may be depressed despite the presence of viable myocardium, because of myocardial stunning [53, 54].

The first data on the prognostic value of MCE in reperfused AMI to predict functional recovery were stated in the classical study by Ito et al. In 39 patients with anterior AMI, intracoronary ioxaglate was administered before and immediately after successful reflow. The residual contrast defect in the risk area demonstrated immediately after reflow was a predictor of poor functional recovery of the postischemic myocardium [41].

All these data confirm that the easiest approach to assess infarct size and predict recovery of regional function during follow-up is to perform MCE at a time outside the window of dynamic changes in myocardial blood flow that take place immediately after reperfusion. Although the optimal time to perform MCE is not determined, it is generally accepted that reactive hyperemia after reflow has disappeared 24-48 h after AMI [55]. Of course, the only limitation of this strategy is that MCE cannot help to decide any intervention immediately after reperfusion therapy, which could be especially useful in the case of thrombolytic therapy. The alternative of using dypiridamole in the acute phase of AMI to assess infarct size is generally not pursued for safety reasons. Moreover, if a significant stenosis persisted after thrombolysis it would also not be an accurate technique. If exogenous hyperemia was induced in this situation, severe hypoperfusion would be induced in the entire infarct-related area perfusion bed which would overestimate infarct size.

Many studies performing MCE after reperfusion have confirmed its ability to predict recovery of regional function during follow-up. Ragosta et al. evaluated 105 patients with a recent AMI using intracoronary MCE and two-dimensional echocardiography more than a day after admission, when these patients were referred to the cardiac catheterization laboratory. A contrast score index was derived by assigning a semiquantitative score to individual segments within the infarct zone (0 = no contrast effect, 0.5 = intermediate contrast effect and 1 = homogeneous contrast effect) and deriving the average score within the infarct bed. In the 90 patients with an open IRA, a strong correlation was noted between wall motion score 1 month later and the contrast score index [56].These data suggest that the presence of perfusion in MCE studies can be used as a surrogate for myocardial viability in patients with recent infarction.

However, the real interest of MCE as a predictor of myocardial viability is using it as a noninvasive technique. The development of new contrast agents with more persistance and nonlinear imaging technologies that can be administered in a peripheral vein has allowed MCE studies to be performed outside the catheterization laboratory. More recent studies performed with intravenous contrast agents have also demostrated the value of MCE in predicting systolic function recovery.

The first study assessing the prognostic value of MCE for systolic function recovery performed with an intravenous contrast agent was published 2 years ago by Rocchi et al [47]. MCE was performed with power Doppler and PESDA (perfluorocarbon-exposed sonicated dextrose albumin) via continuous infusion in 30 patients, 2 days after their first myocardial infarction. Two-dimensional echocardiography was repeated after 6 weeks and segments recovering wall motion in the follow-up echocardiographic study were defined as stunning myocardium. The most interesting finding of this study is that akinetic but perfused myocardium on the second day after the infarction showed a better late recovery of wall motion compared with dysfunctional and nonperfused myocardium. A good correlation with SPECT for the assessment of normal and abnormal perfusion was also described.

Other studies performed with intravenous contrast agents confirm the prognostic value of MCE. In the previously mentioned study performed by Kamp et al. consisting of patients treated with primary PTCA, multiple regression analysis in patients with an anterior AMI revealed that the only independent predictors for left ventricular recovery at 4 weeks follow-up were TIMI flow grade 3 after primary PTCA and the extent of the perfusion defect evaluated 12–24 h after symptom onset [19]. In another type of population, consisting mainly in AMI patients treated with thrombolysis, the predictive value of MCE for functional recovery was also studied. Swinburn et al. evaluated 96 patients with MCE 4.8±1.7 days after AMI and correlated the perfusion data with long-term contractile function during a mean follow-up of 179 days. Optison was intravenously administered in slow boluses and pulse inversion harmonic imaging with a mechanical index of 0.9. MCE was scored semiquantitatively (1: homogeneous contrast opacification, 2: reduced or heterogeneous contrast opacification, 3: no contrast opacification). The median contrast defect index was significantly higher in segments that did not recover than in those that did. Results were better using delayed triggers (1:5 and 1:10 cardiac cycles), which is not surprising taking into account that 74% of the patients had infarct-related stenosis of more than 90% and thus low myocardial blood flow was very frequent. The most important result of the study was the high negative predictive value of MCE for functional recovery (84%). Positive predictive value in revascularized patients was acceptable (78%), whereas it was rather poor in nonrevascularized patients (34%) in whom hibernating myocardium is not expected to recover [48].

More recently, some information has become available regarding utility of real-time techniques for post-AMI prediction of functional recovery. Main et al. assessed perfusion patterns with real-time pulse inversion power Doppler imaging in 34 patients 2 days after AMI, most of them with TIMI grade 3 in angiography before or immediately after MCE. The presence of perfusion in the MCE study predicted recovery of regional systolic function during follow-up (55±20 days) with a positive predictive value of 90%, negative predictive value of 63% and overall accuracy of 79%. Demonstration of MCE flow 2 days after AMI was a strong predictor of functional recovery: 90% of segments showing MCE improved function at follow-up evaluation;

on the contrary, most segments with no reflow showed no functional recovery at follow-up [57]. However, the rather poor negative predictive value described in this study indicates that artifactual defects secondary to attenuation and rib shadowing are still a problem in real-time techniques and require additional experience.

Comparison Between MCE and Other Techniques for Prediction of Systolic Functional Recovery in Reperfused AMI

The limited value of the TIMI angiographic classification of coronary blood flow patterns in assessing microvascular function has led to the definition of new invasive parameters that could be more accurate for assessing the final result of PTCA and short- and long-term prognosis. The most spread parameters are corrected TIMI frame count and TIMI myocardial perfusion grade ("myocardial blush"). TIMI frame count is a parameter that corresponds to the number of cineframes needed for the dye to reach standardized distal landmarks [58]. TIMI myocardial perfusion grade (TMPG) is defined from 0 to 3: TMPG 0, minimal or no myocardial blush; TMPG 1, dye stains the myocardium and this stain persists on the next injection; TMPG 2, dye enters the myocardium but washes out slowly so that dye is strongly persistent at the end of the injection; and TMPG 3, there is normal entrance and exit of dye in the myocardium so that dye is mildly persistent at the end of the injection [59].

Interestingly, MCE has been compared with these new invasive measurements for predicting myocardial systolic function recovery. Lepper et al. assessed the predictive value of postprimary PTCA MCE (performed with intravenous injections of Sonazoid and harmonic intermittent imaging) for follow-up left ventricular function in 38 patients with AMI. The predictive value of MCE was compared with ST-segment elevation index and invasive measurements (angiographic myocardial perfusion grade, corrected TIMI frame count and coronary flow reserve). In an analysis of variance MCE after PTCA was the best parameter for predicting left ventricular function 4 weeks after AMI [60]. A recently published study confirms that the new parameters obtained from angiography are not good predictors of post-MI wall motion recovery during follow-up [61]. This finding may be explained by the fact that all invasive parameters reflect the microvascular function of a given perfusion bed, irrespective of the size of the myocardial territory supplied by the evaluated coronary artery, whereas MCE also assesses the size of the no-reflow area.

Measurement of coronary flow reserve with intracoronary Doppler is an established tool for assessment of microvascular function, although it reflects a different aspect of regional microcirculation compared to MCE and, as TIMI frame count and MPG, it does not take into account the size of the territory supplied by the evaluated coronary artery. However, it is interesting to note that in AMI, an increase of coronary flow reserve is observed in the majority of patients within 24 h after infarct-related artery recanalization and these changes are associated with reduction of MCE perfusion defects. In a study, immediately after angioplasty, no significant differences were observed between the groups with no reflow and reflow. After 24 h, however, patients with reflow had a significantly higher coronary flow reserve than patients with no-reflow [62]. MCE reduction of perfusion defects and coronary flow reserve recovery develop in a parallel fashion after AMI, which is not surprising, because capillaries play a crucial role in the regulation of coronary blood flow [63].

MCE has also been compared with dobutamine echo to analyze their predictive value for contractile function recovery. As previously mentioned, the basis of the use of MCE to evaluate myocardial viability is that areas with severe microcirculation damage have suffered the most severe injury and are probably nonviable. However, in MCE studies, microvascular integrity is used as a surrogate of myocardial contractile function, whereas dobutamine echocardiography assesses viability in an absolutely different manner, exploring the myocardial contractile reserve. Iliceto et al. performed MCE studies and low-dose dobutamine echocardiography in 24 patients before hospital discharge and re-evaluated them 3 months later. MCE had 100% sensitivity and 46% specificity in identifying viable myocardial segments, whereas low-dose dobutamine echocardiography had 71% sensitivity and 88% sensitivity [64]. Other studies have confirmed that microvascular integrity is a prerequisite for myocardial viability [65]. Whereas normal perfusion is not always associated with late functional improvement, persistently impaired perfusion has been consistently associated with lack of functional improvement during follow-up. MCE and low-dose dobutamine echocardiography could be useful as complimentary techniques for the detection of myocardial viability.

Relationship Between MCE Data and Post-AMI Complications

The presence of no-reflow on MCE is predictive of acute complications after AMI. This phenomenon is probably due to the fact that the extent of no-reflow parallels infarct size. Predictive factors for development of the no-reflow phenomenon have been widely studied. In a study that included 199 patients with anterior AMI treated successfully with primary PTCA (TIMI flow grade 3), intracoronary contrast was administered to assess MCE-derived no-reflow area after PTCA and predictive factors were determined. Absence of preinfarction angina, number of Q-waves on ECG, wall motion score, and TIMI flow grade 0 at initial coronary angiography were the independent predictors of no-reflow. In conclusion, the occurrence of no-reflow is related to the infarct size (number of Q-waves), the size of the risk area (assessed in this case with the wall motion score) and the occlusion state of the infarct-related artery before starting any reperfusion therapy.

Ito et al. were the first to evaluate the clinical prognostic value of no-reflow by studying complications, left ventricular morphology, and in-hospital survival after AMI. In total, 126 patients with first anterior AMI treated with reperfusion therapy within 24 h of onset of symptoms underwent intracoronary MCE before and shortly after coronary reflow. Of the 126 patients, 47 (37%) showed MCE no-reflow. Pericardial effusion and early congestive heart failure were observed more frequently in patients with MCE no-reflow than in those with MCE reflow, and heart failure tended to be prolonged in those with MCE no-reflow. Three patients of the subset with no-reflow died of pump failure. Left ventricular end-diastolic volume progressively increased at 1-month follow-up in patients with MCE no-reflow whereas it decreased in those with MCE reflow. These results suggest that the presence of no-reflow correlates with the occurrence of adverse left ventricular remodeling [5].

These data have been confirmed with intravenous MCE. Porter observed that a persistent contrast defect in the infarct zone demonstrated with PESDA following restoration of TIMI grade 3 flow in the IRA identified patients likely to show an increase in left ventricular end-systolic volume and a decrease in ejection fraction during follow-up [49].

In conclusion, the relationship between no reflow and deterioration of regional and global systolic function is well established. It has been suggested that even partial subepicardial myocardial perfusion, which would probably not be sufficient to allow systolic motion recovery, could protect against adverse remodeling [48].

Postprocessing and Image Analysis of Intravenous MCE in AMI: Semiquantitative and Quantitative Methods

Technology developed for MCE is rapidly evolving. From the initial intracoronary studies, the development of new contrast agents more resistant to high pressures and nonlinear imaging technology has allowed use of intravenous contrast agents. The machine settings used in the different MCE studies focused on AMI are dependent on the technology used and the contrast agents applied [66]. It is not easy to set up a study protocol in a field in which knowledge of how to use an evolving technology is continuously changing. These factors make it difficult to compare the results from different studies and MCE still lacks adequate standardization.

Most MCE perfusion studies have been evaluated with visual analysis and semiquantitative scores. The most simple score consists of two categories: absence of perfusion and any degree of myocardial perfusion. Due to the limited information obtained in this way, another score which differentiates three categories has been defined [48, 49]: bright contrast enhancement, patchy or subepicardial contrast enhancement, no contrast enhancement. Visual semiquantitative analysis has several advantages: it is easy and at least can provide some information very quickly regarding probability of recovery of systolic function. However, several drawbacks must be noted: visual analysis is subjective and information obtained is rather incomplete. It is not clear whether patchy and subendocardial contrast enhancement have the same meaning. Semiquantitative scores do not take into account the dynamic information provided by the rate of microcirculation replenishment, but only a global information about brightness of contrast enhancement.

These limitations have stimulated the research related to quantitative methods for intravenous MCE. In 1998, Wei et al. defined a method to assess myocardial blood flow using ultrasound-induced microbubble destruction followed by microbubble replenishment during a continuous venous infusion of contrast agent. This method is based on the measurement of the microbubble reappearance rate after destruction, which provides an estimation of mean myocardial microbubble velocity (B), and the measurement of plateau video intensity at long pulsing intervals, which reflects the microvascular cross-sectional area (A). Hence, with this method both components of myocardial blood flow, blood volume and blood flow velocity, are measured and therefore myocardial blood flow itself is assessed with a combined index, which corresponds to the product of blood volume and blood flow velocity AxB. MCE-derived blood flow velocity and myocardial blood flow index obtained with this method show an excellent correlation with radiolabeled microspheres-derived myocardial blood flow. This study has been the cornerstone of MCE quantitative analysis [67].

The initial study by Wei was performed with intermittent triggered imaging and different pulsing intervals. The myocardial video intensity versus pulsing interval plots were fitted to an exponential function ($y=A(1-e^{-bt})$). More recently, similar replenishment curves plotting video intensity versus time after microbubble destruction have been obtained for real-time MCE studies [68]. Good correlation has also been observed between myocardial blood velocity and myocardial blood flow index and microsphere-derived myocardial blood flow in real-time MCE [69].

It is possible that quantitative techniques using video densitometric analysis might improve overall accuracy of MCE for post-MI assessment. However, most data related to quantitative MCE analysis correspond to experimental studies. Little information has been obtained from a clinical setting. A study focused on identification of hibernating myocardium with quantitative intravenous MCE has been recently published by Shimoni et al [70]. In this study, 20 patients with coronary artery disease and ventricular dysfunction underwent MCE with Optison infusion and intermittent pulse inversion harmonics. MCE replenishment curves were constructed and fitted to an exponential curve to calculate A, B and AxB. The best MCE parameter for predicting functional recovery was AxB. A cut-off point of AxB>1.5 dB/s showed 90% sensitivity for recovery of systolic function. Though not focused on post-MI patients, this study suggests that quantitative analysis of MCE studies could actually play a role in the detection of viable tissue in other clinical studies.

Our echocardiography laboratory has started a quantitative MCE protocol in AMI patients. MCE studies have been performed on 22 patients admitted to hospital for AMI, before and shortly after primary PTCA. MCE studies were performed with SonoVue continuous infusion and CPS (contrast pulse sequence), a new real-time technology implemented in Acuson-Siemens Sequoia equipment. Quantitative analysis was performed on 15 patients with successful primary angioplasty (final result TIMI flow grade 3) in the IRA and good or acceptable acoustic window. In each patient, VDI plateau (A), slope of VDI ascending curve (B), and product AxB were calculated in an akinetic segment with patchy or homogeneous opacification and compared to the normokinetic segment with the highest VDI in the same echocardiographic view (four-chamber or two-chamber apical views), as can be seen in figures 12.11, 12.12. Mean VDI plateau was higher in normokinetic than in akinetic segments (19.6±1.8 dB and 11.6±1.6 dB, p=0.003) and so was the mean VDI slope of replenishment curve (1.08±0.24 and 0.70±0.23, p=0.04). Three flow patterns could be defined: in 40% of the cases, akinetic segments showed acceptable A and B values (>50% from corresponding values in normokinetic segments); in 40% of the cases, the VDI slope of the replenishment curve was severely impaired (B <50% from control values); in the remaining 20% of cases, both A and B were depressed (<50% from control values). These results suggest that in spite of successful primary PTCA, different grades of impairment of microvascular perfusion can be identified with MCE quantitative analysis in AMI patients. It is also interesting to note the limitations of a semiquantitative score, because a large range of impairment was observed within normal or intermediate ("patchy") categories of the semiquantitative score. These differences probably have prognostic implications

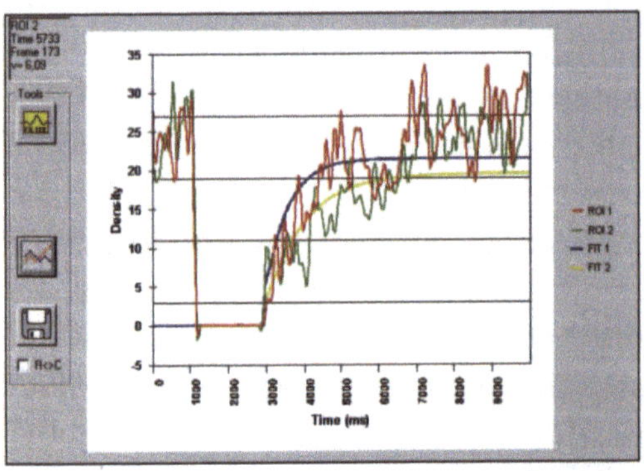

Fig. 12.11. Quantitative analysis of myocardial perfusion in acute myocardial infarction after primary angioplasty. The curve in red corresponds to a normokynetic segment and the curve in green corresponds to an akynetic segment of the risk area. Exponential fitting has been performed for both curves. In this case, only slight differences exist between both segments

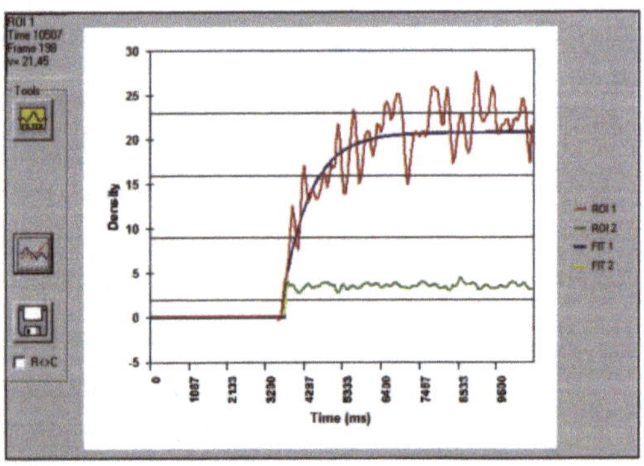

Fig. 12.12. A different example of myocardial perfusion after myocardial infarction, with the same colour coding for both curves. Myocardial perfusion is nulled in the pathological region of interest, whereas the control segment shows a nice perfusion curve. Very large differences in perfusion patterns can be seen among patients in spite of a good angiographic result in all cases

regarding myocardial function recovery during follow-up.

Feasibility of MCE analysis, whether qualitative or quantitative, depends on the quality of the image, which can be a limitation. In a multicenter European study on patients with AMI referred for primary PTCA, feasibility of evaluation of myocardial perfusion defects before primary angioplasty was exellent in patients with anterior AMI (24 of 24 patients, 100%), but lower in those with inferior MI (26 of 31 patients, 84%) [19]. The experience of Shimoni et al. indicates a slighty lower feasibility for quantitative analysis compared with qualitative analysis: 74% of segments with quantitative analysis and 80% with qualitative. In their study, inability to evaluate myocardial perfusion was predominantly seen in basilar segments, mostly because of attenuation [70].

Our experience with real-time MCE is in agreement with these results. Clinical feasibility of CCI (coherent contrast imaging, a pulse cancellation method) was evaluated in our laboratory in 547 segments, using a semiquantitative score that ranged from 0 to 3 (0: not visualized; 1: suboptimal; incomplete definition of endocardium; 2: acceptable, complete definition of endo cardium and incomplete of epicardial boundary; 3: optimal, complete definition of endo-and epicardium). Acceptable or optimal images could generally be obtained (average score of all segments was 2.5) except for basal lateral and mid-basal anterior segments in which feasibility of MCE was lower (average score of 1.4, 1.3 and 0.8, Fig. 12.13) [71].

Other questions in image analysis require a special comment in the case of AMI. The effect of background myocardial backscatter can seriously affect MCE studies. During B-mode second harmonic imaging without contrast enhancement, infarcted regions tend to appear brighter than normal myocardium, thus video intensity in the infarct bed is higher than the remaining myocardium before contrast administration and this may produce "false-negative" studies (i.e., non-identified perfusion defects) if not adequately corrected. Two approaches can be used, background substraction or technologies with good tissue supressor (power Doppler, cancellation pulse-based techniques).

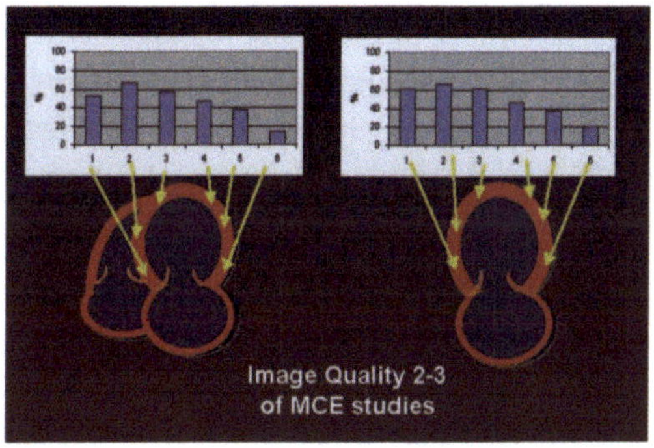

Fig. 12.13. Feasibility of a real-time MCE technique in a non-selected population (CCI, a cancellation pulse technique). Apical segments, septum and inferior wall show good image quality. In some patients it is difficult to obtain images of the basal segments of lateral and anterior wall

Another critical point in MCE analysis is the measurement of slow blood flow velocities associated with collateral myocardial blood flow. In intermittent triggered imaging and intravenous MCE in continuous infusion, it has been demostrated that high pulsing intervals (1:8 to 1:10), which allow identification of low flow to the infarct territory, are more appropriate for the prediction of infarct size and myocardial recovery than low pulsing intervals [72]. The ideal method to acquire long imaging sequences for this purpose in real-time imaging is not yet defined.

Conclusions

Perfusion imaging with MCE in AMI can provide useful information on admission and after reperfusion therapy. MCE can define the area at risk during coronary occlusion, with especially high sensitivity in anterior AMI, and can be useful in the emergency room for the diagnosis of equivocal cases and to help in immediate risk stratification. In nonreperfused infarcts, it can also provide information regarding collateral circulation to the infarct-related artery.

MCE perfusion patterns after primary PTCA give more complete information about restoration of flow at the microcirculation level than both angiographic patency data and even new invasive parameters recently developed such as myocardial blush. It allows the diagnosis of no-reflow and the evaluation of dynamic changes that take place in myocardial perfusion after reflow. A consistent finding in several studies is that a large number of patients have microvascular damage in spite of IRA patency. This phenomenon has prognostic relevance, because the presence of perfusion defects related to no-reflow is related to less recovery in left ventricular systolic function, adverse ventricular remodeling and acute complications after AMI.

MCE after thrombolysis could be very useful to noninvasively confirm the recanalization of the infarct artery, although clinical studies are needed to evaluate the results of this approach since information is lacking in this area.

No-reflow is a complex phenomenon related to severe ischemia but also to microembolism after reperfusion therapy. Treatments aimed at reducing microvascular damage are currently under investigation and could be evaluated with MCE, such as verapamil, nicorandil, adenosine and catheter-based techniques against microembolism.

In the last few years, MCE has seen an increasing field of application in AMI, especially related to changing the administration technique of the contrast agent. Intravenous MCE is a truly noninvasive technique and allows serial studies with minimal risk to the patient, which makes this technique increasingly attractive. However, there is still room for improvement, especially regarding the quality of images (particularly basal segments), standardization of the technique, and accurate analysis of the imaging sequences.

References

1. FTT. Indications for fibrinolytic therapy in suspected acute myocardial infarction. Collaborative overview of early mortality and major morbidity results from all randomised trials of more than 1000 patients. Lancet 1994; 343: 311-322
2. Zijlstra F, Hoorntje JC, de Boer MJ, Reiffers S, Miedema K, Ottervanger JP, et al. Long-term benefit of primary angioplasty as compared with thrombolytic therapy for acute myocardial infarction. N Engl J Med 1999; 341 (19): 1413-9
3. Schomig A, Kastrati A, Dirschinger J, Mehilli J, Schricke U, Pache J, et al. Coronary stenting plus platelet glycoprotein IIb/IIIa blockade compared with tissue plasminogen activator in acute myocardial infarction. Stent versus Thrombolysis for Occluded Coronary Arteries in Patients with Acute Myocardial Infarction Study Investigators. N Engl J Med 2000; 343 (6): 385-91
4. GISSI. Gruppo Italiano per lo studio della streptochinasi nell'Infarto miocardico (GISSI). Effectiveness of intravenous thrombolytic treatment in acute myocardial infarction. Lancet 1986 (1): 397-401
5. Ito H, Maruyama A, Iwakura K, Takiuchi S, Masuyama T, Hori M, et al. Clinical implications of the 'no reflow' phenomenon. A predictor of complications and left ventricular remodeling in reperfused anterior wall myocardial infarction. Circulation 1996; 93 (2): 223-8
6. Topol EJ, Yadav JS. Recognition of the importance of embolization in atherosclerotic vascular disease. Circulation 2000; 101 (5): 570-80
7. Reimer KA, Jennings RB. The "wavefront phenomenon" of myocardial ischemic cell death. II. Transmural progression of necrosis within the framework of ischemic bed size (myocardium at risk) and collateral flow. Lab Invest 1979; 40 (6): 633-44
8. Kloner RA, Ganote CE, Jennings RB. The "no-reflow" phenomenon after temporary coronary occlusion in the dog. J Clin Invest 1974; 54 (6): 1496-508
9. Kemper AJ, O'Boyle JE, Cohen CA, Taylor A, Parisi AF. Hydrogen peroxide contrast echocardiography: quantification in vivo of myocardial risk area during coronary occlusion and of the necrotic area remaining after myocardial reperfusion. Circulation 1984; 70 (2): 309-17
10. Lindner JR, Ismail S, Spotnitz WD, Skyba DM, Jayaweera AR, Kaul S. Albumin microbubble persistence during myocardial contrast echocardiography is associated with microvascular endothelial glycocalyx damage. Circulation 1998; 98 (20): 2187-94
11. Kaul S, Glasheen W, Ruddy TD, Pandian NG, Weyman AE, Okada RD. The importance of defining left ventricular area at risk in vivo during acute myocardial infarction: an experimental evaluation with myocardial contrast two-dimensional echocardiography. Circulation 1987; 75 (6): 1249-60
12. Sabia PJ, Powers ER, Jayaweera AR, Ragosta M, Kaul S. Functional significance of collateral blood flow in patients with recent acute myocardial infarction. A study using myocardial contrast echocardiography. Circulation 1992; 85 (6): 2080-9
13. Kaul S, Pandian NG, Guerrero JL, Gillam LD, Okada RD, Weyman AE. Effects of selectively altering collateral driving pressure on regional perfusion and function in occluded coronary bed in the dog. Circ Res 1987; 61 (1): 77-85
14. Kemper AJ, Force T, Perkins L, Gilfoil M, Parisi AF. In vivo prediction of the transmural extent of experimental acute myocardial infarction using contrast echocardiography. J Am Coll Cardiol 1986; 8 (1): 143-9
15. Coggins MP, Sklenar J, Le DE, Wei K, Lindner JR, Kaul S. Noninvasive prediction of ultimate infarct size at the time of acute coronary occlusion based on the extent and magnitude of collateral-derived myocardial blood flow. Circulation 2001; 104 (20): 2471-7
16. Feiring AJ, Johnson MR, Kioschos JM, Kirchner PT, Marcus ML, White CW. The importance of the determination of the myocardial area at risk in the evaluation of the outcome of acute myocardial infarction in patients. Circulation 1987; 75 (5): 980-7
17. Touchstone DA, Nygaard TW, Kaul S. Correlation between left ventricular risk area and clinical, electrocardiographic, hemodynamic, and angiographic variables during acute myocardial infarction. J Am Soc Echocardiogr 1990; 3 (2): 106-17
18. Kaul S. Assessment of myocardial perfusion with contrast echocardiography. In: Principles and practice of echocardiography, A Weyman. Ed Lea &Febiger 1994: 687-719
19. Kamp O, Lepper W, Vanoverschelde JL, Aeschbacher BC, Rovai D, Assayag P, et al. Serial evaluation of perfusion defects in patients with a first acute myocardial infarction referred for primary PTCA using intravenous myocardial contrast echocardiography. Eur Heart J 2001; 22 (16): 1485-95
20. Vernon SM, Camarano G, Kaul S, Sarembock IJ, Gimple LW, Powers ER, et al. Myocardial contrast echocardiography demonstrates that collateral flow can preserve myocardial function beyond a chronically occluded coronary artery. Am J Cardiol 1996; 78 (8): 958-60
21. Sabia PJ, Powers ER, Ragosta M, Sarembock IJ, Burwell LR, Kaul S. An association between collateral blood flow and myocardial viability in patients with

recent myocardial infarction. N Engl J Med 1992; 327 (26): 1825-31

22. Puma JA, Sketch MH, Jr., Thompson TD, Simes RJ, Morris DC, White HD, et al. Support for the open-artery hypothesis in survivors of acute myocardial infarction: analysis of 11,228 patients treated with thrombolytic therapy. Am J Cardiol 1999; 83 (4): 482-7
23. Ambrosio G, Weisman HF, Mannisi JA, Becker LC. Progressive impairment of regional myocardial perfusion after initial restoration of postischemic blood flow. Circulation 1989; 80 (6): 1846-61
24. Kloner RA. Does reperfusion injury exist in humans? J Am Coll Cardiol 1993; 21 (2): 537-45
25. Rezkalla SH, Kloner RA. No-reflow phenomenon. Circulation 2002; 105 (5): 656-62
26. Kondo M, Nakano A, Saito D, Shimono Y. Assessment of "microvascular no-reflow phenomenon" using technetium-99m macroaggregated albumin scintigraphy in patients with acute myocardial infarction. J Am Coll Cardiol 1998; 32 (4): 898-903
27. Bremerich J, Wendland MF, Arheden H, Wyttenbach R, Gao DW, Huberty JP, et al. Microvascular injury in reperfused infarcted myocardium: noninvasive assessment with contrast-enhanced echoplanar magnetic resonance imaging. J Am Coll Cardiol 1998; 32 (3): 787-93
28. Jeremy RW, Links JM, Becker LC. Progressive failure of coronary flow during reperfusion of myocardial infarction: documentation of the no reflow phenomenon with positron emission tomography. J Am Coll Cardiol 1990; 16 (3): 695-704
29. Iliceto S, Marangelli V, Marchese A, Amico A, Galiuto L, Rizzon P. Myocardial contrast echocardiography in acute myocardial infarction. Pathophysiological background and clinical applications. Eur Heart J 1996; 17 (3): 344-53
30. Lindner JR, Firschke C, Wei K, Goodman NC, Skyba DM, Kaul S. Myocardial perfusion characteristics and hemodynamic profile of MRX-115, a venous echocardiographic contrast agent, during acute myocardial infarction. J Am Soc Echocardiogr 1998; 11 (1): 36-46
31. Villanueva FS, Camarano G, Ismail S, Goodman NC, Sklenar J, Kaul S. Coronary reserve abnormalities in the infarcted myocardium. Assessment of myocardial viability immediately versus late after reflow by contrast echocardiography. Circulation 1996; 94 (4): 748-54
32. Johnson WB, Malone SA, Pantely GA, Anselone CG, Bristow JD. No reflow and extent of infarction during maximal vasodilation in the porcine heart. Circulation 1988; 78 (2): 462-72
33. Vanhaecke J, Flameng W, Borgers M, Jang IK, Van de Werf F, De Geest H. Evidence for decreased coronary flow reserve in viable postischemic myocardium. Circ Res 1990; 67 (5): 1201-10
34. Porter TR, Xie F, Kricsfeld A, Kilzer K. Noninvasive identification of acute myocardial ischemia and reperfusion with contrast ultrasound using intravenous perfluoropropane-exposed sonicated dextrose albumin. J Am Coll Cardiol 1995; 26 (1): 33-40
35. Meza M, Greener Y, Hunt R, Perry B, Revall S, Barbee W, et al. Myocardial contrast echocardiography: reliable, safe, and efficacious myocardial perfusion assessment after intravenous injections of a new echocardiographic contrast agent. Am Heart J 1996; 132 (4): 871-81
36. Cobb FR, Bache RJ, Rivas F, Greenfield JC, Jr. Local effects of acute cellular injury on regional myocardial blood flow. J Clin Invest 1976; 57 (5): 1359-68
37. Villanueva FS, Glasheen WP, Sklenar J, Kaul S. Characterization of spatial patterns of flow within the reperfused myocardium by myocardial contrast echocardiography. Implications in determining extent of myocardial salvage. Circulation 1993; 88 (6): 2596-606
38. Sklenar J, Camarano G, Goodman NC, Ismail S, Jayaweera AR, Kaul S. Contractile versus microvascular reserve for the determination of the extent of myocardial salvage after reperfusion. The effect of residual coronary stenosis. Circulation 1996; 94 (6): 1430-40
39. Bolli R, Triana JF, Jeroudi MO. Prolonged impairment of coronary vasodilation after reversible ischemia. Evidence for microvascular "stunning". Circ Res 1990; 67 (2): 332-43
40. Kaul S. Myocardial contrast echocardiography. Curr Probl Cardiol 1997; 22(11): 549-635
41. Ito H, Tomooka T, Sakai N, Yu H, Higashino Y, Fujii K, et al. Lack of myocardial perfusion immediately after successful thrombolysis. A predictor of poor recovery of left ventricular function in anterior myocardial infarction. Circulation 1992; 85 (5): 1699-705
42. Ito H, Okamura A, Iwakura K, Masuyama T, Hori M, Takiuchi S, et al. Myocardial perfusion patterns related to thrombolysis in myocardial infarction perfusion grades after coronary angioplasty in patients with acute anterior wall myocardial infarction. Circulation 1996; 93 (11): 1993-9
43. Matetzky S, Novikov M, Gruberg L, Freimark D, Feinberg M, Elian D, et al. The significance of persistent ST elevation versus early resolution of ST segment elevation after primary PTCA. J Am Coll Cardiol 1999; 34 (7): 1932-8
44. Claeys MJ, Bosmans J, Veenstra L, Jorens P, De Raedt H, Vrints CJ. Determinants and prognostic implica-

tions of persistent ST-segment elevation after primary angioplasty for acute myocardial infarction: importance of microvascular reperfusion injury on clinical outcome. Circulation 1999; 99 (15): 1972-7
45. Santoro GM, Valenti R, Buonamici P, Bolognese L, Cerisano G, Moschi G, et al. Relation between ST-segment changes and myocardial perfusion evaluated by myocardial contrast echocardiography in patients with acute myocardial infarction treated with direct angioplasty. Am J Cardiol 1998; 82 (8): 932-7
46. Sakuma T, Leong-Poi H, Fisher NG, Goodman NC, Kaul S. Further insights into the no-reflow phenomenon after primary angioplasty in acute myocardial infarction: The role of microthromboemboli. J Am Soc Echocardiogr 2003; 16 (1): 15-21
47. Rocchi G, Kasprzak JD, Galema TW, de Jong N, Ten Cate FJ. Usefulness of power Doppler contrast echocardiography to identify reperfusion after acute myocardial infarction. Am J Cardiol 2001; 87 (3): 278-82
48. Swinburn JM, Lahiri A, Senior R. Intravenous myocardial contrast echocardiography predicts recovery of dysynergic myocardium early after acute myocardial infarction. J Am Coll Cardiol 2001; 38 (1): 19-25
49. Porter TR, Li S, Oster R, Deligonul U. The clinical implications of no reflow demonstrated with intravenous perfluorocarbon containing microbubbles following restoration of Thrombolysis In Myocardial Infarction (TIMI) 3 flow in patients with acute myocardial infarction. Am J Cardiol 1998; 82 (10): 1173-7
50. Ito H, Iwakura K, Oh H, Masuyama T, Hori M, Higashino Y, et al. Temporal changes in myocardial perfusion patterns in patients with reperfused anterior wall myocardial infarction. Their relation to myocardial viability. Circulation 1995; 91 (3): 656-62
51. Asanuma T, Tanabe K, Ochiai K, Yoshitomi H, Nakamura K, Murakami Y, et al. Relationship between progressive microvascular damage and intramyocardial hemorrhage in patients with reperfused anterior myocardial infarction: myocardial contrast echocardiographic study. Circulation 1997; 96 (2): 448-53
52. Brochet E, Czitrom D, Karila-Cohen D, Seknadji P, Faraggi M, Benamer H, et al. Early changes in myocardial perfusion patterns after myocardial infarction: relation with contractile reserve and functional recovery. J Am Coll Cardiol 1998; 32 (7): 2011-7
53. Braunwald E, Kloner RA. The stunned myocardium: prolonged, postischemic ventricular dysfunction. Circulation 1982; 66 (6): 1146-9
54. Cooper HA, Braunwald E. Clinical importance of stunned and hibernating myocardium. Coron Artery Dis 2001; 12 (5): 387-92
55. Sakuma T, Otsuka M, Okimoto T, Fujiwara H, Sumii K, Imazu M, et al. Optimal time for predicting myocardial viability after successful primary angioplasty in acute myocardial infarction: a study using myocardial contrast echocardiography. Am J Cardiol 2001; 87 (6): 687-92
56. Ragosta M, Camarano G, Kaul S, Powers ER, Sarembock IJ, Gimple LW. Microvascular integrity indicates myocellular viability in patients with recent myocardial infarction. New insights using myocardial contrast echocardiography. Circulation 1994; 89 (6): 2562-9
57. Main ML, Magalski A, Chee NK, Coen MM, Skolnick DG, Good TH. Full-motion pulse inversion power Doppler contrast echocardiography differentiates stunning from necrosis and predicts recovery of left ventricular function after acute myocardial infarction. J Am Coll Cardiol 2001; 38 (5): 1390-4
58. Gibson CM, Cannon CP, Daley WL, Dodge JT, Jr., Alexander B, Jr., Marble SJ, et al. TIMI frame count: a quantitative method of assessing coronary artery flow. Circulation 1996; 93 (5): 879-88
59. Gibson CM, Cannon CP, Murphy SA, Marble SJ, Barron HV, Braunwald E. Relationship of the TIMI myocardial perfusion grades, flow grades, frame count, and percutaneous coronary intervention to long-term outcomes after thrombolytic administration in acute myocardial infarction. Circulation 2002; 105 (16): 1909-13
60. Lepper W, Sieswerda GT, Vanoverschelde JL, Franke A, de Cock CC, Kamp O, et al. Predictive value of markers of myocardial reperfusion in acute myocardial infarction for follow-up left ventricular function. Am J Cardiol 2001; 88 (12): 1358-63
61. Greaves K, Dixon SR, Fejka M, O'Neill WW, Redwood SR, Marber MS, et al. Myocardial contrast echocardiography is superior to other known modalities for assessing myocardial reperfusion after acute myocardial infarction. Heart 2003; 89 (2): 139-44
62. Lepper W, Hoffmann R, Kamp O, Franke A, de Cock CC, Kuhl HP, et al. Assessment of myocardial reperfusion by intravenous myocardial contrast echocardiography and coronary flow reserve after primary percutaneous transluminal coronary angioplasty [correction of angiography] in patients with acute myocardial infarction. Circulation 2000; 101 (20): 2368-74
63. Jayaweera AR, Wei K, Coggins M, Bin JP, Goodman C, Kaul S. Role of capillaries in determining CBF reserve: new insights using myocardial contrast echocardiography. Am J Physiol 1999; 277(6 Pt 2): H2363-72
64. Iliceto S, Galiuto L, Marchese A, Cavallari D, Colonna P, Biasco G, et al. Analysis of microvascular integrity, contractile reserve, and myocardial viability after

acute myocardial infarction by dobutamine echocardiography and myocardial contrast echocardiography. Am J Cardiol 1996; 77 (7): 441-5
65. Bolognese L, Antoniucci D, Rovai D, Buonamici P, Cerisano G, Santoro GM, et al. Myocardial contrast echocardiography versus dobutamine echocardiography for predicting functional recovery after acute myocardial infarction treated with primary coronary angioplasty. J Am Coll Cardiol 1996; 28 (7): 1677-83
66. Pérez-David E, García-Fernández M, Desco M, Malpica N, Puerta P, Odreman R, et al. Relationship between videointensity parameters, mechanical index and dose evaluated with a new contrast agent. Experimental study in model pigs. Eur Heart J 2001; 22: 221 (Abstract)
67. Wei K, Jayaweera AR, Firoozan S, Linka A, Skyba DM, Kaul S. Quantification of myocardial blood flow with ultrasound-induced destruction of microbubbles administered as a constant venous infusion. Circulation 1998; 97 (5): 473-83
68. Masugata H, Peters B, Lafitte S, Strachan GM, Ohmori K, DeMaria AN. Quantitative assessment of myocardial perfusion during graded coronary stenosis by real-time myocardial contrast echo refilling curves. [In Process Citation]. J Am Coll Cardiol 2001; 37 (1): 262-9
69. Pérez-David E, García-Fernández M, Ledesma Carbayo M, Silva J, Pérez de Isla L, Antoranz J, et al. Which is the best quantitative method to analyse regional transmural perfusion gradient with real-time myocardial contrast echocardiography? Circulation 2002; 106(19): pp II-676 (Abstract)
70. Shimoni S, Frangogiannis NG, Aggeli CJ, Shan K, Verani MS, Quinones MA, et al. Identification of hibernating myocardium with quantitative intravenous myocardial contrast echocardiography: comparison with dobutamine echocardiography and thallium-201 scintigraphy. Circulation 2003; 107 (4): 538-44
71. Desco M, Ledesma Carbayo M, Santos A, García-Fernández M, Marcos-Alberca P, Malpica N, et al. Coherent contrast imaging quantification for myocardial perfusion assessment. Journal of American College 2001; 37 (Suppl): 495A
72. Swinburn JM, Senior R. Real time contrast echocardiography--a new bedside technique to predict contractile reserve early after acute myocardial infarction. Eur J Echocardiogr 2002; 3 (2): 95-9

Chapter 13

Can Echocardiography Provide Combined Assessment of Left Ventricular Function and Myocardial Perfusion?

Victor Mor-Avi • R. Parker Ward • Roberto M. Lang

While the relationship between coronary blood flow and myocardial function is complex and multifaceted, it can be summarized in one simplistic statement: reduction in coronary flow results in reduced myocardial perfusion leading to an ischemic cascade, the end-point of which is compromised ventricular function. Different methods used for the diagnosis of coronary heart disease are based on detection of these changes, either at rest or under stress. However, most of them focus on a single parameter, such as wall motion or myocardial perfusion, rather than providing comprehensive diagnosis based on the combined assessment of multiple variables. Thus, coronary angiography focuses on coronary anatomy to estimate coronary flow, nuclear imaging provides information on myocardial perfusion, and the echocardiographic diagnosis of ischemic heart disease is mainly based on the assessment of regional wall motion. It has been recognized that a technique capable of evaluating more than one variable in a single test would likely provide a more accurate and reliable diagnostic tool [1-2], and undoubtedly have an impact on the prognosis and risk stratification of patients with suspected ischemic heart disease. In addition, such a technique would be advantageous for the diagnosis of conditions characterized by a mismatch between blood supply and myocardial function, such as hibernating or stunned myocardium [3-5].

Radionuclide Assessment of Perfusion and Function

The concept of multivariable diagnosis of ischemic heart disease has been extensively explored by nuclear cardiologists, as evidenced by a vast volume of publications over the last quarter of a century. In the late 1970s, Alderson et al. proposed expanding the traditional ^{201}Tl perfusion imaging into a combined perfusion-function test by using multiframe image acquisitions triggered to consecutive multiple phases of the cardiac cycle [6], and concluded that the addition of functional assessment was technically feasible and clinically useful. Subsequently, nuclear perfusion imaging techniques were adapted to generate a dynamic display of the beating ventricle geared toward the assessment of ventricular wall motion [7-11]. The radionuclide-based assessment of left ventricular (LV) function was found to be highly reproducible [12, 13], and its accuracy was confirmed using different "gold standard" techniques, including echocardiography [9-11] and magnetic resonance imaging [14, 15]. These validation studies established the basis for the use of combined radionuclide assessment of myocardial perfusion and function in a variety of situations where it could provide useful information on either normal cardiac physiology [16], progression of disease [17-20] and diagnosis of various pathologies [21-24], or the effects of treatment [25]. Naturally, many investigators focused on stress-based applications of this technique as a more accurate tool for the diagnosis of ischemic heart disease [16-18, 21, 26-28].

Everaert and colleagues tested the ability of gated single photon emission computed tomography (SPECT) to detect the effects of low-dose dobutamine on LV systolic wall thickening, and concluded that this technique may be useful in distinguishing viable myocardium from scar tissue by demonstrating a preserved inotropic response in the hypoperfused myocardium [16]. They also showed that stress-induced changes indicative of myocardial viability can be detected using low-dose dobutamine gated SPECT despite the confounding effects of concomitant use of beta-blockers [22]. Flamen et al. demonstrated the value of combined perfusion and function evaluation during exercise for the identification of high-risk patients recovering from uncomplicated acute myocardial infarction [17]. Another recent study described the clinical value of technetium-MIBI imaging of perfusion and function under dipyridamole stress for the identification of patients with multivessel disease and extensive areas of myocardium at risk [26]. Danias et al. reported that this technique allowed the differentiation between patients with ischemic from non-ischemic cardiomyopathy [23]. Dendale and coworkers found that combined evaluation of perfusion and function helped them predict the recurrence of angina pectoris after successful angioplasty [25]. While most investigators used traditional subjective image interpretation, others attempted automated computer analysis to obtain more objective, quantitative measures of myocardial perfusion as well as global and regional ventricular function [29, 30]. All these studies and many others have demonstrated that simultaneous or combined assessment of myocardial perfusion and function enhances the clinical value of nuclear cardiac imaging in the diagnosis of heart disease.

Multimodality Combined Assessment of Perfusion and Function

For several decades, the ability to provide dynamic images of the beating heart in real time has been unique to echocardiography.

Since this ability is a prerequisite for the assessment of regional wall motion, echocardiography is considered the reference method for such assessment, similar to the role of nuclear imaging in assessing myocardial perfusion. Several investigators interested in exploring the possibility of multivariable diagnosis of ischemic heart disease used the combination of these two modalities for the simultaneous assessment of myocardial perfusion and function [18, 20, 24, 28, 31, 32]. Bouvier et al. used this methodology to study elderly endurance athletes and were able to demonstrate the superiority of the athletes' cardiac performance over age-matched untrained control subjects, despite the high incidence of myocardial perfusion defects noted in the athletes [31]. Elhendy and colleagues have recently used combined perfusion and function assessment by simultaneous sestamibi SPECT and two-dimensional echocardiography to establish the relationship between the grade of dobutamine-induced worsening in regional function and the extent of the underlying perfusion defect [18]. Similarly, Khattar et al. described their observation in 100 consecutive patients that the combined assessment of myocardial perfusion and contractile function using inotropic stress Tc-99m sestamibi SPECT imaging and echocardiography significantly improved the accuracy of the noninvasive diagnosis of multivessel disease [24]. Using similar methodology in a 3-month post-revascularization follow-up study, Bax and colleagues were able to demonstrate that normal perfusion irrespective of wall motion abnormalities was predictive of functional recovery [32]. Similar findings were reported in a group of patients recovering from coronary artery bypass grafting (CABG) surgery [28].

In the experimental animal setting, simultaneous assessment of myocardial perfusion and function has also been achieved using techniques other than echocardiography and nuclear imaging. Fuchs and coworkers used radiolabeled microspheres to quantify myocardial tissue blood flow in conjunction with echocardiography in a study aimed at determining angiogenic effects of intramyocardial injection of autologous bone marrow [33]. This methodology was also recently used by Kaul et al. to study the effects of selective alterations in collateral driving pressure on regional perfusion and function in the territory of distribution of the occluded coronary artery in dogs [34]. Sherrer-Crosbie et al. used this methodology in a sheep model of chronic myocardial infarction to demonstrate that the reduced wall motion frequently noted in infarct border zone is a result of mechanical tethering rather than abnormal perfusion [35]. While radiolabeled microspheres are considered the ultimate quantitative "gold standard" for myocardial tissue blood flow, this technique is limited to nonsurvival animal studies.

Kraitchman et al. tested the feasibility of using magnetic resonance imaging (MRI) to simultaneously assess myocardial perfusion and function during dobutamine-induced ischemia in a closed-chest dog model of moderate coronary stenosis [36]. In another animal study, this methodology was used to study the relationship between the size of dipyridamole-induced perfusion defects and wall motion abnormalities in a canine model of nonocclusive coronary stenosis [37]. The combination of MRI and echocardiography was used to study the relationship between myocardial perfusion and function in patients at early phases of recovery from acute myocardial infarction [38]. A combined stress MRI protocol for one-stop evaluation of perfusion and function was recently successfully tested as a clinical guide for coronary revascularization [39]. Similar methodology was successfully used in a clinical study designed to evaluate the effects of laser myocardial revascularization [21, 40]. With the recent development of advanced MRI pulse sequences that allow high-frame-rate imaging during enhancement with gadolinium contrast agents, this technique will undoubtedly play a major role in multivariable cardiac evaluation.

Several studies utilized positron emission tomography (PET) imaging to simultaneously assess myocardial perfusion and function [41]. Rechavia et al. used PET imaging to study the relationship between contractile function and perfusion in remote uninvolved hypercontractile myocardial regions in patients with myocardial infarction and single-vessel coronary artery disease [42]. Maes and colleagues studied a group of patients after acute myocardial infarction who underwent successful thrombolysis, and showed that functional recovery occurs only when adequate tissue blood flow is restored [43]. This finding was subsequently confirmed by other investigators who used gated SPECT imaging to predict recovery following coronary revascularization [28, 32].

Echocardiographic Evaluation of Myocardial Perfusion and Function

While two-dimensional echocardiographic imaging has been playing a pivotal role in the clinical assessment of cardiac function for several decades, its ability to assess myocardial perfusion is not yet as well established. Perfusion imaging relies on the availability of two products: (1) stable, uniform, biodegradable contrast agents capable of transpulmonary passage, and (2) equipment capable of consistent and reproducible imaging of myocardial contrast. Although the development of ideal contrast agents and imaging equipment tailored to visualize their transmyocardial passage has been pursued by a variety of manufacturers, each of these goals turned out to be a major technological challenge that has yet to be fully resolved despite the multiple breakthroughs that we have witnessed in recent years.

Since the initial reports on the use of primitive ultrasound contrast media, such as agitated saline or renografin, to visualize myocardial perfusion in the 1980s [44-48], a tremendous number of research studies and scientific publications has been dedicated to this cause. A quick literature search on this subject today yields over a thousand published papers. The evaluation of myocardial perfusion using ultrasound contrast enhancement has been frequently referred to as the "holy grail" of echocardiography. This term, commonly used in the context of the crusades, reflects the difficulties encountered by the investigators who dedicate their efforts to pursuing this elusive goal. The different aspects of this "crusade" have been previously discussed by others in over 60 review papers in the English language alone [49, 59], and this topic is covered with great attention elsewhere in this volume.

Briefly, the major advances in the field of myocardial contrast echocardiography over the past decade include the development of stable perfluorocarbon-filled microbubbles, frequently referred to as second-generation contrast agents, and the development of perfusion targeted nonlinear imaging modes, such as harmonic imaging, pulse inversion and power modulation, which allow more consistent real-time visualization of intramyocardial contrast enhancement. Despite multiple difficulties and limitations that have yet to be resolved, this technology is gaining broader recognition as a basis for clinical evaluation of myocardial perfusion. Nevertheless, only a few published reports described the use of echocardiography for combined assessment of myocardial perfusion and function [60-64].

In one of the earlier studies, Meza and colleagues tested the value of myocardial contrast echocardiography in combination with dobutamine stress testing in predicting regional functional recovery after revascularization in patients with resting wall motion abnormalities [60]. Thirty-nine patients with significant coronary disease and resting wall motion abnormalities were studied before and after either coronary angioplasty or coronary bypass surgery. Prior to revascularization, each patient underwent a dobutamine stress test for the evaluation of LV wall motion, and intracoronary contrast injections for the assessment of myocardial perfusion. Echocardiographic images obtained after revascularization were used to determine the degree of functional recovery, which was correlated with the results of the initial dobutamine stress and myocardial contrast echocardiographic study. Importantly, the combined use of these techniques significantly improved the accuracy of the prediction of functional recovery over the use of each technique alone: from sensitivity ~80% to >90% and from specificity in the 20%–30% range to ~50%. This study is an excellent example of how combined assessment of perfusion and function can provide more accurate diagnosis than the stand-alone evaluation of each variable.

In a more recent study, Leong-Poi and colleagues used contrast echocardiography in an animal model of stress-induced acute ischemia to study the relationship between perfusion defects and functional abnormalities caused by different degrees of coronary stenosis and different doses of dobutamine [63] under conditions of single-vessel as well as multivessel stenosis. Regional LV function was evaluated by measuring myocardial wall thickening, and perfusion was assessed by examining myocardial contrast replenishment after a variable time interval following a destructive high-energy ultrasound pulse (Fig. 13.1). In single-vessel stenosis, abnormal perfusion characterized by lower replenishment rates was seen at the lowest dose of dobutamine irrespective of the degree of stenosis, whereas functional abnormalities were seen only at high doses of dobutamine and correlated with the degree of stenosis. Interestingly, the spatial

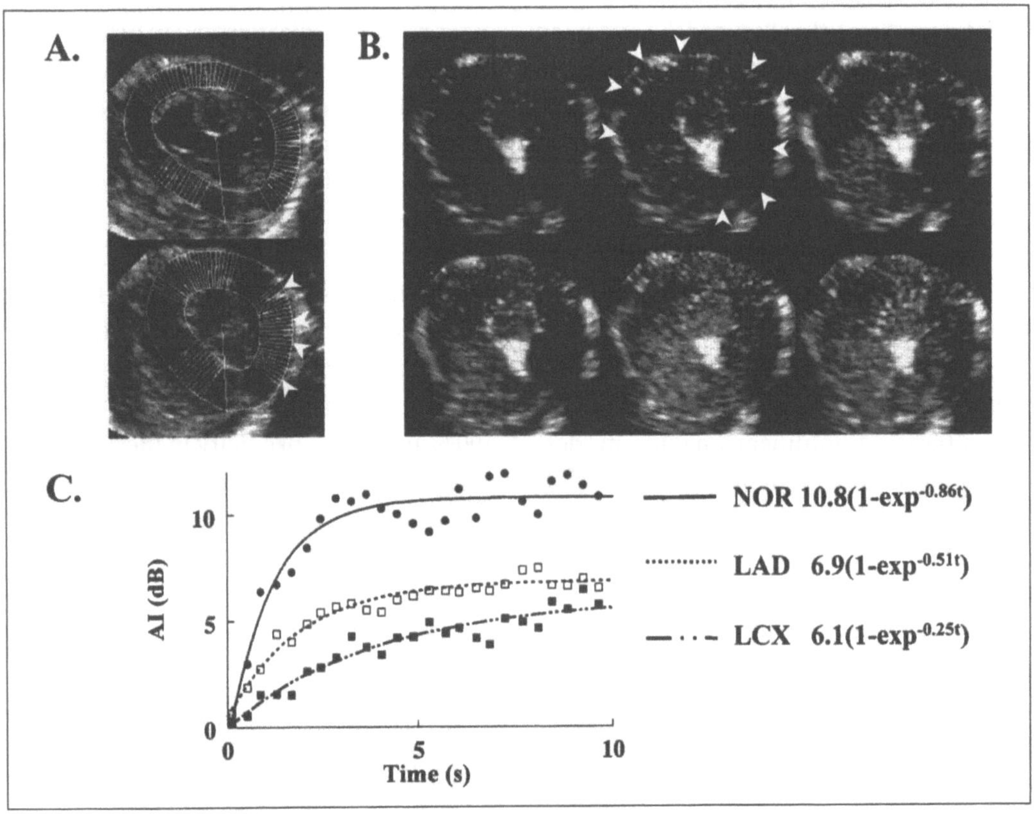

Fig. 13.1. Images from a dog with a moderate left anterior descending artery (*LAD*) and a severe left circumflex artery (*LCx*) stenosis during dobutamine infusion (10 μg/kg/min). **A** End-diastolic and end-systolic images showing reduced wall thickening in the LCx bed. **B** End-systolic MCE images at increasing time points after the destructive flash showing slower filling of both the LAD and LCx bed (the latter filling the slowest) compared with the normal bed. **C** Corresponding time versus acoustic intensity (*AI*) curves. *NOR* indicates normal bed (Reproduced with permission from [63])

extent of abnormal perfusion exceeded that of wall motion abnormality at all but the highest dobutamine dose. This spatiotemporal discordance between abnormal perfusion and function was significantly less pronounced in multivessel stenosis, where it was possible to identify separate regions with abnormal function at lower doses of dobutamine. These findings were used to explain the higher sensitivity of abnormal perfusion compared with abnormal function for the detection of coronary stenosis as well as the higher sensitivity of dobutamine echocardiography for multivessel compared with single-vessel disease [63].

Oraby and coworkers recently evaluated a new imaging technique referred to as coherent contrast imaging, for simultaneous assessment of LV wall motion and myocardial perfusion during dipyridamole stress in 42 patients with known or suspected coronary artery disease [62]. This imaging technique was designed for real-time visualization of myocardial contrast during imaging at low mechanical index, as a way to avoid ultrasound-induced microbubble destruction, and allowed simultaneous visualization of cardiac dynamics necessary for analysis of regional wall motion. Contrast replenishment in the different perfusion territories after a short high-energy pulse was used as an index of regional tissue perfusion. This technique is frequently referred to as flash-echocardiography. The results were compared with those of dipyridamole thallium-201 SPECT study performed in the same setting (Fig. 13.2). These comparisons yielded high correlations, thus providing the necessary validation for the use of combined echocardiographic assessment of myocardial perfusion and function in the evaluation of patients with ischemic heart disease.

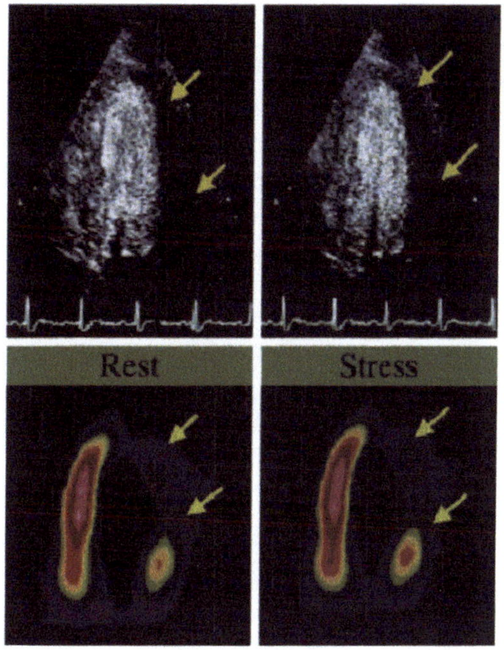

Fig. 13.2. Coherent contrast perfusion imaging. Abnormal myocardial perfusion from the apical four-chamber view at rest (*left*) and at stress (*right*), myocardial contrast echocardiography (*top*), and SPECT uptake (*bottom*). Note the fixed lateral wall perfusion defect in the distribution of the left anterior descending (*upper arrows*) and the left circumflex artery (*lower arrows*); the entire lateral wall was severely hypokinetic from base to apex at rest and remained so after dipyridamole injection (Reproduced with permission from [62])

Garot et al. recently described the results of an animal study aimed at accurate detection and characterization of "stunned myocardium" following repeated episodes of severe ischemia [64]. To achieve this goal, they used myocardial contrast enhancement in combination with Doppler tissue imaging. They measured the transmural distribution of myocardial blood flow across the LV wall and quantified intramural myocardial velocities and strain rates during ischemia and reperfusion, as indices of regional perfusion and function, respectively. Coronary flow restriction resulted in a significant decrease in peak contrast intensity ratio between ischemic and non-ischemic walls, associated with a decrease in peak systolic velocities and strain rates (Fig. 13.3). Interestingly, during reperfusion, while myocardial velocities increased dramatically, strain rate remained markedly reduced despite normal coronary flow. Based on these intriguing findings, the authors suggested that the combination of myocardial contrast and Doppler tissue imaging could be used to distinguish ischemic from postischemic regional wall dysfunction,

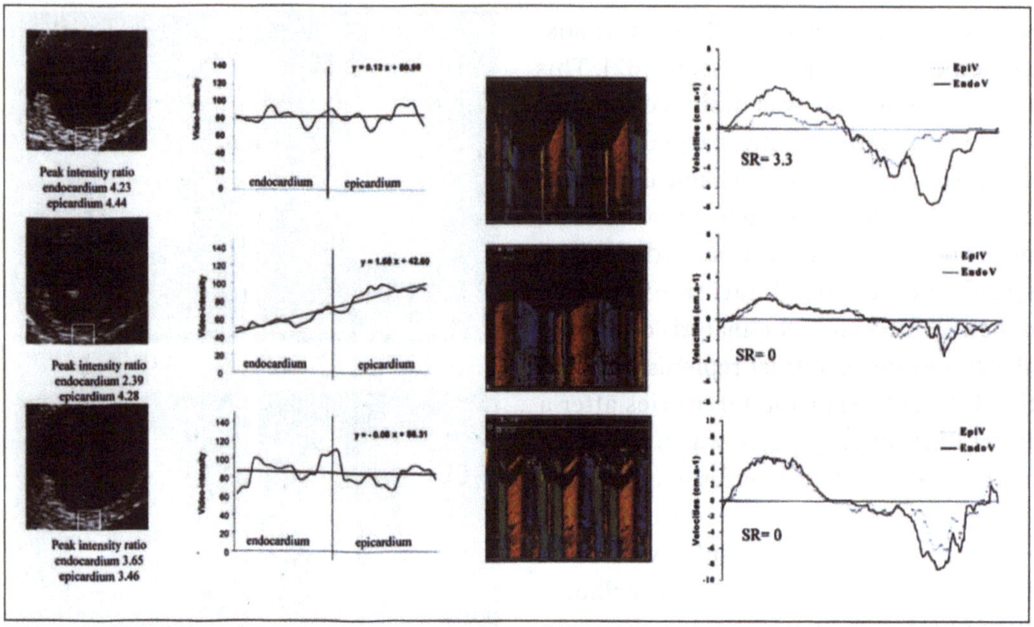

Fig. 13.3. Example of perfusion data obtained from contrast-enhanced gray-scale images (*left*) and myocardial velocities obtained with Doppler tissue imaging (*right*) in a pig. Basal video intensity gradient was small, indicating homogeneous transmural contrast enhancement (*left, top*). Coronary blood flow restriction resulted in impaired subendocardial enhancement along with increase in video intensity gradient (*left, middle*). Recovery of homogenous transmural enhancement was observed after reperfusion (*left, bottom*). Peak systolic velocities at baseline were different in subendocardium and subepicardium (*right, top*). During coronary flow restriction, a decrease in systolic velocities, and consequently in strain rate (*SR*), was noted, predominantly in the subendocardium (*right, middle*). While velocities increased significantly during reperfusion, the strain rate remained unchanged despite normal perfusion (*right, bottom*) (Reproduced with permission from [64])

which may be helpful for evaluating the effects of revascularization in patients with acute coronary syndrome [64].

We recently tested the feasibility of using contrast-enhanced power modulation images for combined assessment of myocardial perfusion and regional LV function in a pig model of acute ischemia and reperfusion [61]. Power modulation is another relatively new perfusion-oriented echocardiographic imaging mode, based on the use of the nonlinear properties of the microbubbles. This mode allows real-time visualization of myocardial contrast enhancement at low mechanical indices and without significant microbubble destruction. In addition, power modulation provides uniform LV cavity opacification essential for automated endocardial border detection. Flash-echocardiography was used to assess myocardial perfusion, which was characterized by the rate of postimpulse replenishment in different perfusion beds. Myocardial function was quantified by calculating regional fractional area changes using endocardial borders, which were automatically detected throughout the cardiac cycle. These measurements were performed under control conditions, as well as during coronary occlusion and reperfusion. All ischemic episodes caused detectable and reversible changes in perfusion and function. Perfusion defects, validated with fluorescent microspheres, were visualized in real time and confirmed by a significant decrease in the calculated perfusion indices. These findings were reversed during reperfusion. In parallel, fractional area changes significantly decreased in ischemic segments, and were restored to normal during reperfusion. These findings obtained in a highly controlled model of reversible myocardial ischemia allowed us to establish a clear causal relationship between ischemia and regional changes in power modulation images, presumably reflecting abnormal perfusion, and substantiated the use of this technique in the diagnosis of ischemic heart disease.

More recently, automated border detection from contrast-enhanced power modulation images has been implemented in a prototype imaging system, which allows the use of color kinesis for real-time color-encoding of endocardial motion during contrast infusion, suitable for quantitative segmental analysis of LV wall motion [65-67]. In addition, we have recently developed a technique for translation-free analysis of myocardial perfusion using automated frame-by-frame identification of myocardial regions of interest from automatically detected endocardial borders [68]. We combined these concepts and used color-encoding information not only for regional analysis of wall motion but also for quick endocardial border detection as a basis for automated identification of myocardial regions of interest and translation-free analysis of myocardial perfusion (Fig. 13.4). This approach allows automated, simultaneous, quantitative analysis of myocardial perfusion and regional wall motion, without the need for manual tracing or frame-by-frame adjustment of myocardial regions of interest.

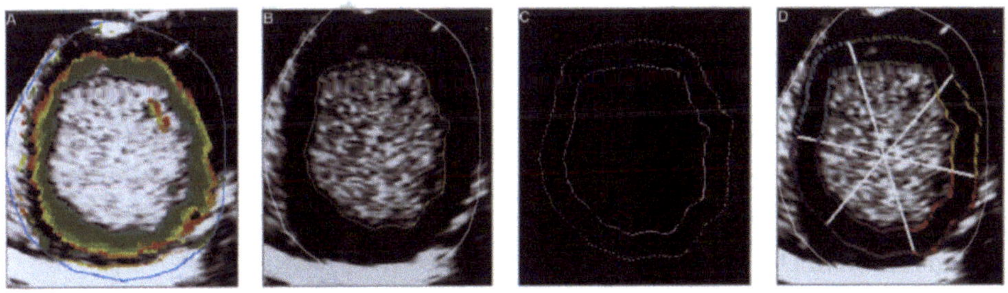

Fig. 13.4. Automated identification of myocardial regions of interest for perfusion analysis from color-encoded, contrast-enhanced, power modulation images (**A**) was achieved by extracting the end-systolic endocardial border (**B**), which was used to generate a band of fixed width around the left ventricular cavity (**C**), and then divided into six wedge-shaped myocardial segments (**D**)

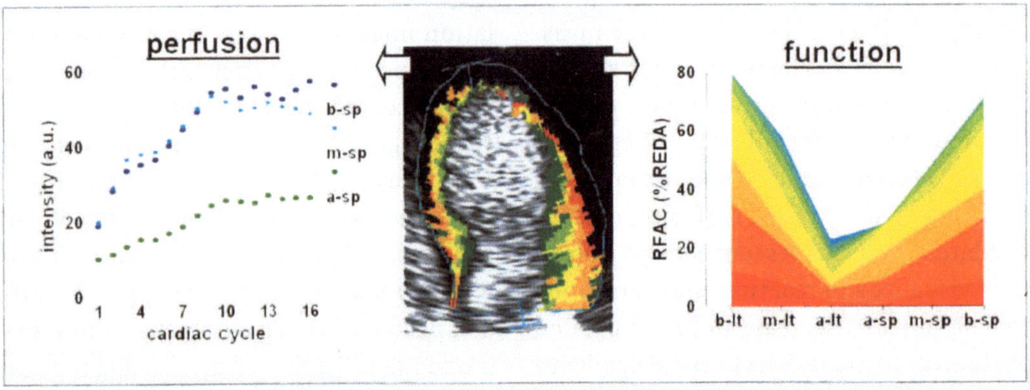

Fig. 13.5. Contrast-enhanced power modulation image (*center*) obtained in a patient after myocardial infarction due to obstruction of the distal LAD artery with color-encoding of endocardial motion. Note the differences between the postimpulse contrast replenishment curves (*left*) obtained in the apical septal (*a-sp*) segment where perfusion defect was noted and the control mid- and basal-septal (*m-sp* and *b-sp*) segments. Note also the concomitant reduction in fractional area change (*RFAC*) in this segment (*right*) reflecting the wall motion abnormality

Following validation in experimental animals, this approach proved feasible in a small group of patients with acute myocardial infarction (Fig. 13.5) by demonstrating the known variety of postintervention scenarios reflecting variable degrees of success of coronary revascularization and myocardial viability. We have also tested the applicability of this technique in dipyridamole stress testing and found that it can be used to detect inducible ischemia in patients with suspected coronary artery disease (Fig. 13.6). Further investigation in a larger patient population is needed to determine the diagnostic accuracy of this combined echocardiographic assessment of myocardial perfusion and function. The availability of this information may prove clinically useful to predict functional recovery in patients after myocardial infarction.

These studies indicate that today's echocardiographic technology is capable of real-time imaging and automated on-line quantification of both myocardial perfusion and regional function. As cardiologists learned through their experience with combined assessment of perfusion and function with other techniques, such multivariable diagnosis promises to improve the accuracy of echocardiographic diagnosis of heart disease and to allow the detection and accurate characterization of pathological conditions that may be very difficult to diagnose otherwise.

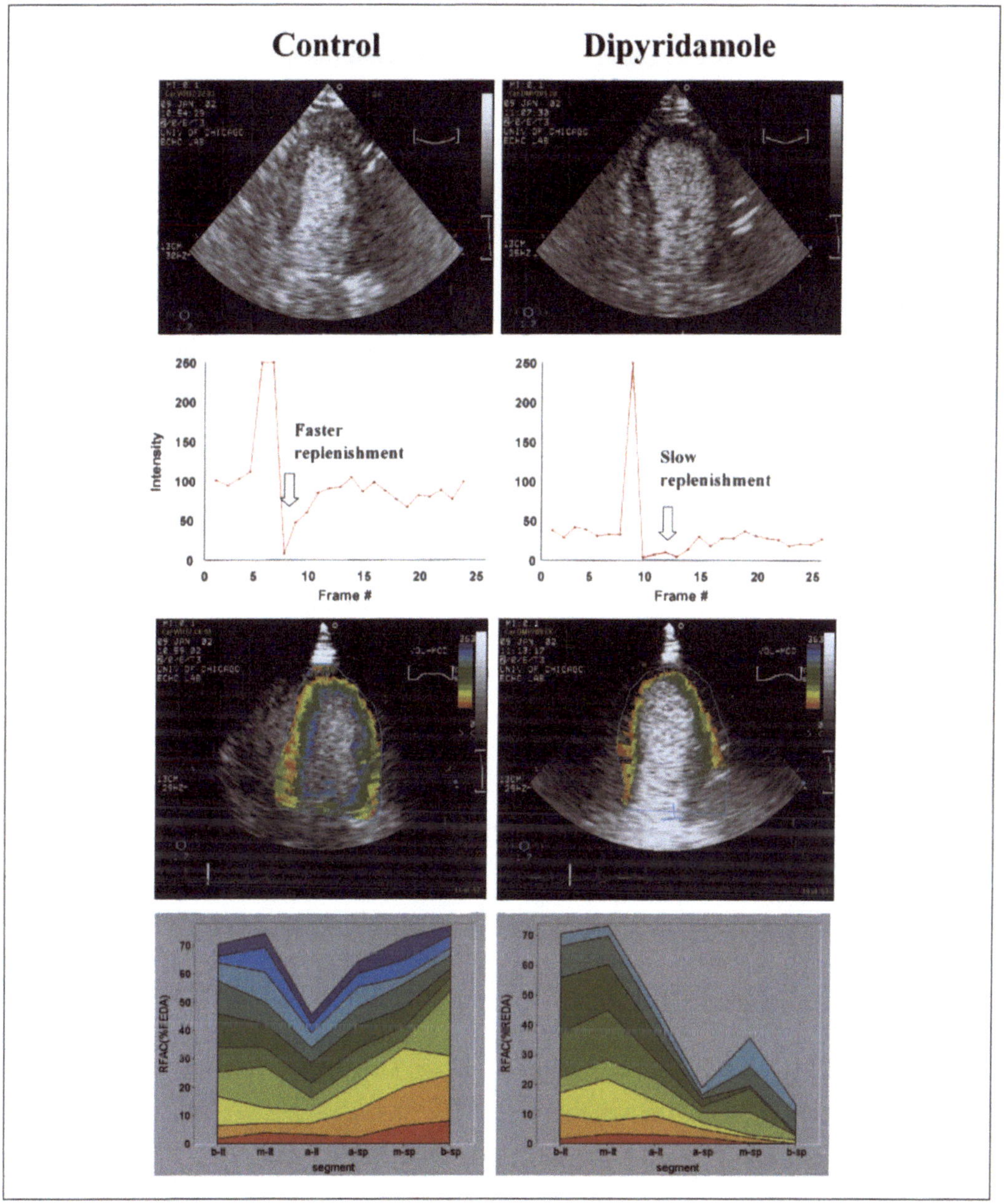

Fig. 13.6. Example of simultaneous quantitative assessment of myocardial perfusion and function during dipyridamole stress in a patient with angina and coronary angiography evidence of total LAD occlusion and collaterals from the right coronary artery The presence of uniform intramyocardial contrast enhancement, with rapid replenishment following high-energy impulse and color bands of uniform thickness, indicated normal myocardial perfusion and function at rest, respectively During dipyridamole stress, an inducible apical perfusion defect and wall motion abnormality were noted, as indicated by a decrease in intramyocardial contrast with a regional delay in postimpulse replenishment and thinning of the color bands in the affected region

References

1. Borges-Neto S, Shaw LK. The added value of simultaneous myocardial perfusion and left ventricular function. *Curr Opin Cardiol.* 1999; 14: 460-463
2. Anagnostopoulos C, Underwood SR. Simultaneous assessment of myocardial perfusion and function: how and when? *Eur J Nucl Med.* 1998; 25: 555-558
3. Braunwald E, Kloner RA. The stunned myocardium: prolonged, postischemic ventricular dysfunction. *Circulation.* 1982; 66: 1146-1149
4. Schulz R, Heusch G. Characterization of hibernating and stunned myocardium. *Eur Heart J.* 1995; 16 Suppl J: 19-25
5. Kloner RA, Arimie RB, Kay GL, Cannom D, Matthews R, Bhandari A, Shook T, Pollick C, Burstein S. Evidence for stunned myocardium in humans: a 2001 update. *Coron Artery Dis.* 2001; 12: 349-356
6. Alderson PO, Wagner HN, Jr., Gomez-Moeiras JJ, Rehn TG, Becker LC, Douglas KH, Manspeaker HF, Schindledecker GR. Simultaneous detection of myocardial perfusion and wall motion abnormalities by cinematic 201Tl imaging. *Radiology.* 1978; 127: 531-533
7. Bonow RO. Gated myocardial perfusion imaging for measuring left ventricular function. *J Am Coll Cardiol.* 1997; 30: 1649-1650
8. Constantinesco A, Mertz L, Brunot B. Myocardial perfusion and function imaging at rest with simultaneous thallium-201 and technetium-99m blood-pool dual-isotope gated SPECT. *J Nucl Med.* 1997; 38: 432-437
9. Cwajg E, Cwajg J, He ZX, Hwang WS, Keng F, Nagueh SF, Verani MS. Gated myocardial perfusion tomography for the assessment of left ventricular function and volumes: comparison with echocardiography. *J Nucl Med.* 1999; 40: 1857-1865
10. Todino V, Rubini G, Cuocolo A. Assessment of left ventricular function by ECG-gated myocardial perfusion scintigraphy with image inversion technique: comparison with equilibrium radionuclide angiography. *J Nucl Cardiol.* 1999; 6: 605-611
11. Chua T, Yin LC, Thiang TH, Choo TB, Ping DZ, Leng LY. Accuracy of the automated assessment of left ventricular function with gated perfusion SPECT in the presence of perfusion defects and left ventricular dysfunction: correlation with equilibrium radionuclide ventriculography and echocardiography. *J Nucl Cardiol.* 2000; 7: 301-311
12. Hyun IY, Kwan J, Park KS, Lee WH. Reproducibility of Tl-201 and Tc-99m sestamibi gated myocardial perfusion SPECT measurement of myocardial function. *J Nucl Cardiol.* 2001; 8: 182-187
13. Danias PG, Ahlberg AW, Travin MI, Mahr NC, Abreu JE, Marini D, Mann A, Mather JF, Boden WE, Heller GV. Visual assessment of left ventricular perfusion and function with electrocardiography-gated SPECT has high intraobserver and interobserver reproducibility among experienced nuclear cardiologists and cardiology trainees. *J Nucl Cardiol.* 2002; 9: 263-270
14. Bremerich J, Buser P, Bongartz G, Muller-Brand J, Gradel C, Pfisterer M, Steinbrich W. Noninvasive stress testing of myocardial ischemia: comparison of GRE-MRI perfusion and wall motion analysis to 99 mTc-MIBI-SPECT, relation to coronary angiography. *Eur Radiol.* 1997; 7: 990-995
15. Aaberge L, Rootwelt K, Smith HJ, Nordstrand K, Forfang K. Effects of transmyocardial revascularization on myocardial perfusion and systolic function assessed by nuclear and magnetic resonance imaging methods. *Scand Cardiovasc J.* 2001; 35: 8-13
16. Everaert H, Vanhove C, Franken PR. Effects of low-dose dobutamine on left ventricular function in normal subjects as assessed by gated single-photon emission tomography myocardial perfusion studies. *Eur J Nucl Med.* 1999; 26: 1298-1303
17. Flamen P, Dendale P, Bossuyt A, Franken PR. Combined left ventricular wall motion and myocardial perfusion stress imaging in the initial assessment of patients with a recent uncomplicated myocardial infarction. *Angiology.* 1995; 46: 461-472
18. Elhendy A, van Domburg RT, Bax JJ, Poldermans D, Nierop PR, Geleijnse ML, Roelandt JR. The grade of worsening of regional function during dobutamine stress echocardiography predicts the extent of myocardial perfusion abnormalities. *Heart.* 2000; 83: 35-39
19. Everaert H, Vanhove C, Franken PR. Assessment of perfusion, function, and myocardial metabolism after infarction with a combination of low-dose dobutamine tetrofosmin gated SPECT perfusion scintigraphy and BMIPP SPECT imaging. *J Nucl Cardiol.* 2000; 7: 29-36
20. Gazarian M, Feldman BM, Benson LN, Gilday DL, Laxer RM, Silverman ED. Assessment of myocardial perfusion and function in childhood systemic lupus erythematosus. *J Pediatr.* 1998; 132: 109-116
21. Palmas W, Friedman JD, Diamond GA, Silber H, Kiat H, Berman DS. Incremental value of simultaneous assessment of myocardial function and perfusion with technetium-99m sestamibi for prediction of extent of coronary artery disease. *J Am Coll Cardiol.* 1995; 25: 1024-1031
22. Everaert H, Vanhove C, Franken PR. Effect of beta-blockade on low-dose dobutamine-induced changes in left ventricular function in healthy volunteers: assessment by gated SPECT myocardial perfusion scintigraphy. *Eur J Nucl Med.* 2000; 27: 419-424

23. Danias PG, Ahlberg AW, Clark BA, III, Messineo F, Levine MG, McGill CC, Mann A, Clive J, Dougherty JE, Waters DD, Heller GV. Combined assessment of myocardial perfusion and left ventricular function with exercise technetium-99m sestamibi gated single-photon emission computed tomography can differentiate between ischemic and nonischemic dilated cardiomyopathy. *Am J Cardiol.* 1998; 82: 1253-1258
24. Khattar RS, Senior R, Lahiri A. Assessment of myocardial perfusion and contractile function by inotropic stress Tc-99m sestamibi SPECT imaging and echocardiography for optimal detection of multivessel coronary artery disease. *Heart.* 1998; 79: 274-280
25. Dendale PA, Franken PR, Van Den HP, Van den BF, Bossuyt A. Exercise myocardial perfusion and wall motion imaging to predict recurrence of angina pectoris after successful angioplasty. *Acta Cardiol.* 1996; 51: 409-423
26. Zafrir N, Bassevitch R, Shimoni A, Teplitsky I, Lubin E. Effect of dipyridamole on myocardial perfusion and function using technetium-99m MIBI. *Int J Cardiol.* 1995; 49: 25-31
27. Kumita S, Cho K, Nakajo H, Toba M, Kijima T, Mizumura S, Oshina T, Kumazaki T, Sano J, Sakurai K, Munakata K. Serial assessment of left ventricular function during dobutamine stress by means of electrocardiography-gated myocardial SPECT: combination with dual-isotope myocardial perfusion SPECT for detection of ischemic heart disease. *J Nucl Cardiol.* 2001; 8: 152-157
28. Paluszkiewicz L, Kwinecki P, Jemielity M, Szyszka A, Dyszkiewicz W, Cieslinski A. Myocardial perfusion correlates with improvement of systolic function of the left ventricle after CABG. Dobutamine echocardiography and Tc-99m-MIBI SPECT study. *Eur J Cardiothorac Surg.* 2002; 21: 32-35
29. Germano G, Kavanagh PB, Berman DS. An automatic approach to the analysis, quantitation and review of perfusion and function from myocardial perfusion SPECT images. *Int J Card Imaging.* 1997; 13: 337-346
30. Nakata T, Katagiri Y, Odawara Y, Eguchi M, Kuroda M, Tsuchihashi K, Hareyama M, Shimamoto K. Two- and three-dimensional assessments of myocardial perfusion and function by using technetium-99m sestamibi gated SPECT with a combination of count- and image-based techniques. *J Nucl Cardiol.* 2000; 7: 623-632
31. Bouvier F, Saltin B, Nejat M, Jensen-Urstad M. Left ventricular function and perfusion in elderly endurance athletes. *Med Sci Sports Exerc.* 2001; 33: 735-740
32. Bax JJ, Visser FC, Elhendy A, Poldermans D, Cornel JH, van Lingen A, Boersma E, Sloof GW, Fioretti PM, Visser CA. Prediction of improvement of regional left ventricular function after revascularization using different perfusion-metabolism criteria. *J Nucl Med.* 1999; 40: 1866-1873
33. Fuchs S, Baffour R, Zhou YF, Shou M, Pierre A, Tio FO, Weissman NJ, Leon MB, Epstein SE, Kornowski R. Transendocardial delivery of autologous bone marrow enhances collateral perfusion and regional function in pigs with chronic experimental myocardial ischemia. *J Am Coll Cardiol.* 2001; 37: 1726-1732
34. Kaul S, Pandian NG, Guerrero JL, Gillam LD, Okada RD, Weyman AE. Effects of selectively altering collateral driving pressure on regional perfusion and function in occluded coronary bed in the dog. *Circ Res.* 1987; 61: 77-85
35. Scherrer-Crosbie M, Liel-Cohen N, Otsuji Y, Guerrero JL, Sullivan S, Levine RA, Picard MH. Myocardial perfusion and wall motion in infarction border zone: assessment by myocardial contrast echocardiography. *J Am Soc Echocardiogr.* 2000; 13: 353-357
36. Kraitchman DL, Wilke N, Hexeberg E, Jerosch-Herold M, Wang Y, Parrish TB, Chang CN, Zhang Y, Bache RJ, Axel L. Myocardial perfusion and function in dogs with moderate coronary stenosis. *Magn Reson Med.* 1996; 35: 771-780
37. Schwitter J, Saeed M, Wendland MF, Sakuma H, Bremerich J, Canet E, Higgins CB. Assessment of myocardial function and perfusion in a canine model of non-occlusive coronary artery stenosis using fast magnetic resonance imaging. *J Magn Reson Imaging.* 1999; 9: 101-110
38. Lombardi M, Kvaerness J, Torheim G, Soma J, Cellerini F, Consalvo M, Landini MC, Cecchi CA, Michelassi C, Skjaerpe T, Jones RA, Rinck PA, L'Abbate A. Relationship between function and perfusion early after acute myocardial infarction. *Int J Cardiovasc Imaging.* 2001; 17: 383-393
39. Sensky PR, Jivan A, Hudson NM, Keal RP, Morgan B, Tranter JL, de Bono D, Samani NJ, Cherryman GR. Coronary artery disease: combined stress MR imaging protocol one-stop evaluation of myocardial perfusion and function. *Radiology.* 2000; 215: 608-614
40. Laham RJ, Simons M, Pearlman JD, Ho KK, Baim DS. Magnetic resonance imaging demonstrates improved regional systolic wall motion and thickening and myocardial perfusion of myocardial territories treated by laser myocardial revascularization. *J Am Coll Cardiol.* 2002; 39: 1-8
41. Leppo JA. An approach to myocardial viability based on perfusion, function and metabolic substrates. *Isr J Med Sci.* 1996; 32: 800-803
42. Rechavia E, de Silva R, Nihoyannopoulos P, Lammertsma AA, Jones T, Maseri A. Hyperdynamic performance of remote myocardium in acute infarc-

tion. Correlation between regional contractile function and myocardial perfusion. *Eur Heart J*. 1995; 16: 1845-1850

43. Maes A, Van de WF, Nuyts J, Bormans G, Desmet W, Mortelmans L. Impaired myocardial tissue perfusion early after successful thrombolysis. Impact on myocardial flow, metabolism, and function at late follow-up. *Circulation*. 1995; 92: 2072-2078
44. Tei C, Sakamaki T, Shah PM, Meerbaum S, Shimoura K, Kondo S, Corday E. Myocardial contrast echocardiography: a reproducible technique of myocardial opacification for identifying regional perfusion deficits. *Circulation*. 1983; 67: 585-593
45. Santoso T, Roelandt J, Mansyoer H, Abdurahman N, Meltzer RS, Hugenholtz PG. Myocardial perfusion imaging in humans by contrast echocardiography using polygelin colloid solution. *J Am Coll Cardiol*. 1985; 6: 612-620
46. Lang RM, Feinstein SB, Feldman T, Neumann A, Chua KG, Borow KM. Contrast echocardiography for evaluation of myocardial perfusion: effects of coronary angioplasty. *J Am Coll Cardiol*. 1986; 8: 232-235
47. Feinstein SB, Lang RM, Dick C, Neumann A, Al Sadir J, Chua KG, Carroll J, Feldman T, Borow KM. Contrast echocardiography during coronary arteriography in humans: perfusion and anatomic studies. *J Am Coll Cardiol*. 1988; 11: 59-65
48. Cheirif J, Zoghbi WA, Raizner AE, Minor ST, Winters WL, Jr., Klein MS, De Bauche TL, Lewis JM, Roberts R, Quinones MA. Assessment of myocardial perfusion in humans by contrast echocardiography. I. Evaluation of regional coronary reserve by peak contrast intensity. *J Am Coll Cardiol*. 1988; 11: 735-743
49. Vandenberg BF. Myocardial perfusion and contrast echocardiography: review and new perspectives. *Echocardiography*. 1991; 8: 65-75
50. Rovai D, Lombardi M, Distante A, L'Abbate A. Myocardial perfusion by contrast echocardiography. From off-line processing to radio frequency analysis. *Circulation*. 1991; 83: III97-103
51. Feinstein SB. Myocardial perfusion: contrast echocardiography perspectives. *Am J Cardiol*. 1992; 69: 36H-41H
52. Jayaweera AR, Kaul S. Quantifying myocardial blood flow with contrast echocardiography. *Am J Card Imaging*. 1993; 7: 317-335
53. Kaul S. Myocardial contrast echocardiography in coronary artery disease: potential applications using venous injections of contrast. *Am J Cardiol*. 1995; 75: 61D-68D
54. Villanueva FS, Kaul S. Assessment of myocardial perfusion in coronary artery disease using myocardial contrast echocardiography. *Coron Artery Dis*. 1995; 6: 18-28
55. Main ML, Grayburn PA. Clinical applications of transpulmonary contrast echocardiography. *Am Heart J*. 1999; 137: 144-153
56. Mulvagh SL, DeMaria AN, Feinstein SB, Burns PN, Kaul S, Miller JG, Monaghan M, Porter TR, Shaw LJ, Villanueva FS. Contrast echocardiography: current and future applications. *J Am Soc Echocardiogr*. 2000; 13: 331-342
57. Porter TR, Cwajg J. Myocardial contrast echocardiography: a new gold standard for perfusion imaging? *Echocardiography*. 2001; 18: 79-87
58. Wei K. Assessment of myocardial blood flow and volume using myocardial contrast echocardiography. *Echocardiography*. 2002; 19: 409-416
59. Zoghbi WA. Evaluation of myocardial viability with contrast echocardiography. *Am J Cardiol*. 2002; 90 Suppl 10A: 65J-71J
60. Meza MF, Ramee S, Collins T, Stapleton D, Milani RV, Murgo JP, Cheirif J. Knowledge of perfusion and contractile reserve improves the predictive value of recovery of regional myocardial function post revascularization: a study using the combination of myocardial contrast echocardiography and dobutamine echocardiography. *Circulation*. 1997; 96: 3459-3465
61. Mor-Avi V, Caiani EG, Collins KA, Korcarz CE, Bednarz JE, Lang RM. Combined assessment of myocardial perfusion and regional left ventricular function by analysis of contrast-enhanced power modulation images. *Circulation*. 2001; 104: 352-357
62. Oraby MA, Hays J, Maklady FA, El Hawary AA, Yaneza LO, Zabalgoitia M. Comparison of real-time coherent contrast imaging to dipyridamole thallium-201 single-photon emission computed tomography for assessment of myocardial perfusion and left ventricular wall motion. *Am J Cardiol*. 2002; 90: 449-454
63. Leong-Poi H, Rim SJ, Le DE, Fisher NG, Wei K, Kaul S. Perfusion versus function: the ischemic cascade in demand ischemia: implications of single-vessel versus multivessel stenosis. *Circulation*. 2002; 105: 987-992
64. Garot P, Pascal O, Simon M, El Amine S, Benacerraf S, Champagne S, Benaiem N, Mazoit JX, Hittinger L, Garot J, Dubois-Rande JL, Gueret P, Teiger E. Usefulness of combined quantitative assessment of myocardial perfusion and velocities by myocardial contrast and Doppler tissue echocardiography during coronary blood flow reduction. *J Am Soc Echocardiogr*. 2003; 16: 1-8
65. Mor-Avi V, Vignon P, Koch R, Weinert L, Spencer KT, Lang RM. Segmental analysis of Color Kinesis images: New method for quantitative assessment of left ventricular contraction and relaxation. *Circulation*. 1997; 95: 2082-2097

66. Lang R, Vignon P, Weinert L, Bednarz J, Korcarz C, Sandelski J, Koch R, Prater D, Mor-Avi V. Echocardiographic quantification of regional left ventricular wall motion using Color Kinesis. *Circulation.* 1996; 93: 1877-1885
67. Koch R, Lang RM, Garcia M, Weinert L, Bednarz J, Korcarz C, Coughlan B, Spiegel A, Kaji E, Spencer KT, Mor-Avi V. Objective evaluation of regional left ventricular wall motion during dobutamine stress echocardiographic studies using segmental analysis of color kinesis images. *J Am Coll Cardiol.* 1999; 34: 409-419
68. Caiani EG, Lang RM, Caslini S, Collins KA, Korcarz CE, Mor-Avi V. Quantification of regional myocardial perfusion using semiautomated translation-free analysis of contrast-enhanced power modulation images. *J Am Soc Echocardiogr.* 2003; 16: 116-123

Chapter 14

From a Toy with Lots of Potential to a Useful Clinical Tool - The Oxford Way of Doing Contrast Echocardiography

Jonathan Timperley • Helene Thibault • Harald Becher

Why Are There Still Problems in Translating the Potential Benefits of Contrast Echocardiography into Clinical Echocardiography?

There have been a large number of experimental and clinical studies demonstrating a variety of applications of ultrasound contrast agents. Although there has been a convergence of opinions over the last few years, there is still some debate on the practical clinical issues including indications, choice of contrast agent, best imaging modality etc. Many papers and presentations conclude that the use of contrast has huge potential (Table 14.1) [1], but concrete guidelines on how to integrate the technology into a busy clinical echocardiography laboratory are lacking. There are only a few well-controlled multicentre studies which are based on good blind reads, but the protocols of these studies performed in academic (tertiary) centres are not suitable for echocardiography laboratories in district general hospitals. Unfortunately most of these research groups use contrast echocardiography mainly for research studies rather than for "bread and butter" echocardiography. Thus there are no large quality series of contrast echocardiography studies, which are needed to assess the value of this technology in routine practice.

Sonographers and physicians interested in expanding their echocardiographic skills are dependent on the educational activities of the manufacturers of contrast media or ultrasound equipment. They are often confronted with selected opinions or, at best, with more or less controlled clinical studies often sponsored by one of the manufacturers of contrast media or ultrasound equipment. Participants of contrast echocardiography courses become excited by a multitude of indications demonstrated with ideal cases but often are alone when trying to transfer their training into their clinical work. Currently, there is only one official statement of the American Society of Echocardiography (ASE) [8] on the use of ultra-

Table 14.1. Potential of contrast echocardiography

Improved signal-to-noise ratio of Doppler signals[a]
Improved LV border definition[a] [2, 3]
Automatic analysis of LV function
Improved detection of LV thrombus [4] and masses[a]
Assessment of myocardial perfusion (ischaemia, viability) [3, 6, 7]
Assessment of coronary flow reserve[a]
Detecting vulnerable plaques
Enhanced thrombolysis
Local drug delivery

[a] Covered by approved indications

sound contrast media for left heart disease. Neither the British Society of Echocardiography nor any other European society of echocardiography has established guidelines on the use of contrast echocardiography. The recommendation of the ASE was published in 2001 but does not consider the important new contrast specific ultrasound methods and needs to be revised. In this chapter we describe how a busy echocardiography laboratory uses contrast echocardiography for clinical diagnosis.

Integrating Contrast Echocardiography in the Diagnostic Process to Assess Patients with Chest Pain

Prerequisites

Table 14.2 lists the criteria for starting contrast echocardiography in the echocardiography laboratory. The scientific evidence of contrast echo [9] has been demonstrated in previous chapters. Symposia and workshops often include use of contrast for myocardial perfusion imaging although this is not an approved indication but is considered more exciting than left ventricular opacification (LVO) studies. Although safety and tolerance of ultrasound contrast media are extremely favourable, use of ultrasound contrast for perfusion imaging cannot yet be advocated in a clinical echocardiography laboratory. It would only be justified to use contrast for myocardial perfusion imaging when there is no alternative safe method and there is adequate experience (which is often lacking) or there is an approved indication which provides data useful for assessment of myocardial contrast in addition to the findings for the approved indication. Fortunately, new low-power contrast-specific imaging technology allows us to perform a LVO study and a perfusion study simultaneously. Thus, perfusion can be assessed without prolonging a contrast study for LVO and without increasing the amount of contrast infused. Scanning with the new low-power contrast-specific imag-

Table 14.2. Criteria for introducing contrast echocardiography studies in a clinical echocardiography laboratory

- Scientific evidence
- Guidelines
- Safety, tolerance
- Medico-legal (approved indication)
- Funding for contrast agent
- Adequate scanner
- Simple, standardized protocol
- Training programmes

Table 14.3. Infrastructure for modern contrast echocardiography

Space:	No extra space for performing the studies but storage of contrast agent, syringes, lines
Staff:	No extra staff (when pump is used for contrast infusion)
Time slots:	No extra time when used for stress echocardiography[a]
Contrast agent:	Usually 1 vial per patient
Consenting:	Written informed consent is obtained for dobutamine stress echocardiography but not required for additional contrast

[a] In the John Radlcliffe Hospital the time slots for a complete dobutamine stress are 45 min and for a low-dose dobutamine stress 30 min, for resting contrast studies the maximum of 10 min have to be added to the 20 min of a regular transthoracic echocardiogram

ing modalities is currently the only way to obtain myocardial contrast echocardiograms outside clinical trials. In our laboratory, power pulse inversion, power modulation (Philips) or CPS (Acuson) have been successfully used for simultaneous acquisition of wall motion and perfusion imaging.

Cost benefit is another important issue. Although there are convincing data that contrast echocardiography is cost effective [10], this only holds true if it is performed with as little contrast as possible. In many clinical trials, complex protocols have been used including the use of several vials of ultrasound contrast agents. With current pricing of ultrasound contrast media it will be difficult to obtain a budget for more than one vial per patient. This is considered in Figs. 14.3 and 14.5, where we describe the current Oxford approach for clinical contrast echo.

The Infrastructure

Contrast echocardiography can be integrated without major changes. A laboratory which provides stress testing will have no difficulties in introducing contrast echocardiography. Table 14.3 provides a check-list for the infrastructure.

Ultrasound Scanner: Presets for Contrast Imaging

The acquisition of contrast images must be simple and standardized. Most current high-end scanners provide a variety of contrast-specific methods and protocols. The manufacturers say that different contrast agents and indications may require different imaging modalities. This is not acceptable for a busy clinical echocardiography laboratory. It is unrealistic to have several imaging modalities which have to be adjusted in different patients. When introducing contrast echocardiography in a department, one should decide on one or two imaging modalities which have to be programmed as a preset. In Oxford we use power modulation imaging as our standard contrast echocardiographic method. This imaging modality can be used both for LV border definition and assessment of myocardial perfusion. We have programmed a preset on a commercially available system which is activated by pressing a button on the control panel and works in almost very patient without further adjustments (Fig. 14.1).

In combination with an infusion of SonoVue at a rate of 0.8 ml/min using an agitating pump, the contrast preset using power modulation almost always provides suffient LVO to perform wall motion analysis. Usually myocardial contrast enhancement is good but there are some patients in whom myocardial contrast enhancement is unsatisfactory. In these patients, triggered imaging using an alternative preset such as harmonic power Doppler is an alternative and should be available at least as a backup method. It is well known that high-power triggered imaging such as harmonic power Doppler provides the best signal-to-noise ratio and it would be an ideal technique using low-power real-time power modulation with intermittent harmonic power Doppler frames. This would provide optimal real-time imaging of wall motion combined with the most sensitive method for perfusion imaging. There is already a *monitor mode* implemented in some scanners, but this modality combines only low-power *fundamental* imaging with harmonic power Doppler. This technique helps to adjust the scan-plane for the triggered images but the real-time low-power images are not useful for further assessment of wall motion. However, this is not covered by the current indication of the contrast agent and requires additional time and contrast agent for acquisition of the images.

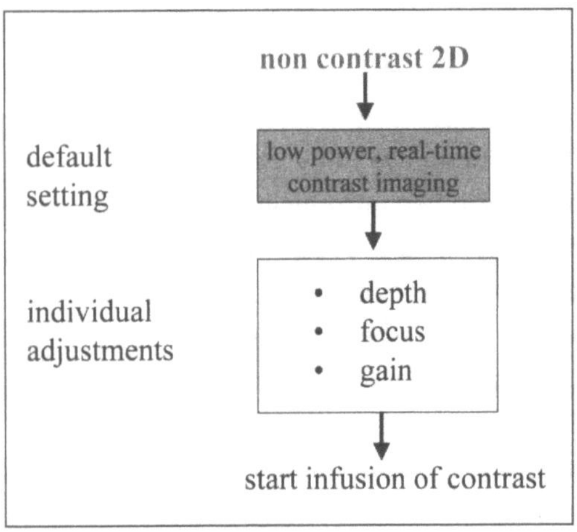

Fig. 14.1. Setting the scanner for contrast echocardiography

Contrast Agent/Infusion Pump

Different contrast agents are available and all work well for the assessment of LV wall motion and perfusion. So far, there are no data available that one of the approved contrast agents is superior to the others. Researchers in contrast echocardiography have used different agents and suggested that different indications may require different agents. If this is true, it will cause confusion in clinical echocardiography laboratories with a requirement to stock different agents and preparations. We believe that all clinically relevant indications can be assessed using a single contrast agent which the echocardiography laboratory needs to select before embarking on contrast echocardiography.

We have based our decision to use SonoVue mainly on the availability of a contrast infusion pump. It has been argued that infusion of contrast is complicated, but in

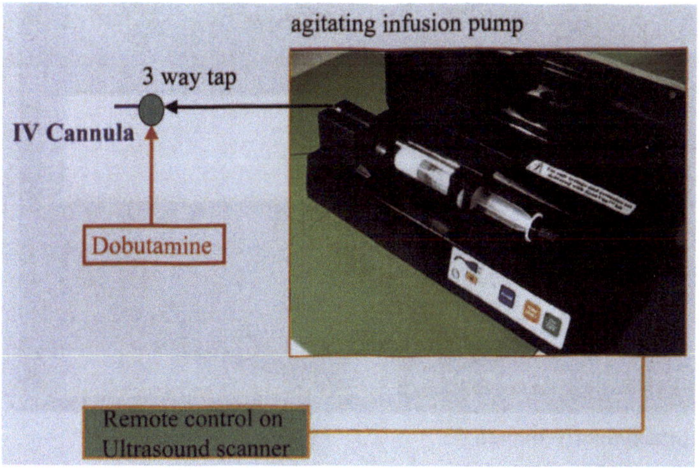

Fig. 14.2. Infusion pump for contrast studies, the line is connected to a three-way tap in stress echocardiography. The three-way tap is not needed for resting contrast studies

reality it simplifies and shortens the time needed for the application of the contrast and provides much longer intervals for image acquisition. A special infusion pump has been developed for SonoVue which provides constant agitation. With the advent of this pump we abandoned repetitive bolus application. The pump can be prepared within 2 min prior to the study while the patient undresses or during an echocardiography study. By an alternating rotating action, the contrast agent is agitated preventing bubbles separating and floating to the surface. The pump is then kept in a *stand-by* mode. The pump is started by the sonographer using a remote control and no additional staff is needed. An infusion of SonoVue at 0.8 ml/min is used and need not be changed in the majority of patients. Continuous infusion over a short time provides stable conditions to acquire loops from different scanplanes without hunting for images in the short period when contrast enhancement is optimal after a bolus injection. In stress echocardiography, infusion can be stopped at any time and resumed when needed. Between infusion periods the contrast agent is continuously agitated. The contrast infusion is connected via a three-way tap at the IV cannula. Thus, contrast can be infused simutaneously or separately during dobutamine stress echocardiography. We now use the infusion pump for every contrast study (Fig. 14.2).

Performing a Resting Contrast Study

Indications for Resting Contrast Echocardiography: John Radcliffe Hospital Oxford

- *Assessment of LV function in patients with suboptimal recordings*

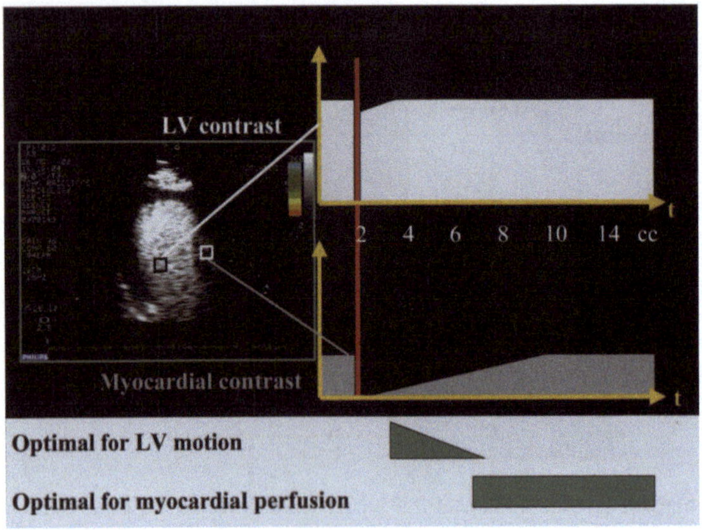

Fig. 14.3. Protocol for peforming a resting contrast study

- *Automatic LV boundary detection and 3D reconstruction**
- *Delineation of LV thrombi and masses in patients with suboptimal windows*
- *Assessment of the vascularity of cardiac masses*
- *Myocardial viability***
- *Assessment of reperfusion in acute transmural myocardial infarction****

* For off-line quantitative analysis of LV volumes and ejection fraction, preliminary data show comparable accuracy to manual tracing but faster performance than manual tracing.
** Currently used in conjunction with dobutamine stress echo, a pure resting contrast study would only be considered in patients with severe ventricular arrhythmia in whom dobutamine infusion would be hazardous.
*** Most promising indication for a resting myocardial contrast echocardiogram, but currently used only in a clinical trial.

Acquisition

Figure 14.3 shows the curent clinical protocol for a pure resting contrast study. First the apical four-chamber view is taken using our standard non-contrast harmonic imaging setting. Then the contrast preset is activated, the depth adjusted and the controls for time and lateral gain are checked. Infusion of contrast is started and within 1 min complete and intensive LVO as well as myocardial contrast enhancement can be found in almost every patient. Single loops of the apical four-chamber view, two-chamber view and long axis are acquired for assessment of LV function and stored on magnetico-optical disc. In each scan-plane, two loops are acquired. After acquisition of apical views, acquisition of parasternal long- and short-axis views should be attempted in all patients. However, these planes are off-axis in many patients and attenuation from contrast in the right ventricle may impair imaging. In most of the resting contrast studies, LV function is the main interest and acquisition of single loops facilitates subsequent automatic analysis using off-line software. During assessment of LV function, myocardial contrast enhancement can sometimes obscure the definition of LV borders, but "clearing" the myocardium with a burst of a few frames with high transmit power results in an optimum display of the borders. In the majority of patients, the myocardial contrast enhancement does not impair analysis. If the assessment of myocardial perfusion is required we use a flash replenishment technique as described in the section on contrast stress study.

Adjustment of the infusion speed or the lateral gain and TCG is usually not necessary. The current preset is quite robust similar to the setting of non-contrast 2D imaging. There are only a few patients in whom the gain has to be adjusted for perfusion imaging.

Reading and Analysis

Visual analysis of LV function is performed in all patients according to ASE guidelines for non-contrast imaging. Myocardial contrast and particularly the enhancement of the epicardial vessels helps in judging wall thickening as well as inward motion of the myocardium. Contrast images are ideal for measuring LV volumes and LV ejection fraction (Fig. 14.4). The post-flash images provide the best contrast between the myocardium and the LV cavity. Manual tracing on still frames is easy and quick and so in every contrast study these measurements should be obtained! The tools for automatic assessment of LV borders (such as colour kinesis) are currently being investigated in clinical trials and may be a useful clinical tool in the future.

Although we currently perform resting studies almost exclusively for assessment of LV wall motion and delineation of suspected thrombi and masses, myocardial contrast signals are judged using visual assessment. A visually evident contrast defect is considered present when there is a relative decrease in contrast enhancement in one region compared with other adjacent regions which have the same or worse imaging conditions. The diagnostic confidence of an observed perfusion defect increases when two contiguous segments fail to exhibit contrast enhancement. A contrast defect usually does not extend over the full thickness of the myocardium. With current contrast-specific low-power imaging, usually signals in the epicardial layers of the myocardium are displayed. Whether this represents real tissue perfusion or just blooming of signals from epicardial vessels has not yet been completely evaluated. For the assessment of a perfusion defect it is probably not relevant. However, we should be cautious when making the diagnosis of subendocardial perfusion defect with the poor spatial resolution of current real-time imaging modalities. An epicardial contrast enhancement increases the diagnostic confidence of a perfusion defect. If a segment is completely black, an imaging artefact such as attenuation or rib shadowing has to be considered.

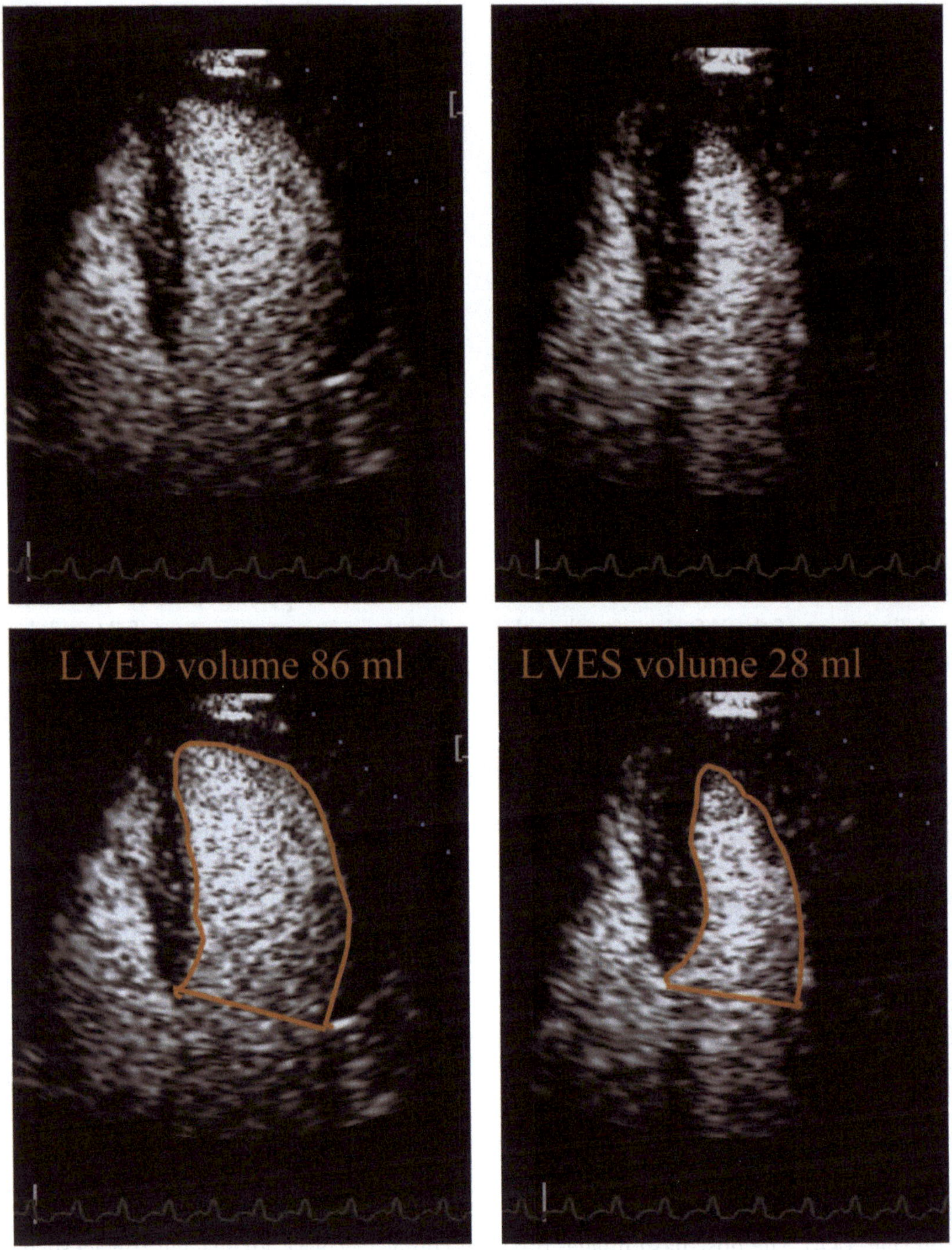

Fig. 14.4. A Four- and two-chamber views, endsystolic and endiastolic contrast echocardiograms for assessment of LV volumes and ejection fraction. Note the excellent endocardial border definition. **B** Tracing of the endocardial borders

Table 14.4. Interpretation of resting contrast echocardiography studies

Wall motion	Myocardial contrast	Diagnostic significance
Normal	Normal	Higher diagnostic confidence
Abnormal	Abnormal	Higher diagnostic confidence
Abnormal	Normal	SCAR vs stunning, hibernation[a]
Normal	Abnormal	Consider imaging artefact[b]

[a] If the indication is myocardial viability we still use a low-dose dobutamine stress in addition

[b] In acute coronary syndromes there may a situation where a perfusion defect preceeds wall motion abnormality, but there are no controlled clinical studies available

Because of the limited experience with real-time perfusion imaging we still use the perfusion data only in conjuction with the findings of visual LV wall motion analysis (see Table 14.4). Generally, concordance of wall motion analysis and perfusion imaging increases the diagnostic confidence. This is particurlarly useful when judgement of LV wall motion is dubious. Probably the most important situation where perfusion imaging makes a difference is in akinetic areas.

Before one tries to assess myocardial contrast enhancement it is important to look at myocardial thickness which often can be seen very well during infusion of contrast. A thin myocardium (<5 mm) usually indicates non-viable tissue. When analysing loops obtained with real-time imaging, judgement of wall motion and myocardial perfusion is often combined. A subendocardial defect makes a wall motion defect much clearer and vice versa. Thus, assessment of myocardial contrast often helps to increase the diagnostic confidence of dubious wall motion analysis. In a resting study, a perfusion defect can be due to ischaemia with a flow-limiting coronary stenosis at rest, a scar or an artefact. Artefacts are most common in the basal lateral and anterior wall and can be easily detected by the typical criteria of attenuation and shadowing or a normal thickening. Other discrepant findings between wall motion and myocardial contrast enhancement occur with stunning and hibernation. Both conditions can be suspected when reduced wall motion and good contrast enhancement are found in a resting perfusion study.

Performing a Stress Contrast Study

Indications for Contrast Stress Contrast Echocardiography: John Radcliffe Hospital Oxford

- *For the assessment of ischaemia*
- *In patients with good acoustic windows at peak stress or when symptoms occur*
- *In patients with poor acoustic window at rest, low stress and peak stress or when symptoms occur*
- *For the assessment of hibernation using low-dose dobutamine*
- *At rest to assess for resting regional abnormality*

- *May be required later to assess for biphasic response depending on acoustic window*

In stress echocardiography it is reasonable not to confine the use of contrast to patients with poor windows. Patients with adequate windows can cause problems in acquiring diagnostic images when they are feeling uncomfortable or short of breath at high doses of dobutamine and particularly when they develop anginal symptoms. In these situations it is extremely useful to have the best imaging modality available.

Acquisition Contrast Stress Echocardiography: John Radcliffe Hospital Oxford

When we integrated contrast echo into our dobutamine protocol it was our aim to use as little contrast as possible (because of the costs) and not to prolong the study particularly at peak stress. Figures 14.5 and 14.6 show the current Oxford protocols. Based on the image quality of the baseline recordings we decide whether contrast agent is infused at rest and peak stress or only at peak stress. In patients with good endocardial border delineation, we perform a dobutamine stress echocardiogram according to the standard protocol without contrast infusion at rest. After acquisition of the peak stress loops, the contrast infusion is started and the dobutamine infusion is stopped (Fig. 14.7). Within 30 s there is sufficient contrast enhancement and the peak contrast images are acquired in the apical views (Fig. 14.8). We do not routinely acquire parasternal contrast views at peak stress. In the recovery period the contrast images are reviewed. If peak myocardial contrast enhancement looks normal (homogeneous contrast enhancement) and wall motion is normal no other contrast recordings are needed. If there is an area with reduced con-

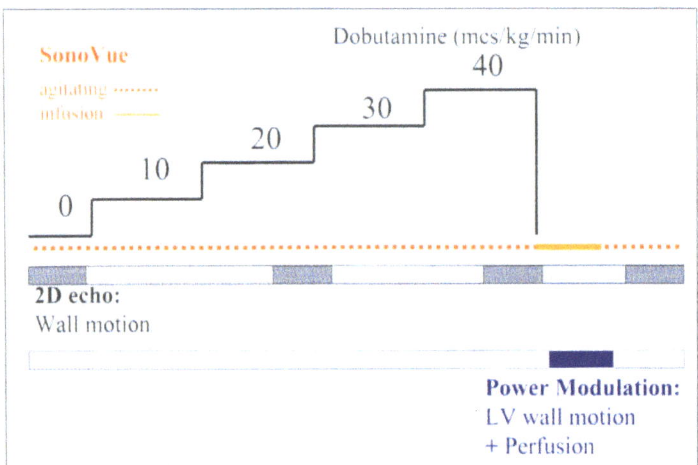

Fig. 14.5. Protocol for peforming a stress contrast study (patient with poor acoustic window)

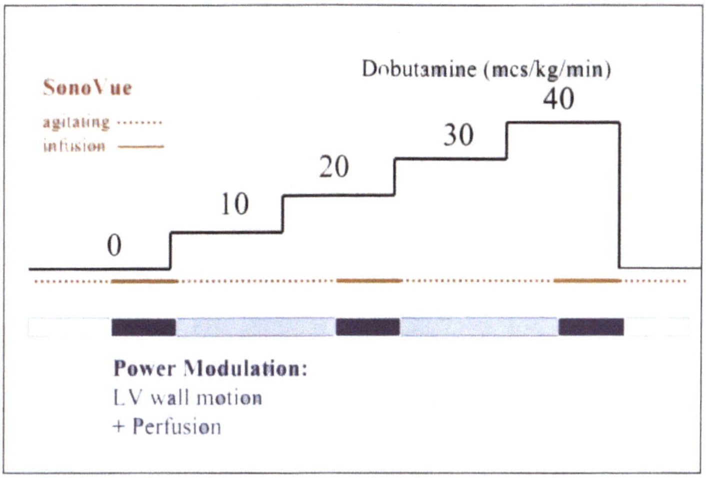

Fig. 14.6. Protocol for peforming a stress contrast study (patient with good acoustic window)

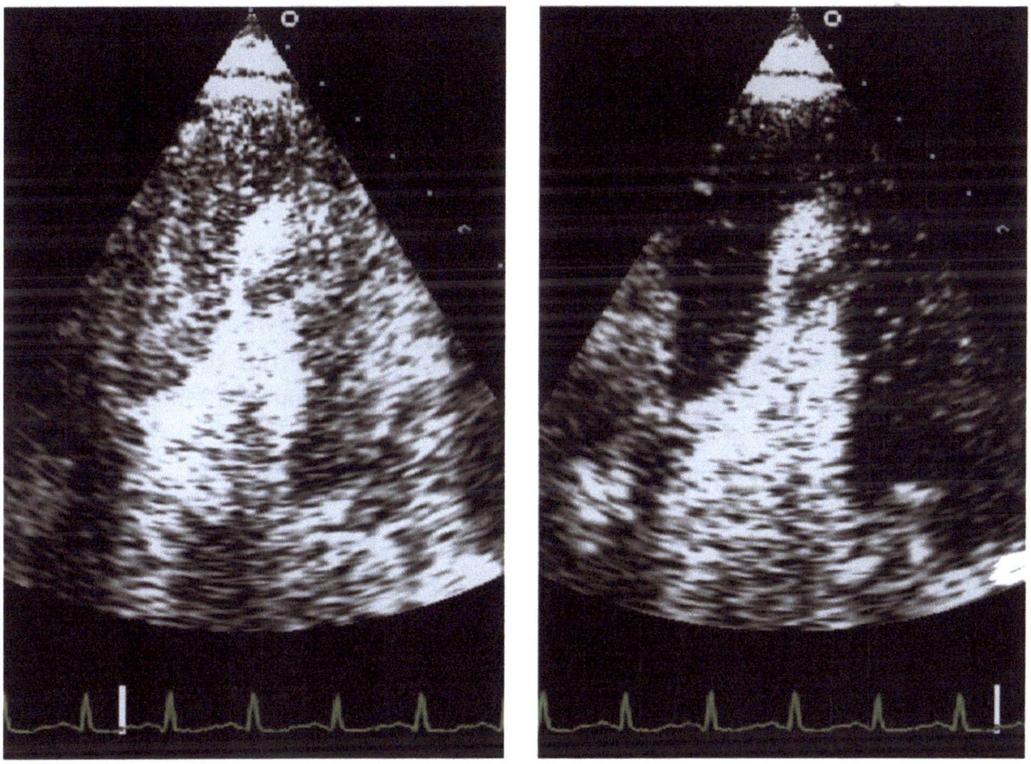

Fig. 14.7. Power modulation, low transmit power (MI 0.2), SonoVue infusion, 0.8 ml/min, four-chamber view, normal myocardial contrast enhancement (*left*), same setting after "clearing" the myocardium provides excellent endocardial definition (*right*)

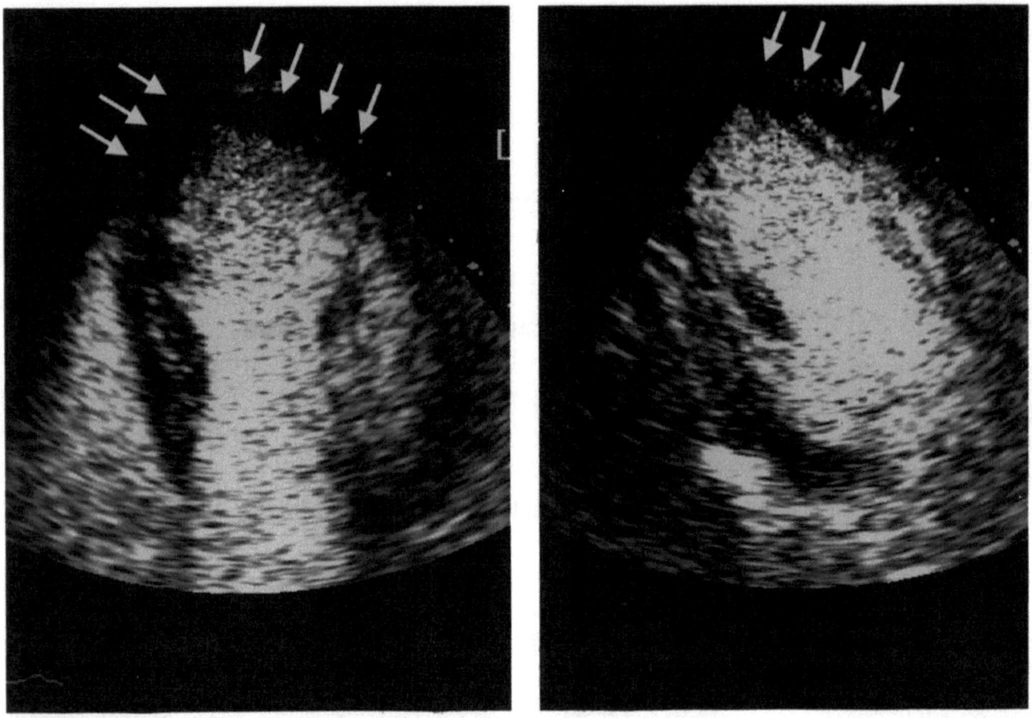

Fig. 14.8. Power modulation, low transmit power (MI 0.2), SonoVue infusion, 0.8 ml/min, apical perfusion defect seen in four-chamber view, (*left, arrows*), and three-chamber view (*right, arrows*)

trast enhancement, resting contrast echocardiography is performed after the heart rate has returned to baseline. This approach allows us to perform most of our contrast studies with a single vial of contrast.

When looking for perfusion defects it is crucial to avoid oversaturation with contrast or inadequate myocardial contrast enhancement. The destruction of myocardial contrast shortly after increasing the transmit power and subsequent contrast replenishment in the myocardium results in different concentrations of contrast and help to obtain the optimum contrast between normally perfused areas and hypoperfused myocardium. Subtle subendocardial defects may be obscured by excess contrast. These may be revealed by alterations in contrast rate or further bubble destruction with intermittent high power.

Reading and Analysis

Visual analysis is performed in the same way as in resting contrast echocardiography (see previous section). No postprocessing is used and no quantitative analysis is performed. We are aware that both can improve analysis but the available data from clinical trials are not robust enough to use these sophisticated and time-consuming tools in a busy echocardiography laboratory. A perfusion defect is diagnosed by comparing the signal enhancement in segments at the same depth in the same view (as we do in a resting study), and by comparing the contrast defect with side-by-side baseline images.

Contrast enhancement facilitates the detection of new wall motion abnormalities and our contrast stress echocardiograms are judged on the wall motion findings. However, the perfusion pattern in an abnormally contracting wall segment is integrated to produce a comprehensive assessment (see Table 14.5). Concordant findings in wall motion and perfusion increase our confidence when assessing a dubious wall motion abnormality. For instance, when asked for the significance of an angiographically determined coronary stenosis, normal wall motion and perfusion in the territory supplied by this vessel should negate the need for coronary intervention. With a questionable wall motion finding, however, either further expensive diagnostic tests are performed or the coronary intervention would be performed. From a medico-legal standpoint it appears more important to diagnose significant inducible ischaemia even at risk of reducing the specificity of the test. With today's minimal risks of coronary angiography (and in the future, further reductions with non-invasive coronary angiography) it seems to be less hazardous for a patient to have an "over-read" rather than "under-read" study. Therefore, it is important that a study reported as "normal" is truly normal.

That does not mean that we have to entirely sacrifice specificity. Combined assessment of wall motion and perfusion can also help to increase the diagnostic confidence of abnormal findings. A new wall motion

Table 14.5. Interpretation of stress contrast studies

Wall motion	Myocardial contrast	Diagnostic significance
Normal	Normal	Higher diagnostic confidence
New WMA	PD at stress	Higher diagnostic confidence, perfusion defect often displays better extent of ischaemia[a]
New WMA[a]	Normal	Consider imaging artefact in perfusion imaging or scan out of plane[b] *use WMA for clinical diagnosis*
Normal	PD at stress	PD reflects better sensitivity of perfusion compared to wall motion analysis[c]

WMA, wall motion abnormality; PD, perfusion defect

[a] The full extent of the hypoperfused area should be assessed during the contrast replenishment following clearance of myocardial contrast by a short period of scanning with higher transmit power

[b] With adequate image quality perfusion overrules questionable wall motion findings. However, perfusion is not yet an approved indication and therefore stress echocardiography cannot be read just using perfusion data

[c] With current acquisition protocol rare in our experience

abnormality should be combined with a perfusion defect if myocardial contrast echocardiography is performed properly.

A new wall motion abnormality without a corresponding perfusion defect is likely to be an artefact, because a perfusion abnormality is the prerequisite of a wall motion abnormality. However, even with optimal endocardial border definition, wall motion may be misinterpreted when out of the optimal scan-plane. Discordant findings of LV function and perfusion do occur. In this setting we use the wall motion abnormality (WMA) and would proceed with invasive testing and accept that we might overdiagnose some patients, but we do not want to miss patients with true wall motion analysis by exclusively trusting an imaging technology which has not been validated fully for this purpose. With more experience with perfusion assessment, we certainly can save those patients with false-positive wall motion analyses from further testing. We will gain this experience from our audits performed every year.

Display of perfusion defects without corresponding wall motion abnormalities is possible, but it is not frequent using this protocol. We are aware that the perfusion defect may be visualized at a stage of stress where wall motion is still normal. This would only be possible when we could use contrast enhancement at lower stages of stress which is currently not performed because of the increased amount of contrast needed for this purpose. It is not that we are concerned about the volume of contrast but of the cost of several vials for every stress echocardiography study.

The Future: Perfusion Imaging Instead of Wall Motion Analysis or Both?

It seems to be reasonable to use all available information from an echocardiographic study to make a clinical diagnosis. Thus, having both the information from LV wall motion analysis and perfusion imaging seems the way forward. Indeed, the imaging modality we use allows us to acquire and analyse function and perfusion qualitatively and quantitatively in many ways. However, it should be clear that the use of quantitative imaging prolongs and complicates contrast echocardiographic studies and in many centres there will not be enough time and resources to acquire and to analyse all the information made available from combined wall motion/perfusion studies.

Numerous convincing studies have shown that perfusion imaging should be more sensitive than LV wall motion analysis and that changes in perfusion preceed wall motion abnormalities in acute ischaemia. Therefere it may be questioned whether we cannot give up assessment of wall motion in many situations. There are several advantages in having a perfusion method for assessment of ischaemia instead of LV wall motion analysis. Judgement of LV wall motion may be challenging at higher heart rates even in patients with good acoustic windows and there is still considerable interoberver variability. Assessment of perfusion images can be performed on still frames which theoretically should facilitate visual judgement in comparison to read loops. If we can rely on myocardial perfusion images, stress using a vasodilator would be preferable and would considerably reduce the time for a single test. Moreover, the amount of contrast needed for a dipyridamole stress echocardiogram is lower than for an exercise or dobutamine protocol. Thus, as soon as there is an approval for perfusion imaging, we will consider abandoning the regular dobutamine protocol and use a vasodilator stress protocol.

References

1. Mulvagh SL, DeMaria A, Feinstein SB et al. Contrast echocardiography: current and future applications. J Am Soc Echocardiogr 2000; 13: 331-42
2. Nanda NC, Wistran DC, Karlsberg RP et al. Multicenter evaluation of SonoVue for improved endocardial border delineation. Echocardiography 2002; 19: 27-36
3. Oraby MA, Hays J, Maklady FA, El-Hawary AA, Yaneza LO, Zabalgoitia M. Comparison of real-time coherent contrast imaging to dipyridamole thallium-201 single-photon emission computed tomography for assessment of myocardial perfusion and left ventricular wall motion. Am J Cardiol. 2002; 90(5): 449-54
4. Thanigaraj S, Schechtman KB, Perez JE et al. Improved echocardiographic delineation of left ventricular thrombus with the use of intravenous second-generation contrast image enhancement. J Am Soc Echocardiogr 1999; 12: 1022-6
5. Lepper W, Shivalkar B, Rinkevich D et al: Assessment of the vascularity of a left ventricular mass using myocardial contrast echocardiography. J Am Soc Echocardiogr 2002; 15(11): 1419-22
6. Porter T, Xie F, Silver M, Kricsfeld et al. Real-time perfusion imaging with low mechanical index pulse inversion Doppler imaging. J Am Coll Cardiol 2001; 37: 748-53
7. Shimoni S, Zoghbi WA, Xie F et al. Real-time assessment of myocardial perfusion and wall motion during bicycle and treadmill exercise echocardiography: Comparison with single photon emission computed tomography. J Am Coll Cardiol 2001; 37: 741-7
8. Waggoner AD, Ehler D, Adams D et al. Guidelines for the cardiac sonographer in the performance of contrast echocardiography: recommendations of the American Society of Echocardiography Council on Cardiac Sonography. J Am Soc Echocardiogr 2001; 14: 417-20
9. Becher H, Burns PN. Handbook of contrast echocardioraphy. Heidelberg: Springer Verlag 2000
10. Tardif JC, Dore A, Chan KL et al. Economic impact of contrast stress echocardiography on the diagnosis and initial treatment of patients with suspected coronary artery disease. J Am Soc Echocardiogr 2002; 15(11): 1335-45

Chapter 15

Clinical Application of Contrast Echocardiography in Critically Ill Patients

William A. A. Foster • Jonathan R. Lindner

Echocardiography and the Critically Ill Patient

Patients managed in the intensive care unit (ICU) setting typically have dysfunction of one or more organ systems, of which the circulatory system is among the most common. Cardiovascular pathology is not only a frequent primary cause for ICU care, but it also is a frequent complication in the critically ill patient presenting with other life-threatening diseases. Due to the tenuous status of most ICU patients, the initial cardiac assessment must be rapid, complete, and precise in defining the underlying pathophysiology. Noninvasive echocardiographic imaging has become an integral part of the evaluation and care of critically ill patients due to its portability, safety, and ability to provide a comprehensive assessment of cardiac performance in a very rapid manner.

Information provided by 2-D and Doppler echocardiography can be potentially lifesaving. Accordingly, guidelines recommending the use of echocardiography in the critically ill patient [1] are liberal despite a paucity of large trials designed to test the incremental value of the test for positively influencing patient outcome. The impact of echocardiography in clinical practice can be appreciated, however, by some of the nonrandomized clinical trials that have been performed to date. For the evaluation of critically ill patients with hypotension or pulmonary edema, echocardiography is extremely sensitive in discerning a cardiac versus noncardiac etiology [2]. Even when cardiac disease is suspected, the assessment of ventricular function, valvular function, or cardiac hemodynamics can play a major role in optimizing therapy. Echocardiographic findings have been shown to produce an objective change in therapy in over half of patients in the ICU in whom the test was requested [3].

Although patients in the ICU have the most to gain from echocardiography, they are also the most challenging to image from a transthoracic approach. Adequate acoustic windows are often difficult to obtain for many reasons (Table 15.1). The technical difficulties in imaging ICU patients has led to increasing use of transesophageal echocardiography (TEE) in these patients. In a prospective study of critically ill patients with unexplained hypotension, 64% of transthoracic studies were inadequate for accurate interpretation whereas only 3% of TEE studies were inadequate [4]. The impact of echocardiography in this study could be appreciated by the change in diagnosis that was made based on TEE findings in 28% of patients [4]. Compared to transthoracic echocardiography, however, TEE requires more time and expertise, is more costly, and is not without risks and patient discomfort. Accordingly, the use of intravenous microbubble contrast agents together with transthoracic ultrasound has been increasingly applied in the ICU setting.

In this chapter, we will discuss the role of contrast echocardiography in critically ill patients for facilitating endocardial border definition, hemodynamic assessment, and identification of potentially catastrophic complications such as ventricular pseudoaneurysms and thrombi. We will also discuss the potential impact of bedside assessment of myocardial perfusion with myocardial contrast echocardiography (MCE) on the management of critically ill patients in the ICU setting.

Table 15.1. Technical challenges for echocardiographic imaging of ICU patients

Positive pressure ventilation
Pressure support ventilation/PEEP
Lung disease
Previous chest surgery
Surgical dressings/surgical drains
Inability to position appropriately

Endocardial Border Definition

The most common reason for performing echocardiography in the ICU is to assess left ventricular systolic function in patients who have either unexplained hypotension, congestive heart failure, or suspected ischemia. Accurate assessment of global function or regional systolic thickening requires visualization of the endocardial borders. Adequate border delineation is not possible in a relatively large percentage of patients in the ICU setting for reasons stated previously. These obstacles persist despite recent advances in technology such as harmonic imaging. While state-of-the-art imaging methods have decreased the frequency of technically inadequate studies in the general population referred for echocardiography to 5%–15%, the frequency of inadequate studies in ICU patients is much higher and, in unselected patients, as many as 1 in 4 myocardial segments are uninterpretable [5]. Left ventricular cavity opacification with stable, encapsulated microbubble agents that can be administered intravenously often improves visualization of the endocardial contours, illustrated by the end-systolic and end-diastolic apical four-chamber images in Fig. 15.1.

Although determination of overall left ventricular function is often possible even when not all segments are well seen, there are many situations in the ICU where optimal visual-

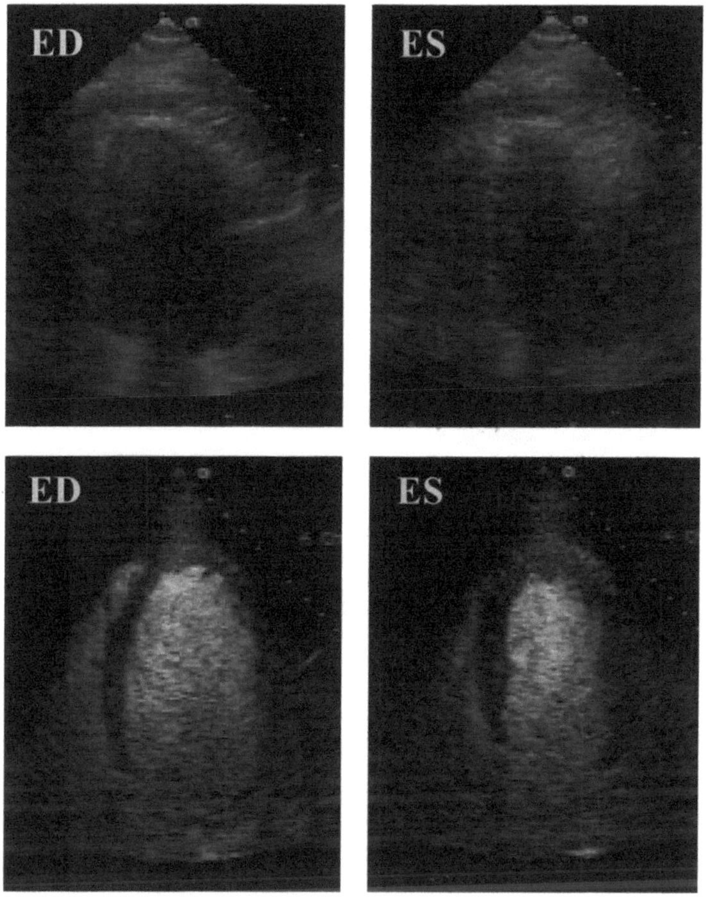

Fig. 15.1. Apical four-chamber images at end-diastole (*ED*) and end-systole (*ES*) from a patient before (*top images*) and after (*bottom images*) administration of an intravenous microbubble contrast agent

ization of systolic thickening for *all* myocardial segments is particularly important. The most common of these circumstances is when echocardiography is performed to evaluate for active ischemia. In a study of patients where transthoracic echocardiography with harmonic imaging was performed in consecutive unselected patients in the ICU, the use of intravenous contrast for left ventricular cavity opacification decreased the number of uninterpretable segments from 28% to 7%, and increased the number of segments that could be interpreted without doubt from 58% to 86% [5]. Accordingly, ejection fraction could be accurately assessed in only 62% without, and 91% with contrast enhancement. In clinical practice, all patients do not necessarily receive microbubble contrast agents. Instead, patients are usually identified based on the inability to adequately assess ventricular performance with non-contrast-enhanced

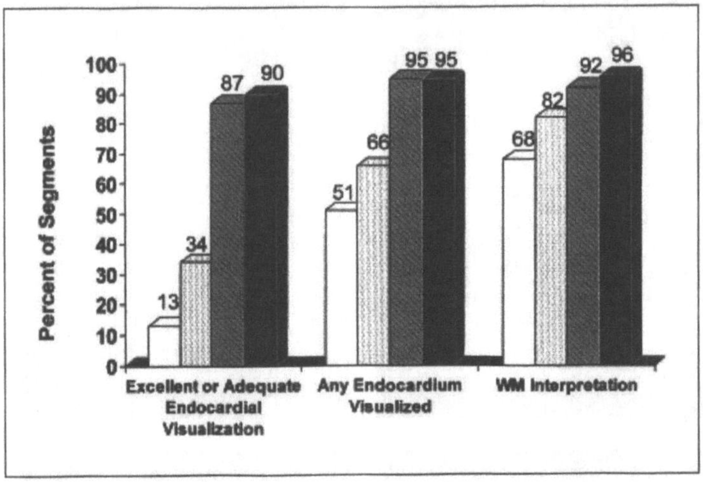

Fig. 15.2. Percentage of segments able to be visualized and interpreted for wall motion (*WM*) by echocardiography in patients with technically difficult studies by transthoracic imaging. Data are shown for fundamental imaging at 2-3.5 MHz (*white bars*), harmonic imaging with transmission frequency of 1.75 MHz (*light gray bars*), contrast-enhanced imaging (*dark gray bars*), and TEE (*black bars*) (Reproduced with permission from Yong et al. [6])

transthoracic imaging. As would be expected, contrast appears to have an even greater impact when ICU patients with technically difficult echocardiograms are selected. In one study, the use of intravenous contrast compared to harmonic imaging alone markedly increased the percentage of segments adequately visualized (Fig. 15.2), and improved the number of patients in whom ejection fraction could be assessed from 50% to 97% [6]. Using TEE as a gold standard, the use of contrast in selected patients with technically difficult windows also improved sensitivity for detecting wall motion abnormalities from 75% to 89% [6].

Contrast enhancement may not only improve diagnostic yield, but also reader confidence [5-8]. Contrast administration appears to have the greatest role for improving confidence of readers with the least clinical experience interpreting echocardiograms [7]. The importance of this issue is underscored by the immediate treatment decisions that must be sometimes made in the ICU by readers with limited expertise in wall motion assessment.

Assessment of right ventricular function is also important in the evaluation of critically ill patients with hypotension or hypoxia. Although relatively uncommon, isolated right ventricular infarction can be a cause of acute circulatory collapse [9]. Identification of right ventricular involvement with an inferior myocardial infarction is also important for optimizing therapy, such as avoidance of vasodilators and diuretics. Echocardiographic evaluation of right ventricular size and function has also increasingly been used to identify patients with acute pulmonary embolism who are hemodynamically stable but likely to benefit from thrombolytic therapy [10]. Although the role of contrast echocardiography in these settings has not been prospectively studied, there are preliminary data implying that assessment of right ventricular size and systolic performance is more accurate when microbubble contrast enhancement is employed [11].

Although microbubble administration for endocardial border enhancement does incur cost, the appropriate use of contrast in selected patients is likely to be a cost-effective strategy. Results from a phase III clinical trial demonstrated that use of contrast agents for left ventricular opacification in patients with suboptimal windows referred for transthoracic echocardiography is economically favorable due to a reduced need for more costly procedures [12]. It is likely that selected use of contrast will be especially advantageous in terms of cost-savings in the ICU setting. Cost and resource-utilization models based on the premise that microbubble administration would preclude the subsequent use of TEE to determine left ventricular function have confirmed the cost benefit of contrast echocardiography in ICU patients with technically difficult studies [6].

Hemodynamic Assessment

The determination of pulmonary artery pressure and left heart filling pressures is routinely used to guide treatment of the critically ill patient. Provided that continuous monitoring is not needed, noninvasive hemodynamic assessment with Doppler echocardiography can prevent the need for invasive right heart catheterization. The use of microbubble contrast agents facilitates acquisition of the raw data needed to make these measurements. Agitated saline contrast is generally sufficient for enhancing Doppler signals from right-sided flows, such as tricuspid regurgitation. Agitated saline contrast does not, however, produce left-sided enhancement because of pulmonary entrapment of large bubbles, and very rapid gas volume loss for the small bubbles. For pulmonary transit and left-sided enhancement, more stable contrast agents are used that are encapsulated or contain high-molecular-weight gases that are less soluble and diffusible. The most common reason for this application of contrast is to enhance pulmonary venous Doppler signals (Fig. 15.3) which can provide potentially important information on the left ventricular diastolic performance [13]. Intravenous contrast administration has been shown to markedly increase the percentage of studies where pulmonary venous Doppler signals are adequate for interpretation from 27% to 92%, and to provide a signal quality that is equivalent to that obtained by TEE [14].

Identification of pulmonary venous flow has also become important in certain patient groups in whom pulmonary vein stenosis or occlusion can occur. In patients undergoing lung transplantation, pulmonary vein thrombosis in the post operative period occurs in 15% of patients, and is associated with an increased mortality rate [15]. Pulmonary venous stricture or thrombosis can also occur in patients undergoing radiofrequency catheter ablation of focal atrial fibrillation, or in patients with congenital heart disease with or without prior surgical correction of pulmonary venous anomaly [16-17]. Although contrast echocardiography has not been studied extensively in these populations, it is likely that enhancement of Doppler signals will facilitate identification of abnormal pulmonary venous flow patterns associated with these potentially catastrophic events.

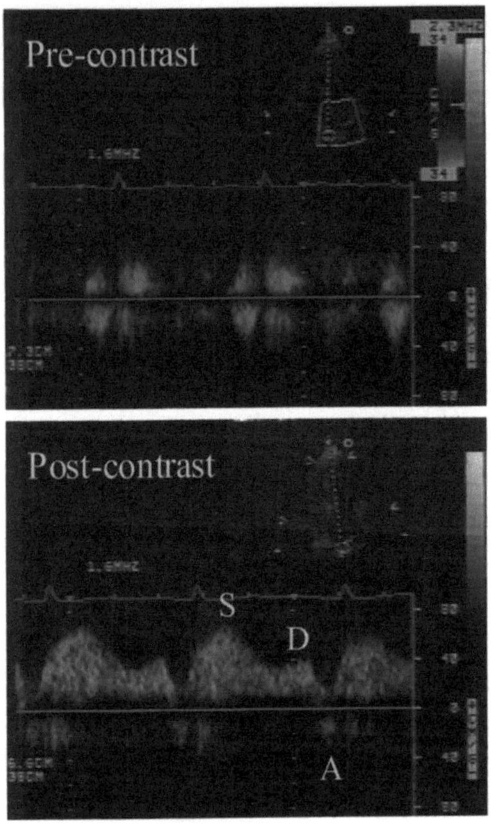

Fig. 15.3. Pulmonary venous Doppler signals obtained from the apical four-chamber imaging plane before and after contrast enhancement with an intravenous microbubble contrast agent. After low-dose contrast administration, there is marked improvement in ventricular systolic (*S*), early diastolic (*D*), and atrial systolic (*A*) velocity signals

Anatomic Complications of Disease

Echocardiography has proven to be invaluable for identifying serious anatomic complications of cardiovascular disease such as ventricular thrombus, pseudoaneurysm, or aortic dissection. The ability to diagnose these conditions promptly and confidently cannot be overstressed since each is an indication for urgent medical or surgical intervention.

Echocardiography has been widely used to identify intracardiac thrombus in patients with recent myocardial infarction or in patients with suspected embolic ischemic events. Provided the images are adequate, transthoracic imaging is quite sensitive and accurate for identifying left ventricular thrombi [18, 19]. TEE can be performed when transthoracic images are less than optimal, although this approach is sometimes limited in its ability to image the left ventricular apex. Contrast enhancement with intravenous agents has become increasingly applied to identify ventricular thrombi with transthoracic imaging when apical structures are unclear because of poor endocardial definition, near-field clutter artifact, or a false tendon [20]. The presence of thrombus is confirmed by an intracavitary filling defect (Fig. 15.4). Contrast enhancement can also potentially be of use to identify apical filling abnormalities caused by inflammatory and thrombotic masses in patients with eosinophilic cardiomyopathies, and for detecting intracardiac tumors [20-21]. Although differentiating tumor from thrombus can sometimes be difficult, perfusion imaging with MCE has been report-

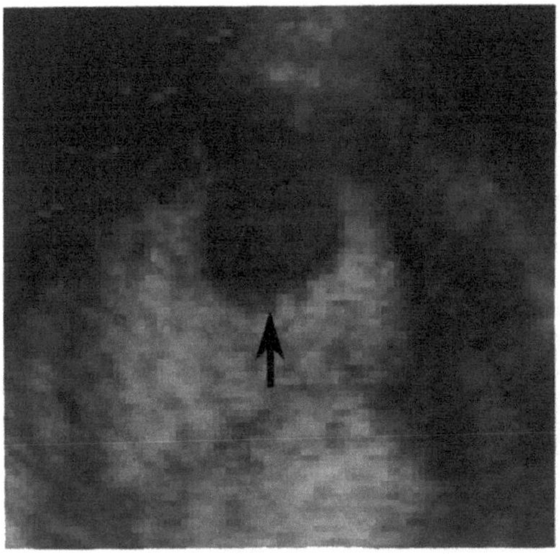

Fig. 15.4. Example of an apical thrombus (*arrow*) on echocardiography in the apical four-chamber imaging plane following intravenous administration of a microbubble contrast agent

ed to provide information on vascularity of intracardiac masses, thereby confirming the diagnosis of tumor (Fig. 15.5).

Ventricular aneurysms have been reported to occur in 5%–15% of patients following myocardial infarction. Although true aneurysms are normally easily detected by transthoracic echocardiography, the use of contrast can be helpful in identifying mural thrombi within the aneurysm. Diagnosis of pseudoaneurysms, caused by partial or complete rupture of the ventricular free wall, tends to be more difficult than with true aneurysms. Pseudoaneurysms often have a very narrow neck and can be difficult to discriminate from a localized pericardial fluid collection. The entry of microbubble contrast agents into a pseudoaneurysm has been shown to facilitate the diagnosis of this ominous complication of ischemic heart disease [20, 22] (Fig. 15.6).

Echocardiographic diagnosis of thoracic aortic dissection relies on the detection of an intimal tear and differential flow in the true

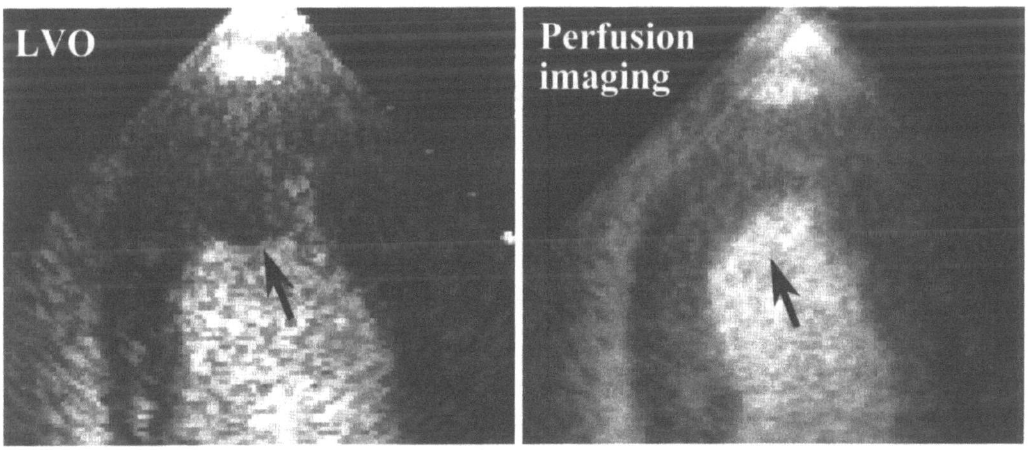

Fig. 15.5. Example of a tumor at the apex of the left ventricular cavity. During imaging for left ventricular opacification (*LVO*), a mass was evident as an intracavitary filling defect (*arrow*). The contrast-enhanced signal during perfusion imaging with high-power intermittent harmonic imaging was very high, making it difficult to discern from the blood in the left ventricular cavity, and indicating the presence of a hypervascular tumor (Reproduced with permission from Lepper et al. [21])

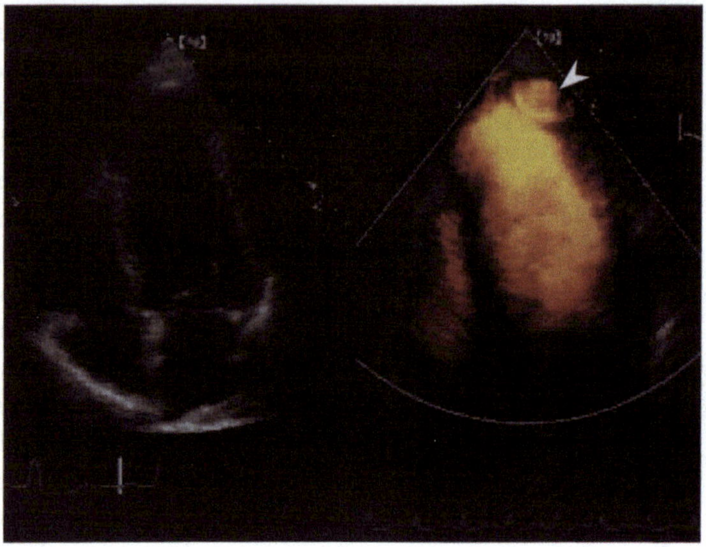

Fig. 15.6. An apical four-chamber view demonstrating an example of an apical-lateral ventricular pseudoaneurysm (*arrow*), which is better seen during contrast enhancement and power-Doppler imaging (Reproduced with permission from Bednarz et al. [20])

and false lumen. TEE has a sensitivity of more than 97% in identifying dissection of the thoracic aorta [23]. Although the specificity has increased in the past decade, there continues to be occasional false-positive TEE studies due largely to reverberation artifacts creating the appearance of an intimal flap. Case reports have demonstrated that contrast administration during TEE can differentiate these artifacts from true dissection [24]. The use of contrast with TEE has also been shown to be useful for distinguishing true lumen from false lumen, which is important for guiding appropriate cardiopulmonary bypass cannula placement during surgical repair [25]. The use of contrast administration to facilitate diagnosis of thoracic aortic dissection with transthoracic echocardiography, which has a sensitivity of 55%–80% without contrast [23, 26], has not been reported. This potential use of contrast may be important in the emergency room setting since the requirement of specially trained personnel to perform TEE can result in a delay in diagnosis.

Myocardial Perfusion and Other Future Applications

Methods for quantifying myocardial perfusion with MCE have been described in other chapters. Several prospective studies are currently underway to determine its relative utility for identifying ischemia at the bedside and for determining prognosis. Preliminary results have indicated that MCE is both sensitive and accurate for this purpose. Since MCE can be performed at the patient's bedside and provides immediate information to the clinician, it will likely have a major impact on treatment in the critically ill patient. Perfusion imaging will be useful for detecting active ischemia in patients with a primary cardiac etiology, or in those with other medical/surgical problems in whom ischemia can be precipitated by hemodynamic instability, tachycardia, and increased coagulable states. In those with acute ischemic injury, MCE performed at the bedside with intravenous administration of microbubbles can provide information on the spatial extent of hypoperfusion [27] and may, therefore, be useful for determining whether acute reperfusion therapy in a high-risk patient is warranted. Similarly, MCE may be useful for excluding ischemia in critically ill patients with left ventricular systolic dysfunction from other causes. Nonischemic ventricular dysfunction is commonly encountered in patients with sepsis due to release of cytokines, increased nitric oxide production, and abnormal calcium handling [28]; and those with increased intracranial pressure due to elevated catecholamines [29].

Targeted microbubble contrast agents have recently been developed that allow noninvasive assessment of cellular or molecular processes. Attachment to thrombus has been achieved by targeting microbubbles to platelet or fibrin components [30, 31]. Recently, in vivo imaging of tissue inflammation has been achieved with microbubbles targeted to activated leucocytes or to endothelial cell adhesion molecules [32, 33]. Although these techniques are far from routine clinical use, they are likely to enhance the capability of echocardiography to diagnose these processes that are common in the critical care patient.

Conclusion

Optimal care of the unstable patient in the ICU depends on prompt and confident diagnosis of cardiovascular pathology. Echocardiography is commonly used in this setting since it is rapid, portable, and widely available. Obtaining images adequate for interpretation is, however, often difficult in the critically ill patient. In individuals with poor echocardiographic windows, microbubble contrast enhancement can provide unequivocal information on ventricular function, ventricular geometry, and the presence of anatomic complications. Although there are few large, prospective trials evaluating the incremental benefit in this patient population, current practice trends indicate that contrast administration is particularly helpful for evaluating the critically ill patient.

References

1. Cheitlin MD, Alpert JS, Armstrong WF, et al. ACC/AHA guidelines for the clinical applications of echocardiography: a report of the American College of Cardiology/American Heart Association Task Force on Practice Guidelines (Committee on Clinical Application of Echocardiography). *Circulation* 1997; 95: 1686-1744
2. Kaul S, Stratienko AA, Pollock SG, Marieb MA, Keller MW, Sabia PJ. Value of two-dimensional echocardiography for determining the basis of hemodynamic compromise in critically ill patients: a prospective study. *J Am Soc Echocardiogr* 1994; 7: 598-606
3. Tam JW, Nichol J, MacDiarmid AL, Lazarow N, Wolfe K. What is the real clinical utility of echocardiography? A prospective observational study. *J Am Soc Echocardiogr* 1999; 12: 689-697
4. Heidenreich PA, Stainback RF, Redberg RF, Schiller NB, Cohen NH, Foster E. Transesophageal echocardiography predicts mortality in critically ill patients with unexplained hypotension. *J Am Coll Cardiol* 1995; 26: 152
5. Reilly JP, Tunick PA, Timmermans RJ, Stein B, Rosenzweig BP, Kronzon I. Contrast echocardiography clarifies uninterpretable wall motion in intensive care unit patients. *J Am Coll Cardiol* 2000; 35: 485-490
6. Yong Y, Wu D, Fernandes V, et al. Diagnostic accuracy and cost-effectiveness of contrast echocardiography on evaluation of cardiac function in technically very difficult patients in the intensive care unit. *Am J Cardiol* 2002; 89: 711-718
7. Lindner JR, Moos SP, Dent JM, Jayaweera AR, Kaul S. Enhancement of left ventricular cavity opacification by harmonic imaging after venous injection of Albunex. *Am J Card*iol 1997; 79: 1657-1662
8. Rainbird AJ, Mulvagh SL, Oh JK, et al. Contrast dobutamine stress echocardiography: clinical practice assessment in 300 consecutive patients. *J Am Soc Echocardiogr* 2001; 14: 378-385
9. Goldstein JA. Right heart ischemia: pathophysiology, natural history, and clinical management. *Prog Cardiovasc Dis* 1998; 40: 325-341
10. Grifoni S, Olivotto I, Cecchini P, et al. Short-term clinical outcome of patients with acute pulmonary embolism, normal blood pressure, and echocardiographic right ventricular dysfunction. *Circulation* 2000; 101: 2817-2822
11. Tokgozöglu SL, Caner B, Kabakçi G, Kes, S. Measurement of right ventricular ejection fraction by contrast echocardiography. *Int J Cardiol* 1997; 59: 71-74
12. Shaw LJ, Gillam L, Feinstein S, Dent J, Plotnick. Use of an intravenous contrast agent (Optison) to enhance echocardiography: efficacy and cost implications. *Am J Managed Care* 1998; 4: SP169-SP176
13. Schiller NB. Hemodynamics derived from transesophageal echocardiography (TEE). *Cardiology Clinics.* 2000; 18: 699-709
14. von Bibra H, Sutherland G, Becher H, Neudert J, Nihoyannopoulos P. Clinical evaluation of left heart Doppler contrast enhancement by a saccharide-based transpulmonary contrast agent. *J Am Coll Cardiol* 1995; 25: 500-508
15. Schulman LL, Anandarangam T, Leibowitz DW, et al. Four-year prospective study of pulmonary venous thrombosis after lung transplantation. *J Am Soc Echocardiogr* 2001; 14: 806-812
16. Gerstenfeld EP, Guerra P, Sparks PB, Hattori K, Lesh MD. Clinical outcome after radiofrequency catheter ablation of focal atrial fibrillation triggers. *J Cardiovasc Electrophysiol* 2001; 12: 900-908
17. Minich LL, Tani LY, Breinholt JP, Tuohy AM, Shaddy RE. Complete follow-up echocardiograms are needed to detect stenosis of normally connecting pulmonary veins. *Echocardiography.* 2001; 18(7): 589-592
18. Visser CA, Kan G, Davis GK, Lie KI, Durrer D. Two dimensional echocardiography in the diagnosis of left ventricular thrombus: a prospective study of 67 patients with anatomic validation. *Chest* 1983; 83: 228-232
19. Stratton JR, Lighty GW, Pearlman AS, Ritchie JL. Detection of left ventricular thrombus by two-dimensional echocardiography: sensitivity, specificity, and causes of uncertainty. *Circulation* 1982; 66: 156-166
20. Bednarz JE, Spencer KT, Weinert L, Sugeng L, Mor-Avi V, Lang RM. Identification of cardiac masses and abnormal blood flow patterns with harmonic power Doppler contrast echocardiography. *J Am Soc Echocardiogr* 1999; 12: 871-875
21. Lepper W, Shivalkar B, Rinkevich D, Belcik T, Wei K. Assessment of the vascularity of a left ventricular mass by myocardial contrast echocardiography. *J Am Soc Echocardiogr* 2002; 15: 1419-1422
22. Moreno R, Zamorano JL, Almeria C. Usefulness of contrast agents in the diagnosis of left ventricular pseudoaneurysm after acute myocardial infarction. *Eur J Echocardiogr* 2002; 3: 111-116
23. Nienaber CA, von Kodolitsch, Y, Nicolas V, et al. The diagnosis of thoracic aortic dissection by non-invasive imaging procedures. *N Engl J Med* 1993; 328: 1-9
24. Kimura BJ, Phan JN, Housman LB. Utility of contrast echocardiography in the diagnosis of aortic dissection. *J Am Soc Echocardiogr* 1999; 12: 155-159
25. Voci P, Testa G, Tritapep L, Menichetti A, Caretta Q. Detection of false lumen perfusion at the beginning

of cardiopulmonary bypass in patients undergoing repair of aortic dissection. *Crit Care Med* 2000; 28: 1841
26. Cigarroa JE, Isselbacher EM, DeSanctis RW, Eagle KA. Medical progress: diagnostic imaging in the evaluation of suspected aortic dissection - old standards and new directions. *N Engl J Med* 1993; 328: 35-43
27. Balcells E, Powers ER, Lepper W, Belcik T, Wei K, Ragosta M, Lindner JR. Detection of myocardial viability by contrast echocardiography in acute myocardial infarction predicts recovery of resting function and contractile reserve. *J Am Coll Cardiol* 2003; 41: 827-833
28. Krishnagopalan S, Aseem K, Parrillo JE, Kumar A. Myocardial dysfunction in the patient with sepsis. *Curr Opinion Crit Care* 2002; 8: 376-388
29. Zaroff JG, Rordorf GA, Ogilvy CS, Picard MH. Regional patterns of left ventricular systolic dysfunction after subarachoid hemorrhage: evidence for neurally mediated cardiac injury. *J Am Soc Echocardiogr* 2000; 13: 774-779
30. Lanza GM, Wallace KD, Scott MJ, et al. A novel site-targeted ultrasonic contrast agent with broad biomedical application. *Circulation* 1997; 95: 3334-3340
31. Unger EC, McCreery TP, Sweitzer RH, Shen D, Wu G. In vitro studies of a new thrombus-specific ultrasound contrast agent. *Am J Cardiol* 1998; 81: 58G-61G
32. Christiansen JP, Leong-Poi H, Xu F, Klibanov AL, Kaul S, Lindner JR. Non-invasive imaging of myocardial reperfusion injury using leucocyte-targeted contrast echocardiography. *Circulation* 2002; 105: 1764-1767
33. Lindner JR, Song J, Christiansen J, Klibanov AL, Xu F, Ley K. Ultrasound assessment of inflammation and renal tissue injury with microbubbles targeted to P-selectin. *Circulation* 2001; 104: 2107-2112

Chapter 16
Therapeutic Application of Ultrasound Contrast Agents

Mario J. García

Introduction

In patients with chronic ischemic heart disease, restoring blood flow is the only means of preventing loss of myocardial function. Not infrequently, myocardial revascularization using surgical placement of bypass grafts or percutaneous angioplasty is either not feasible or fails to provide complete restoration of blood flood to ischemic myocardium. In such cases, the development of collateral vessels can mitigate myocardial ischemia [1]. Collateral circulation can also limit myocyte apoptosis during coronary occlusion [2], reducing infarct size [3]. The extent of collateral development varies among individuals, and until recently, the factors that determine angiogenesis were not understood. Recent advances in the understanding of vascular biology, however, have brought attention to the study of therapeutic angiogenesis, the promotion of new vessel growth using vascular growth factor [4-6] (Fig. 16.1). Angiogenesis is a complex process that involves endothelial cell migration and proliferation, smooth muscle cell proliferation and migration, formation of new vascular structures, and deposition of new matrix [7]. To date, various angiogenic growth factors, such as the fibroblast growth factor (FGF) and vascular endothelial growth factor (VEGF), have been evaluated as potential therapeutic agents in animal models and patients with chronic myocardial ischemia [8, 9]. Although early experience in therapeutic angiogenesis has been quite promising [10, 11], significant limitations remain given the inadequacy of existing delivery methods. Direct myocardial injection or coronary cannulation appears to be necessary to consistently augment blood flow, but is impractical in the clinical setting. Systemic intravenous administration of angiogenic proteins is easier to implement but results in low concentration at the desired site. In the case of FGF, intravenous infusion results in less than 1% deposition of the growth factor in the myocardium [12]. The advantage of giving endothelial growth peptides is the ability to

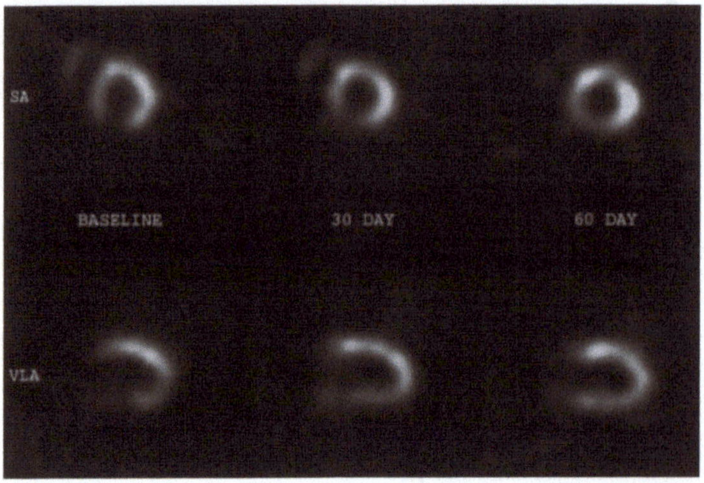

Fig. 16.1. Case study demonstrating improved resting perfusion by SPECT sestamibi in the inferior wall of a patient after VEGF intracoronary administration (Reproduced from [36], with permission)

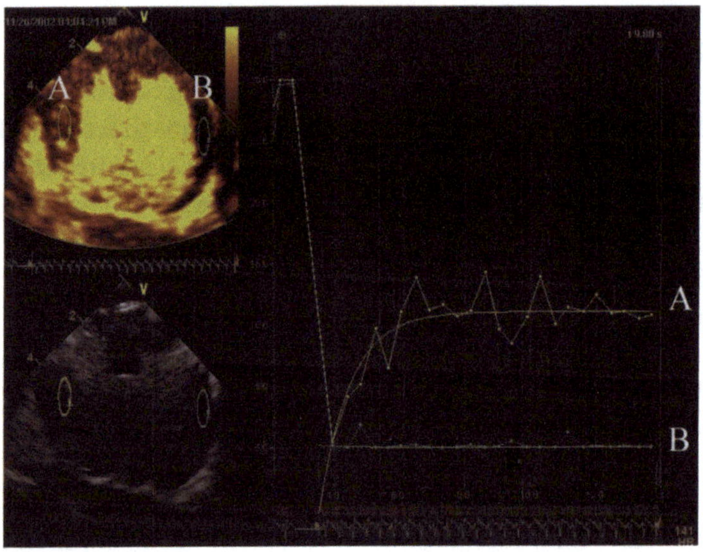

Fig. 16.2. Assessment of myocardial blood flow using flash-high mechanical index destruction followed by real-time imaging at low mechanical index. This image demonstrates marked reduction in blood flow in the lateral wall (**B**) after ligation of the circumflex artery in a dog, compared to the septum (**A**)

achieve precise dosing at known intervals, but large quantities are required because of their short half-life. Unfortunately, administering high doses of either intravenous VEGF or bFGF is limited by nitric oxide (NO)-mediated dose-dependent hypotension [13, 14]. Delivering the genetic material directly to myocardial cells would be therefore desirable in order to increase local concentration and reduce systemic side effects. While numerous issues remain concerning the most efficacious and safest method for packaging and delivering the growth factors [6], ultrasound contrast-enhanced delivery appears promising.

Assessment of Collateral Blood Flow and Efficacy of Therapeutic Angiogenesis

In trials of therapeutic angiogenesis, assessing the efficacy is of utmost importance. Current methods to assess the development of the coronary collateral circulation have limitations. Direct coronary angiography cannot define vessels less than 100 μm in size, and is therefore inadequate to assess the development of collateral flow [15]. Contrast enhanced magnetic resonance imaging (MRI) [16] has been used to assess myocardial perfusion in experimental models of angiogenesis, but MRI contrast agents such as gadolinium extravasate from the intravascular space and are, thus, not pure intravascular tracers. Scintigraphic techniques have limited spatial resolution and their application in serial studies is limited by radiation exposure [17]. Alternatively, myocardial contrast echocardiography allows serial studies to be obtained while providing a noninvasive assessment of the microvasculature [18-20] (Fig. 16.2). Myocardial contrast echocardiography, using peripheral intravenous injection of microbubbles, can track the spatial distribution and time course of coronary collateral development. Ultrasound microbubbles resonate when excited by ultrasound energy, reflecting acoustic signals at a higher frequency that can be detected through harmonic imaging [21-23]. Since most of the intramyocardial blood volume consists of capillaries, the video intensity of the images obtained is predominantly a representation of capillary volume [24]. Myocardial contrast echocardiography also has the potential to provide an assessment of collateral flow reserve through the use of vasodilators such as adenosine or dipyridamole [25]. In a study of patients with recent myocardial infarction and a totally occluded infarct-related artery [2], myocardial contrast echocardiography, using intracoronary and direct aortic root injection of sonicated Renografin, was able to demonstrate the existence of extensive collateral circulation in a significant number of myocardial segments, and to relate the extent of collateral flow with the improvement of myocardial function at follow-up. In the same study, coronary angiography significantly underestimated collateral flow. More recently, Mills et al. [26] demonstrated that the development of these collaterals might be tracked serially with peripheral intravenous injections. Whether this technique will be capable of demonstrating more subtle improvement in resting capillary blood volume in trials of therapeutic angiogenesis remains to be seen. This technique may be more sensitive, particularly if used with continuous intravenous contrast infusion and triggered harmonic imaging [27].

Although already a promising technique,

the utility of myocardial contrast echocardiography in evaluating the effect of therapeutic angiogenesis will probably remain an important area of research in the near future.

Therapeutic Agents

Successful angiogenesis has resulted from delivery of angiogenic proteins, adenoviral vectors or plasmids containing transgenes that encode angiogenic proteins. Among the growth factors involved in the angiogenic response to chronic ischemia and ischemic preconditioning, FGF and VEGF [28] are the angiogenic agents used in most current clinical studies. In addition, other growth promoters and inhibitors that play an important role in vascular biology and could be potentially employed as cardiovascular therapeutic agents are currently under investigation.

Angiogenic Proteins

Vascular endothelial growth factor (VEGF) is a dimeric endothelial cell-specific growth factor. VEGF is synthesized by perivascular cells and acts as a paracrine factor. The expression of VEGF is up-regulated by hypoxia and various cytokines. VEGF stimulates migration, proliferation, and expression of various genes in endothelial cells in culture and in vivo [29-31]. Four isoforms of VEGF differing in numbers of amino acids are known. The isoforms with 121 and 165 amino acids ($VEGF_{121}$ and $VEGF_{165}$) have been used in human investigations. They can be administered directly as a peptide or indirectly as a gene. The expression of VEGF receptors is also up-regulated by hypoxia, thus therapeutic angiogenesis trials have been designed to target under-perfused skeletal muscle and myocardial regions [32]. VEGF has been shown to improve blood flow through collateral development in animal experiments [33-35]. A recent study [36] demonstrated improvement in resting myocardial perfusion in humans after VEGF administration with evidence for a dose-dependent effect.

Basic fibroblast growth factor (FGF) is a 16.5-kDa 146 heparin-binding amino acid. Because of its heparin-binding properties, FGF binds to endothelial cell surface heparan sulfates [37], giving it a relatively long effective tissue half-life [38]. FGF stimulates migration and proliferation of fibroblasts, macrophages, smooth muscle and endothelial cells [39]. FGF can also stimulate endothelial production of plasminogen activator and matrix metalloproteinases, inducing vasodilation through stimulation of nitric oxide release [40, 41]. FGF is present in the myocardium [42] and is also up-regulated by hypoxia [43, 44] or hemodynamic stress [45]. FGF has been shown to induce angiogenesis in animal models of myocardial ischemia in the setting of acute coronary thrombosis [46-48] and during chronic ischemia [49, 50]. In contrast to VGEF, FGF can be administered intravenously in relatively higher doses [51] without significant hemodynamic effects, although dosing is also limited by hypotension [40] caused by NO release inducing arteriolar vasodilation [52]. Slowing the rate of infusion can mitigate the acute hypotensive effects of FGF [53]. Renal insufficiency due to membranous nephropathy accompanied by proteinuria [54] might be also a long-term side effect of FGF-2 administration. Other potential concerns about the long-term use of FGF are the exacerbation of blood malignancies [55] and destabilization of coronary plaque [56, 57] leading to acute coronary syndromes [51]. Endothelial growth factors have been implicated as mediators of intraocular neovascularization [58, 59]. However, in a recent study [53] of patients with normal retinae at baseline and in individuals with mild to moderate nonproliferative retinopathy, FGF did not induce new vessel formation. Mild transient asymptomatic thrombocytopenia has also been reported in FGF-treated patients [50, 10].

Elafin is a 6-kDa peptide found in human skin that has potent and specific inhibitory activity against serine elastases [60]. Serine elastases activate [61] extracellular matrix-bound growth factors [62], critical for smooth muscle cell proliferation and neointimal formation. Elastases activate inflammatory cytokines [63] and degrade the endothelial basement membrane, facilitating the migration of inflammatory cells into the vessel wall [64]. Elastases stimulate elastin synthesis [65]. Elastin is an important component of atherosclerotic plaques, serving as a base for monocyte adhesion [66], lipid accumulation and plaque calcification [67]. The administration of elafin in an animal model of heart transplantation has been shown to limit neointimal formation slowing the appearance of coronary arteriopathy. Elafin reduces the deposition of elastin and protects against cholesterol-induced infiltration of macrophages. Elafin has been shown to successfully reduce the inflammatory response in vein grafts and limit neointimal formation induced by cholesterol feeding [68] with a 50% reduction in cholesterol-induced atherosclerotic plaque formation. The release of peptides by serine elastase-mediated degradation of elastine is prevented by elafin in cultured cells [69]. Whether these findings can be translated to clinical use remains to be seen.

Adenoviral Vectors

Presently, the clinical application of endothelial growth factors requires large doses and frequent administration. As an alternative, in vivo transfection of angiogenic growth factor-encoding genes has been proposed. This technique has been shown to be feasible and effective in patients with chronic lower limb ischemia [70]. Genes can be engineered to generate specific peptides. DNA-encoding VEGF carried by an adenoviral vector has been administered into the myocardium at the time of coronary artery bypass surgery [71] and during angiography by selective infusion into a coronary artery [36], resulting in reduction in angina and improved myocardial perfusion.

Alternatively, native genes from one organ can be transfected to a different target organ for a specific effect. *Vasopressin receptor genes*, usually expressed only in kidney, have been delivered to myocardium using recombinant adenoviruses [72], and their expression converted the basal negative inotropic response to infused vasopressin into a positive response, a potentially beneficial approach for failing myocardial cells.

Gene transfer of *endothelial NO synthase (eNOS)* has been shown to improve vascular function in diabetic vessels. Diabetes mellitus is often associated with impairment of endothelium-dependent relaxation [73, 74]. After gene transfer, expression of endothelial NO synthase is greater in atherosclerotic than normal vessels [75, 76]. Adenovirus-mediated gene transfer of endothelial NO synthase to carotid arteries has been shown to improve impaired NO-mediated responses to acetylcholine in diabetic rabbits [77]. Numerous studies suggest that the mechanism of impaired endothelium-dependent relaxation in diabetes and atherosclerosis may involve inactivation of NO by oxygen-derived free radicals [75, 76, 78-83]. Although several mechanisms may contribute to this response to eNOS, gene transfer provides a revolutionary approach to the treatment of diabetic coronary arteriopathy.

Heat shock proteins are intracellular proteins that protect cells from the effects of environmental stress [84], such as heat stress [85] and ischemia-reperfusion injury [86]. Increased levels of heat shock protein-70 have been shown to be protective against ischemia-reperfusion injury [87] and improved recovery of ventricular and coronary endothelial function in animals after prolonged cardioplegic arrest and reperfusion [88]. A recent study [89] demonstrated significant improvement of postischemic recovery of mechanical function in heat shock protein-70 gene-transfected hearts, in an animal model of heart transplantation. Heat shock protein-70 overexpressing mice had better postischemic recovery of ventricular function after a period of ischemia and reperfusion. Heat shock protein-70 may exert its beneficial effects not only on the myocardium but also on endothelial function. Future advances in transfection techniques may allow a more rapid induction of protein expression, possibly introducing genes into the donor heart by catheter techniques before transplantation [90].

There are, however, potential limitations to adenoviral transfer therapy. Once the gene is administered or activated, it is difficult to modulate its response, resulting in potential under-or overdosing. Viral transfection carries the risk of oncogenesis and triggering autoimmune response.

Plasmid Transfer

Plasmids are small, circular pieces of DNA. These particles are less toxic than complete gene sequences. The effect of plasmids is, however, limited by their greater susceptibility to the host's immune system. Recent trials in patients with peripheral disease have shown, however, that direct limb injection of naked plasmid DNA-encoding VEGF can result in neovascularization [91]. Vascular endothelial growth factor expression peaked from 1 to 3 weeks after the gene transfer. After 4 weeks, the ankle-brachial index increased by 30%. This improvement was sustained at 12 weeks. Blood flow measured by MRI improved in eight of ten limbs with angiographic evidence of new collateral formation observed in seven of ten extremities. In an experimental animal model, intramuscular injection of naked plasmid DNA encoding VEGF has shown to increase capillary formation and blood flow to ischemic limbs [92]. In humans with critical limb ischemia, naked plasmid DNA-encoding VEGF has also shown increased collateral vessel formation, improved limb blood flow, and improvement in symptoms of claudication [70]. More recently, direct myocardial injections of naked plasmid DNA-encoding VEGF were given via a lateral thoracotomy to patients with chronic ischemic heart disease unable to receive complete conventional revascularization [93]. Improved myocardial perfusion has been observed by single photon emission computed tomography (SPECT) imaging. Although these trials demonstrated safety and feasibility in patients with end-stage coronary artery disease, the use of thoracotomy precluded randomization against placebo. In addition to improved perfusion, other investigators have shown improved segmental contractility using electromechanical mapping [94]. This invasive method can be used to determine the extent and location of myocardial ischemia in real time and thus direct the injection of naked plasmid DNA-encoding VEGF using an endovascular percutaneous approach. The relatively short half-life of plasmids and the direct delivery may minimize long-term consequences, such as retinopathy and tumor growth [33]. The used of naked plasmid DNA, however, is not effective for intra-arterial or intravenous administration because plasmid DNA is rapidly degraded in circulating blood.

Delivery Methods

The delivery of angiogenic factors to the myocardium has been achieved either by intracoronary injection of the angiogenic factor at catheterization, by direct intramyocardial injection after thoracotomy, or by intravenous administration. Currently, however, it is unknown which is the safest and most effective delivery strategy to induce clinically important therapeutic angiogenic responses in ischemic myocardium. Direct myocardial injection can be performed via thoracotomy at the time of bypass surgery or during catheterization, but is inconvenient, as it requires repetitive use. Single intracoronary doses have been effective in the enhancement of collateral blood flow in pigs [95], as was a series of two local injections via a balloon catheter, 3-or 4-week periadventitial infusion via minipump [96]. Several uncontrolled phase I clinical trials of intracoronary VEGF protein infusion appeared to demonstrate less angina and improved exercise time as well as improvement of MRI perfusion and left ventricular (LV) function [36, 97]. However, this method is also limited by the apparent requirement for invasive arterial cannulation or invasive direct myocardial injection. In general, systemic administration of angiogenic proteins results in low concentration at the desired site. In the case of FGF, intravenous infusion results in less than 1% deposition of the growth factor in the myocardium [12]. Intravenous VEGF is also limited by NO-mediated hypotension [13, 14]. In this section, we will review the relative advantages and disadvantages of existing delivery methods.

Intramyocardial Injection

The greatest advantage of direct intramyocardial injection of angiogenic growth factors or genes is that the angiogenic factor will be primarily used by the targeted myocardium and not delivered to other tissues [98-99]. As previously discussed, this approach has resulted in improved myocardial perfusion and function in an animal model with adenoviral vectors containing the VEGF transgene [35]. More recently, recombinant FGF was injected directly into the myocardium just distal to the anastomotic site of the left internal mammary and anterior descending coronary artery [100] (Fig. 16.3). Angiography performed 12 weeks later demonstrated arterial collaterals in the area of the FGF injection. However, no long-term follow-up or objective evidence of improved myocardial perfusion was reported in this study. Intramyocardial injection of naked DNA-encoding VGEF has also been performed successfully via a minimally invasive chest wall incision [93]. This approach appears to be safe according to these and other preliminary studies, but it requires general anesthesia therefore being impractical for patients who otherwise do not need a thoracotomy. An alternative approach consists

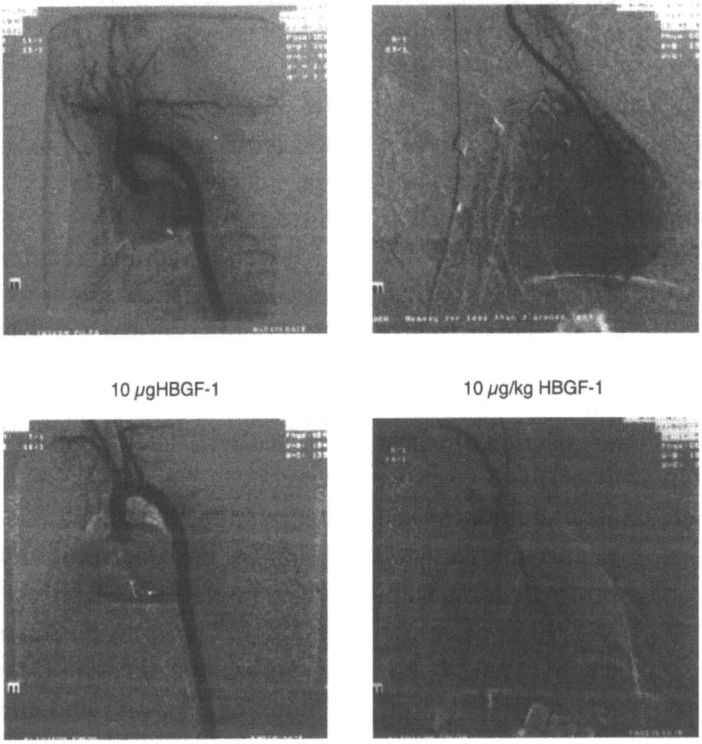

Fig. 16.3. Angiographic demonstration of increased collateral development following administration of human growth factors (*bottom*) vs. controls (*top*). *Left images* obtained from rats, *right images* from humans after bypass grafting of the left anterior descending artery (Reproduced from [100], with permission)

of transendocardial injection during cardiac catheterization [101, 102]. Using electromechanical mapping, investigators have shown the feasibility and safety of this approach in patients with chronic ischemic heart disease, demonstrating improved perfusion and segmental contractility. The electromechanical mapping system allows determining, in real time, the regions where electromechanical dissociation exists, representing ischemic myocardium, thus permitting precise local delivery [102, 103]. Studies are needed to determine whether transendocardial and transepicardial administrations are equally effective. One advantage of direct intramyocardial injection is that it permits the effective use of naked DNA avoiding the potential toxicities that might result from the use of viral vectors. Compared to viral vectors, naked DNA carries a lower risk of provoking an immune response, allowing repetitive dosing. In a randomized, double-blind, placebo-controlled, dose-escalating clinical trial [104], naked plasmid DNA-encoding VEGF was injected into the LV myocardium of patients with class III or IV angina. A total of 114 LV injections were delivered without documented hemodynamic alterations, sustained ventricular arrhythmias, ECG evidence of infarction, or ventricular perforation. In this trial, anginal symptoms and exercise tolerance significantly improved when compared to placebo. In addition, many hypoperfused hypokinetic segments demonstrated improvement in contractility at follow-up, suggesting that this approach may be useful in treating myocardial hibernation. Optimizing the anatomic site, number, and dose of intramyocardial injections will require further investigation. Furthermore, the choice of appropriate formulation or vector in the case of VEGF remains to be determined. Although feasible, the long-term effects of direct intramyocardial injection are unknown (Fig. 16.4). If multiple dosing intervals are required to sustain a meaningful result, these methods may become less practical.

Intrapericardial Delivery

This mode of delivery offers the potential advantage of prolonged exposure of myocardial tissue to the administered drug stored in the pericardial sac [105-108]. Pericardial administration results in substantial cardiac bFGF delivery, with 19% extraction after 2 hours [109]. Sustained-release polymers for extravascular elution of FGF have been safely implanted in the pericardial space in patients undergoing coronary bypass surgery [110]. Sustained release intrapericar-

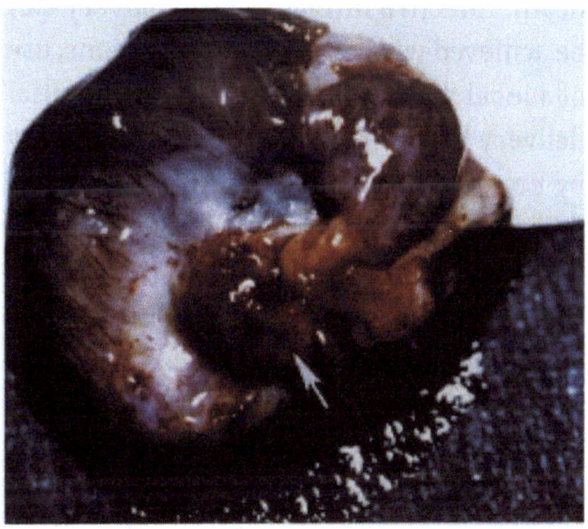

Fig. 16.4. Development of a large angioma following direct myocardial injection of VGEF in a rat following a myocardial infarction (From [104a])

dial delivery of FGF has been shown to improve myocardial blood flow, regional LV function in the ischemic myocardium and to increase exercise tolerance [12, 111, 112]. Customized needle systems have been designed to permit pericardial puncture using a percutaneous approach with safety features to minimize the risk of trauma [113]. This approach, however, may not be feasible in patients with lung disease or with previous pericardiotomy and adhesions.

Endovascular Administration

Intracoronary administration of adenoviral vectors expressing FGF has been shown to improve regional myocardial perfusion and contractility in ischemic myocardial regions [114]. In an animal model of chronic ischemia [13], a low-dose of VEGF resulted in greater collateral perfusion compared to untreated controls, while higher doses were associated to severe hypotension and death. Effective intracoronary delivery can be achieved with direct bolus injections, use of a local delivery catheter, or periadvential delivery [96]. Direct intracoronary delivery by bolus injection appears to require multiple administrations, however, in order to be effective [34]. In human trials, the magnitude of improvement in symptoms, quality of life, and exercise tolerance was similar to that seen following percutaneous coronary interventions and bypass surgery in patients with ischemic heart disease [115, 116]. Compared to the intra-arterial route, the efficacy of intravenous administration of angiogenic growth factors appears to be limited. Intravenous bolus injection of basic FGF has been shown to be ineffective in inducing an angiogenic response in a canine model of myocardial ischemia [117]. Uptake of FGF and VGEF is dependent on the local concentration at the delivery site. Both these growth factors bind to heparan sulfate receptors in the lungs, resulting in a reduced concentration delivered to the myocardium when administered intravenously. Studies have shown that only 0.5% of intravenously injected radiolabeled FGF is localized in the myocardium, compared to 3%–5% delivered via direct intracoronary injection [109]. Unfortunately, maximal intravenous doses of VEGF and FGF are limited by hypotension [13, 49, 50, 118-120]. Hypotension is primarily mediated by VEGF-induced release of NO [13, 120, 121] and therefore might be circumvented effectively by pretreatment with a nitric oxide synthase inhibitor [122] (Fig. 16.5). Unfortunately, NO is essential for

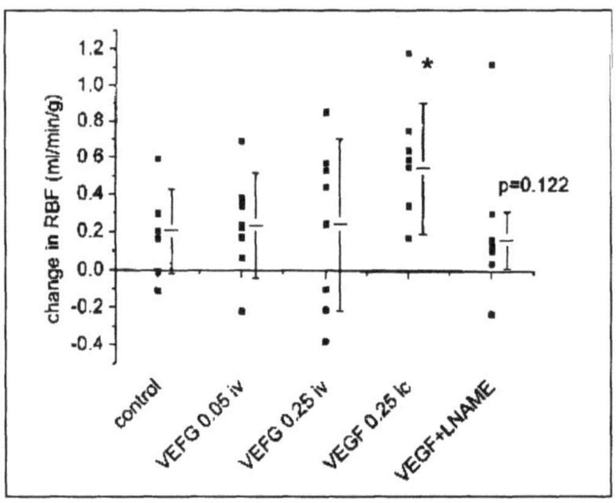

Fig. 16.5. Comparison of regional blood flow between various intravenous doses and intracoronary administration of VGEF in a pig model of chronic myocardial ischemia. Only intracoronary injection resulted in a significant increase in blood flow (From [122], with permission American College of Cardiology Foundation)

VEGF-induced angiogenesis, and NO synthase blockade may inhibit angiogenic effects of VEGF therapy [123-125]. In addition, an important concern with the pharmacological use of angiogenic growth factors is the potential acceleration of malignancies or proliferative retinopathy. The mitogenic effects of angiogenic growth factors may also accelerate atherosclerotic lesion growth and may lead to plaque destabilization and acute coronary syndromes [126-128]. A phase I open-label study of intravenous VEGF reported improvements in both angina class and exercise performance. However, a larger double-blind study of a single intracoronary infusion of VEGF followed by serial intravenous infusions over 7 days failed to demonstrate any improvement in symptoms, exercise testing, or nuclear perfusion imaging at day 60 compared with placebo controls [97]. Although the lack of benefit may reflect the route of administration chosen, the improvement in the nontreated patients noted in this study reinforces the need for a placebo-controlled group in clinical studies of therapeutic angiogenesis.

Thus, it is apparent that one of the most important obstacles is the lack of an effective delivery system that can be targeted to specific organs or tissues.

Therapeutic Cardiovascular Applications of Ultrasound

The therapeutic applications of using ultrasound relate to the direct mechanical properties of acoustic energy through its interaction with tissue. In cardiovascular medicine, ultrasound energy has been used to enhance direct endogenous and therapeutic thrombolysis [129]. Ultrasound energy has been shown to permeabilize plasma membranes and reduce the thickness of the unstirred layer at the cell surface [33, 130]. Several investigators have recently reported ultrasound enhancement of transfection using plasmids or liposomes with and without the addition of stabilized gas bubbles [131, 132]. Ultrasound energy can also potentiate gene delivery in proportion to the delivered energy [133]. Ultrasound-mediated enhancement of transfection has been reported in the literature [134-137] and is attributed to ultrasonic cavitation of cells. Many lipofection reagents contain dioleoylphosphatidylethanolamine, which encourages DNA release from endosomes through a physicochemical transition that may be accelerated by ultrasound [138-139]. Recent studies in nonvascular cell cultures confirm transfection rates of up to 15% using naked DNA and 2- to 1,000-fold enhancements in reporter gene expression after lipofection [131, 136, 140-142]. A recent study demonstrated that ultrasound may enhance transgene expression after naked DNA and/or liposome-mediated transfection of primary vascular cells [137]. Ultrasound energy increases permeability to large macromolecules, including plasmid DNA [143] and high-molecular-weight dextrans. Studies performed to date have not specifically defined all the possible mechanisms of ultrasound action. In addition to its influence on cell entry by the mechanical effect, which increases the porosity of the cell membrane, ultrasound could also increase intracellular traffic, lysosomal degradation, nuclear translocation, RNA transcription, or protein translation. Laurie et al. [137] demonstrated that low-intensity ultrasound energy is associated with substantial enhancements in reporter gene expression without significant acute cell death or damage. In their study, ultrasound treatment also had an inhibitory effect on vascular smooth muscle cell counts. Other studies have also shown cell-type specific effects of ultrasound energy on cell proliferation in vitro, including stimulation of rat fibroblast proliferation [144] and inhibition of human [145] vascular smooth muscle cell proliferation. Investigators [146] have shown that catheter-mediated intravascular ultrasound can enhance blue fluorescent protein gene delivery in a rabbit model of arterial mechanical overdilation injury. In their study, ultrasound exposure after balloon angioplasty increased 12-fold in in vivo plasmid-mediated subjects over plasmid controls and adenoviral-mediated expression increased 19-fold over adenoviral controls.

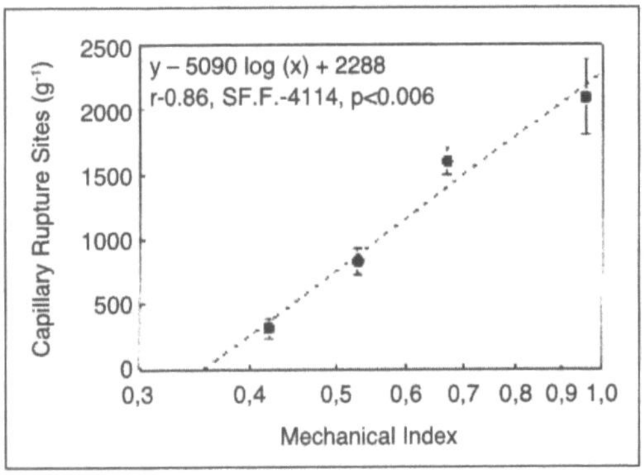

Fig. 16.6. Capillary rupture as a function of the mechanical index after direct application of ultrasound to skeletal muscle (Reproduced from [148], with permission)

All these studies [144] have used low to intermediate levels of ultrasound energy, but have not specifically addressed whether there is a dose–effect relationship. Future studies are needed to further address the biological effects of intensity, frequency, and ultrasound energy exposure time in order to optimize its therapeutic angiogenesis potential.

Contrast Ultrasound Enhancement of Therapeutic Angiogenesis

Peripheral intravenous injection without myocardial targeting may induce undesirable angiogenesis in other organs, as angiogenesis with VEGF has also been described in the absence of ischemia [147]. Targeting angiogenesis factors to specific tissue allows the systemic administration of lower doses of these agents with a decreased risk of side effects such as hypotension or neovascularization in nontargeted tissues.

Ultrasound-mediated microbubble destruction has been proposed as a method for delivering drugs or genes to specific tissues, including the heart [27, 131, 148-151] (Fig. 16.6). Ultrasonic destruction of gas-filled microbubbles has been shown to cause capillary rupture, leading to local extravasation of red blood cells and local delivery of polymer microspheres directly into striated muscle [149]. Ultrasound-mediated disruption of gas-filled microbubbles has also been used to direct transgene expression in the myocardium [152]. In this study, the authors demonstrated a tenfold increase in the transgene expression of β-galactosidase in the contrast-ultrasound treated animals (Fig. 16.7). VGEF is known to bind serum proteins [153] and thus can be incubated and attached to the albumin layer in ultrasound contrast agents [154]. Therefore, by destroying microbubbles containing VEGF with high ultrasound energy in the coronary microcirculation, a large amount of VEGF can be released into the myocardium. Using this approach, Mukherjee et al. [155] at our laboratory proposed that VGEF injected via a peripheral vein may be targeted to the myocardium using ultrasound and an albumin-based ultrasonic contrast agent (perfluorocarbon exposed sonicated dextrose albumin, PESDA). This study showed a significant increase in endothelial uptake of VEGF with ultrasound alone or a combination of ultrasound and PESDA. A tenfold increase in endothelial uptake of oligonucleotides with ultrasound alone [156] has been previously reported. In isolated heart (Langendorff) preparations, the optimum acoustic power for enhancement of VEGF uptake was 0.6–0.8 W/cm^2. Currently available diagnostic echocardiography equipment can deliver an acoustic output up to 0.44 W/cm^2 [157], but even at that level our study demonstrated an eightfold increase in VEGF uptake.

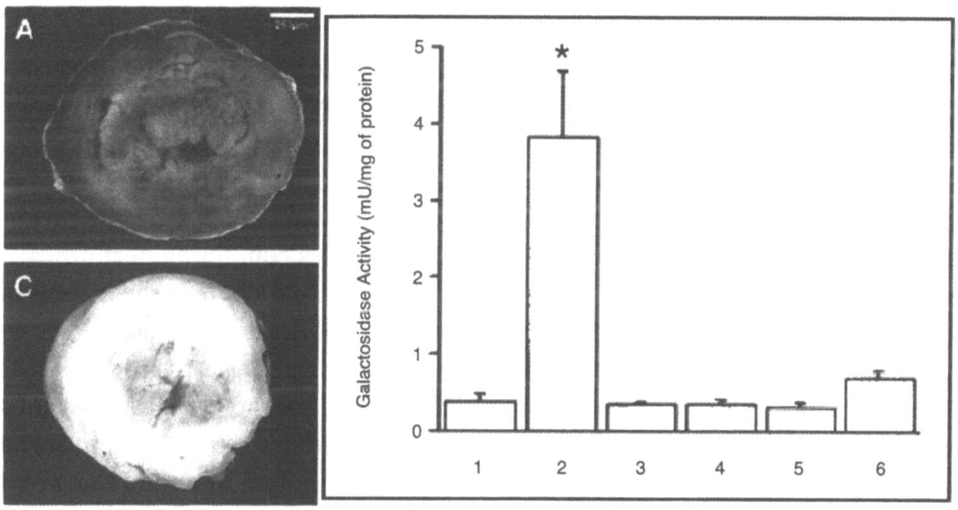

Fig. 16.7. Expression of galactosidase after gene transfection. The rat ventricle stained in *blue* demonstrates increased expression after ultrasound destruction of gene–microbubble mixture. Galactosidase expression is much greater in animals. Echocardiographic destruction of microbubbles containing AdCMV-β-Gal (*2*), compared to other groups. *1:* Ultrasound destruction of microbubbles without AdCMV-β-Gal; *3:* Microbubbles containing AdCMV-β-Gal without ultrasound; AdCMV-β-Gal (no microbubbles) without ultrasound; Ultrasound during infusion of AdCMV-β-Gal (no microbubbles); Ultrasound destruction of microbubbles followed by AdCMV-β-Gal infusion (Reproduced from [152], with permission)

One important concern about ultrasound biological effects is its potential for causing cell membrane lysis. Consistent with prior data [136], this study confirmed that high acoustic power was associated with destruction of the cell membranes. Above certain thresholds for intensity and duration, ultrasound has been found to induce breaks in DNA [158], apoptosis [159], membrane damage [160], and enhanced free radical delivery [161]. Electron microscopy revealed disruption of the membrane of the endothelial cells as well as an increased gap between endothelial cells with an acoustic power of > 0.8 W/cm^2. It appears that lower acoustic power increases permeability that facilitates endothelial VEGF uptake. Other investigators [146] have quantitatively evaluated cell viability in animals exposed to intravascular ultrasound during gene transfection. Although ultrasound exaggerated the toxicity of low-dose adenovirus, possibly through additive injury achieved by increased viral delivery, it did not increase apoptosis or macrophage infiltration in plasmid-mediated transfected animals.

The mechanism of contrast microbubble enhancement is still unclear. Investigators [148] have demonstrated rupture of capillaries with microbubble destruction during ultrasound exposure and have been able to deliver colloidal particles and red blood cells [149] to the tissue. Others [152] have shown that albumin-coated microbubbles could be used to effectively deliver an adenoviral transgene containing β-galactosidase to rat myocardium by ultrasound-mediated microbubble destruction. Enhancement of transfection of a plasmid DNA into cultured cells using albumin encapsulated air microbubbles exposed to ultrasound, suggests that microbubbles may play a role in reversible pore formation during the process of cavitation [136]. It is conceivable that the incremental effect of PESDA with ultrasound seen in these studies is due to more efficient sonoporation rather than binding of VEGF. It is also possible that VEGF combines with the albumin on the surface of the microbubble, facilitating its adhesion to the endothelial surface [162], and/or that this binding protects VGEF destruction in the capillary beds. However, this mechanism is less likely, since in our experiments we were unable to demonstrate actual binding of VEGF to PESDA.

Contrast-Fluorescein-Labeled VEGF Preparation

Perfluorocarbon-exposed sonicated dextrose albumin (PESDA) is a solution of microbubbles containing perflurocarbon enveloped in an albumin shell. Sonicating a solution of dextrose containing albumin and perflurocarbon gases produces PESDA [153]. Three parts of 5% dextrose and one part of 5% human serum albumin are hand agitated with 8 ml of a fluorocarbon gas (decafluorobutane), and the sample is then exposed to electromechanical sonication at 20 kHz for 80 s. During this process, the albumin-formed bubbles create a relatively rigid shell. The mean size of the PESDA microbubbles produced in this manner is about 5 mm. The safety of PESDA has been

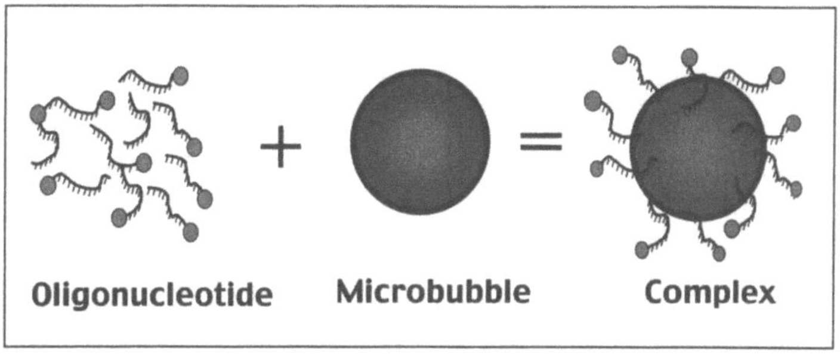

Fig. 16.8. Diagram illustrating the process of incubation of oligonucleotides to a contrast microbubble. Oligonucleotides may encode the expression of therapeutic proteins and/or may be labeled (fluorescein, radioactive isotopes) in order to determine cellular uptake

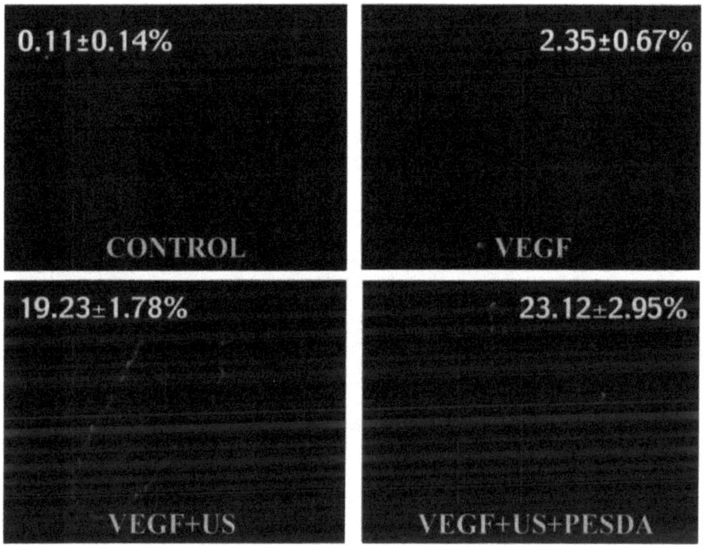

Fig. 16.9. Endothelial deposition of a fluorescein labeled VGEF on rat capillaries after saline, VGEF alone, VGEF + ultrasound and VGEF + microbubbles + ultrasound (From [155], with permission American College of Cardiology Foundation)

demonstrated in humans [153]. One hundred micrograms of fluorescein isothiocyanate (FITC) mixture (Cal-biochem) is mixed with 500 mg of rhVEGF (recombinant human VEGF, Genentech, CA) to achieve a conjugation ratio of 5:1 (protein: FITC) and incubated at room temperature for 2 h. The mixture is then dialyzed overnight with a dispodialyzer in order to remove free FITC molecules. Fluorescein-labeled VEGF is then mixed with PESDA at room temperature for 60 min prior to injection into animals (Fig. 16.8).

In the hypertensive rat model, after four weekly injections of VEGF, Mukherjee demonstrated a fourfold increase in endothelial and smooth muscle cell count, probably caused by increased cell migration [163, 164], demonstrating that VEGF delivered using this technique is biologically active (Figs. 16.9, 16.10). With the application of continuous wave Doppler ultrasound (0.6 W/cm^2 at 1 MHz for 15 min) to the chest wall, there was an eightfold increase in VEGF uptake in the heart by ultrasound alone, and a 13-fold increase with ultrasound and echo contrast compared with control rats. One limitation of this study was that the animals were spontaneously hypertensive rats. Although myocardial ischemia has been reported in hypertensive rats, the magnitude of ischemia is unpredictable. This is important, since studies in a variety of animal models using VEGF have shown angiogenesis only in the presence of ischemia [165]. In addition, the ultrasound energy that is delivered to the myocardial tissue in rats using a surface transducer may vary from that to be expected in a larger animal or human. We therefore tested this approach of tissue-directed VEGF delivery in combination with ultrasound and ultrasonic contrast (NC100100-Sonazoid) in dogs subjected to coronary ischemia [166]. We performed gradual occlusion of the circumflex coronary artery using an ameroid constrictor in 18 mongrel dogs, who were then randomized to either saline, VEGF alone, VEGF + ultrasound, and VEGF + ultrasound + contrast. Using radiolabeled microspheres,

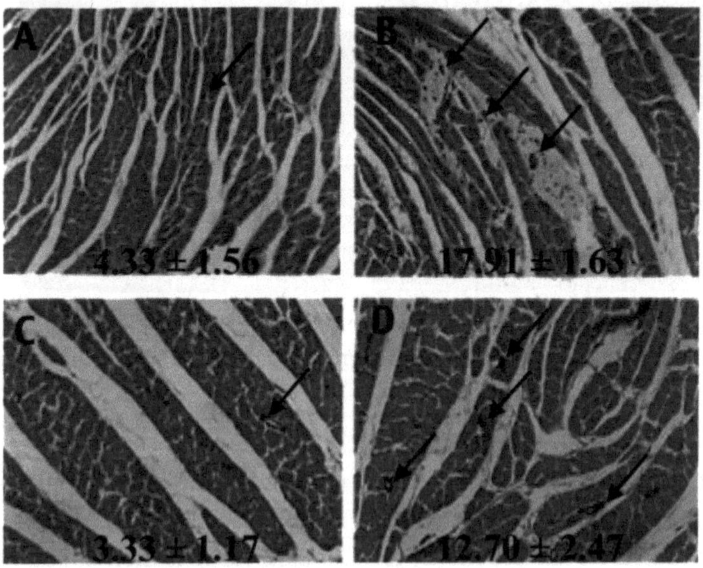

Fig. 16.10. Immunohistochemistry showed marked increase in endothelial cell and smooth muscle cell count (not associated with a vascular lumen) in groups treated with ultrasound (US) during administration of VEGF compared with groups treated with VEGF alone. **A** Endothelial cells as shown by von-Willebrand Factor staining in a rat heart from an animal treated with VEGF alone and **B** endothelial cells in a rat heart treated with VEGF + US. **C** Smooth muscle cells in a rat heart from an animal treated with VEGF alone and **D** a rat heart from an animal treated with VEGF + US (From [155], with permission American College of Cardiology Foundation)

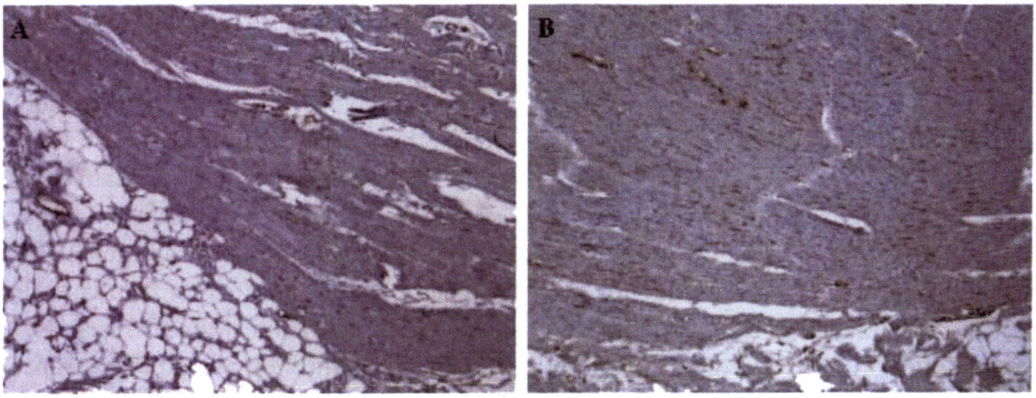

Fig. 16.11. **A** Endothelial cells as shown by factor VIII staining in the ischemic area from an animal in saline group. **B** Endothelial cells as shown by factor VIII staining in the ischemic area from an animal in the VEGF+US+contrast group (Reproduced from [166], with permission)

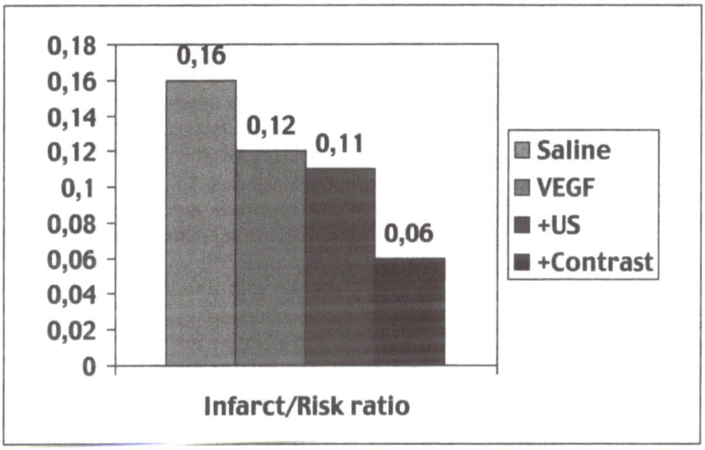

Fig. 16.12. The infarct/risk area ratio is significantly decreased in VEGF+US+contrast treatment group compared with other treatment group ($p < 0.05$) (Reproduced from [166], with permission)

we found a 60% increase from baseline in regional myocardial blood flow in the ischemic territory of animals treated with the combination of VEGF + ultrasound + contrast, but no significant increase in the other three groups. Interestingly, regional myocardial blood flow in the left anterior descending artery territory was also increased in the VEGF + ultrasound + contrast group. Endothelial cell count per field also increased, as measured by factor VIII immunostaining in this group (33.23 ± 4.51) compared to the VGEF only group (17.27 ± 2.48 $p = 0.04$, Fig. 16.11). There was also a decrease in infarct/risk area in VEGF + ultrasound + contrast group, compared with

VEGF + ultrasound (11.22 ± 1.29% p = 0.22), VEGF alone (12.68 ± 3.68% $p = 0.18$) or saline group (6.48 ± 2.31% vs 16.58 ± 1.99%, $p = 0.02$, Fig. 16.12).

Further work is needed to optimize the echocardiographic parameters for microbubble destruction, to maximize the amount of VEGF-encoded plasmid or adenovirus that can be attached to the microbubbles, and to determine the range of reagents amenable to ultrasound-mediated microbubble delivery. The efficacy of other angiogenesis factors, such as FGF, using this approach also needs to be determined. Finally, long-term safety issues need to be addressed, particularly those related to ultrasound local injury, neoangiogenesis in nontargeted tissues, and risk of carcinogenesis. Nevertheless, the future of therapeutic echocardiography is very promising and we anticipate that this field will rapidly advance in the upcoming years.

References

1. Levin DC. Pathways and functional significance of coronary collateral circulation. Circulation 1974; 50: 831-7
2. Sabia RJ, Powers ER, Jayaweera AR, et al. Functional significance of collateral blood flow in patients with recent acute myocardial infarction: a study using myocardial contrast echocardiography. N Engl J Med 1992; 327: 1825-31
3. Hirai T, Fujita M, Nakajima H, et al. Importance of collateral circulation for prevention of left ventricular aneurysm formation on acute myocardial infarction. Circulation 1989; 79: 791-6
4. Lewis BS, Flugelman MY, Weisz A, et al. Angiogenesis by gene therapy: a new horizon for myocardial revascularization? Cardiovasc Res 1997; 35: 490-7
5. Folkman J. Angiogenic therapy of the human heart. Circulation 1998; 97: 628-9
6. Kornowski R, Fuchs S, Leon M, et al. Delivery strategies to achieve therapeutic myocardial angiogenesis. Circulation 2000; 101: 454-8
7. Schaper W, Ito W. Molecular mechanisms of collateral vessel growth. Circ Res 1996; 79: 911-9
8. Freedman SB and Isner JM. Therapeutic angiogenesis for ischemic cardiovascular disease. J Mol Cell Cardiol 2001; 33: 379-393
9. Epstein SE, Fuchs S, Zhou YF, et al. Therapeutic interventions for enhancing collateral development by administration of growth factors: basic principles, early results and potential hazards. Cardiovasc Res 2001; 49: 531-542
10. Lazarous DF, Shou M, Scheinowitz M, et al. Comparative effect of basic fibroblast growth factor and vascular endothelial growth factor on coronary collateral development and the arterial response to injury. Circulation 1996; 94: 1074-1082
11. Harada K, Friedman M, Lopez JJ, et al. Vascular endothelial growth factor administration in chronic myocardial ischemia. Am J Physiol 1996; 270: H1791-H1802
12. Laham RJ, Rezaee M, Post M, et al. Intracoronary and intravenous administration of basic fibroblast growth factor: myocardial and tissue distribution. Drug Metab Dispos 1999; 27: 821-826
13. Hariawala MD, Horowitz JJ, Esakof D, et al. VEGF improves myocardial blood flow but produces EDRF-mediated hypotension in porcine hearts. J Surg Res 1996; 63: 77-82
14. Ku DD, Zaleski JK, Liu S, Brock TA. Vascular endothelial growth factor induces EDGF-dependent relaxation in coronary arteries. Am J Physiol 1993; 265: H586-H592
15. Jochem W, Soto B, Karp RB, et al. Radiographic anatomy of the coronary collateral circulation. Am J Roent Rad Ther Nuc Med 1972; 116: 50-61
16. Pearlman JD, Hibberd MG, Chuang ML, et al. Magnetic resonance mapping demonstrates benefits of VEGF-induced myocardial angio-genesis. Nature Med 1995; 1: 1085-9
17. Beller GA. Clinical Nuclear Cardiology. Philadelphia: W.B. Saunders Co, 1995
18. Jayaweera AR, Edwards N, Glasheen WP, et al. In vivo myocardial kinetics of air-filled albumin microbubbles during myocardial contrast echocardiography. Comparison with radio-labeled red blood cells. Circ Res 1994; 74: 1157-65
19. Ragosta M, Camarano G, Kaul S, et al. Microvascular integrity indicates myocellular viability in patients with recent myocardial infarction. New insights using myocardial contrast echocardiography. Circulation 1994; 89: 2562-9

20. Villanueva FS, Glasheen WP, Sklenar J, et al. Characterization of spatial patterns of flow within the re perfused myocardium by myocardial contrast echocardiography. Implications in determining extent of myocardial salvage. Circulation 1993; 88: 2596-606
21. Lindner JR, Firschke C, Wei K, et al. Myocardial perfusion characteristics and hemodynamic profile of MRX-115, a venous echocardiographic contrast agent, during acute myocardial infarction. J Am Soc Echo 1998; 11: 36-46
22. Porter TR, Xie F. Transient myocardial contrast after initial exposure to diagnostic ultrasound pressures with minute doses of intravenously injected microbubbles. Demonstration and potential mechanisms. Circulation 1995; 92: 2391-5
23. Mulvagh SL, Foley DA, Aeschbacher BC, et al. Second harmonic imaging of an intravenously administered echocardiographic contrast agent: visualization of coronary arteries and measurement of coronary blood flow. J Am Coll Cardiol 1996; 27: 1519-2525
24. Wei K, Jayaweera AR, Firoozan S, et al. Quantification of myocardial blood flow with ultrasound-induced destruction of microbubbles administered as a constant venous infusion. Circulation 1998; 97: 473-83
25. Villanueva FS, Camarano G, Ismail S, et al. Coronary reserve abnormalities in the infarcted myocardium. Assessment of myocardial viability immediately versus late after reflow by contrast echocardiography. Circulation 1996; 94: 748-54
26. Mills JD, Fischer D, Villanueva FS. Coronary collateral development during chronic ischemia: Serial assessment using harmonic myocardial contrast Echocardiography. J Am Coll Cardiol 2000; 36: 618-24
27. Wei K, Skyba DM, Firschke C, et al. Interactions between microbubbles and ultrasound: in vitro and in vivo observations. J Am Coll Cardiol 1997; 29: 1081-8
28. Folkman J. Seminars in Medicine of the Beth Israel Hospital, Boston. Clinical applications of research on angiogenesis. N Engl J Med 1995; 333: 1757-63
29. Leung DW, Cachianes G, Kuang WJ, et al. Vascular endothelial growth factor is a secreted angiogenic mitogen. Science 1989; 246: 1306-1309
30. Plate KH, Breier G, Weich HA, et al. Vascular endothelial growth factor is a potential tumour angiogenesis factor in human gliomas in vivo. Nature 1992; 359: 845-848
31. Ferrara N, Houck K, Jakeman L, et al. Molecular and biological properties of the vascular endothelial growth factor family of proteins. Endocrinol Rev 1992; 13: 18-32
32. Tuder R, Flook B, Voekel N. Increased gene expression for VEGF and the VEGF receptors KDR/flk and flt in lungs exposed to acute or chronic hypoxia. J Clin Invest 1995; 95: 1798-1807
33. Takeshita S, Zheng L, Brogi E, et al. Therapeutic angiogenesis: a single intra-arterial bolus of vascular endothelial growth factor augments revascularization in a rabbit ischemic hindlimb model. J Clin Invest 1994; 93: 662-670
34. Banai S, Jaklitsch M, Shou M, et al. Angiogenic-induced enhancement of collateral blood flow to ischemic myocardium by vascular endothelial growth factor in dogs. Circulation 1994; 89: 2183-2189
35. Mack C, Patel S, Schwarz E, et al. Biologic bypass with the use of adenovirus-mediated gene transfer of the complementary deoxyribonucleic acid for vascular endothelial growth factor 121 improves myocardial perfusion and function in the ischemic porcine heart. J Thorac Cardiovasc Surg 1998; 115: 168-176
36. Hendel RC, Henry TD, Rocha-Singh K, et al. Effect of intracoronary recombinant human vascular endothelial growth factor on myocardial perfusion: Evidence for a dose-dependent effect. Circulation 2000; 101: 118-121
37. Faham S, Hileman RE, Fromm JR, et al. Heparin structure and interactions with basic fibroblast growth factor. Science 1996; 271: 1116-20
38. Rosenberg RD, Shworak NW, Liu J, et al. Heparan sulfate proteoglycans of the cardiovascular system. J Clin Invest 1997; 99: 2062-70
39. Slavin J. Fibroblast growth factors: at the heart of angiogenesis. Cell Biol Int 1995; 19: 431-44
40. Cuevas P, Carceller F, Ortega S, et al. Hypotensive activity of fibroblast growth factor. Science 1991; 254: 1208-10
41. Sellke FW, Wang SY, Friedman M, et al. Basic FGF enhances endothelium-dependent relaxation of the collateral-perfused coronary microcirculation. Am J Physiol 1994; 267: H1303-11
42. Casscells W, Speir E, Sasse J, et al. Isolation, characterization, and localization of heparin-binding growth factors in the heart. J Clin Invest 1990; 85: 433-41
43. Bernotat-Danielowski S, Sharma HS, Schott RJ, et al. Generation and localisation of monoclonal antibodies against fibroblast growth factors in ischaemic collateralised porcine myocardium. Cardiovasc Res 1993; 27: 1220-8
44. Padua RR, Sethi R, Dhalla NS, et al. Basic fibroblast growth factor is cardioprotective in ischemia- reperfusion injury. Mol Cell Biochem 1995; 143: 129-35
45. Schneider H, Huse K. Arterial gene therapy. Lancet 1996; 348: 1380-1; discussion 1381-2

46. Yanagisawa-Miwa A, Uchida Y, Nakamura F, et al. Salvage of infarcted myocardium by angiogenic action of basic fibroblast growth factor. Science 1992; 257: 1401-3
47. Battler A, Scheinowitz M, Bor A, et al. Intracoronary injection of basic fibroblast growth factor enhances angiogenesis in infarcted swine myocardium. J Am Coll Cardiol 1993; 22: 2001-6
48. Horrigan MC, Malycky JL, Ellis SG, et al. Reduction in myocardial infarct size by basic fibroblast growth factor following coronary occlusion in a canine model. Int J Cardiol 1999; 68 Suppl 1: S85-91
49. Unger EF, Banai S, Shou M, et al. Basic fibroblast growth factor enhances myocardial collateral flow in a canine model. Am J Physiol 1994; 266: H1588-95
50. Lazarous DF, Scheinowitz M, Shou M, et al. Effects of chronic systemic administration of basic fibroblast growth factor on collateral development in the canine heart. Circulation 1995; 91: 145-53
51. Laham RJ, Chronos NA, Pike M et al. Intracoronary basic fibroblast growth factor (FGF-2) in patients with severe ischemic heart disease: Results of a phase I open-label dose escalation study. J Am Coll Cardiol 2000; 36: 2132-9
52. Laham RJ, Simons M, Tofukuji M, et al. Modulation of myocardial perfusion and vascular reactivity by pericardial basic fibroblast growth factor: insight into ischemia-induced reduction in endothelium-dependent vasodilatation. J Thorac Cardiovasc Surg 1998; 116: 1022-8
53. Lazarous DF, Unger EF, Epstein SE et al. Basic fibroblast growth factor in patients with intermittent claudication: results of a phase I trial. J Am Coll Cardiol 2000; 36: 1239-44
54. Mazue G, Bertolero F, Jacob C, et al. Preclinical and clinical studies with recombinant human basic fibroblast growth factor. Ann N Y Acad Sci 1991; 638: 329-40
55. Bertolini F, Paolucci M, Peccatori F, et al. Angiogenic growth factors and endostatin in non-Hodgkin's lymphoma. Br J Haematol 1999; 106: 504-9
56. Cuevas P, Gonzalez AM, Carceller F, et al. Vascular response to basic fibroblast growth factor when infused onto the normal adventitia or into the injured media of the rat carotid artery. Circ Res 1991; 69: 360-9
57. Edelman ER, Nugent MA, Smith LT, et al. Basic fibroblast growth factor enhances the coupling of intimal hyperplasia and proliferation of vasa vasorum in injured rat arteries. J Clin Invest 1992; 89: 465-73
58. Casey R, Li WW. Factors controlling ocular angiogenesis. Am J Ophthalmol 1997; 124: 521-9
59. Sharp PS. The role of growth factors in the development of diabetic retinopathy. Metabolism 1995; 44: 72-5
60. Wiedow O, Schroder JM, Gregory H, et al. Elafin: an elastase-specific inhibitor of human skin: purification, characterization, and complete amino acid sequence. J Biol Chem 1990; 265: 14791-14795
61. Cappelluti E, Strom SC, Harris RB. Potential role of two novel elastase- like enzymes in processing pro-transforming growth factor-alpha. Biochemistry 1993; 32: 551-560
62. Thompson K, Rabinovitch M. Exogenous leucocyte and endogenous elastases can mediate mitogenic activity in pulmonary artery smooth muscle cells by release of extracellular-matrix bound basic fibroblast growth factor. J Cell Physiol 1996; 166: 495-505
63. Hazuda DJ, Strickler J, Kueppers F, et al. Processing of precursor inter-leukin 1 beta and inflammatory disease. J Biol Chem 1990; 265: 6318-6322
64. Watanabe H, Hattori S, Katsuda S, et al. Human neutrophil elastase: degradation of basement membrane components and immunolocalization in the tissue. J Biochem (Tokyo) 1990; 108: 753-759
65. Foster JA, Rich CB, Miller MF. Pulmonary fibroblasts: an in vitro model of emphysema: regulation of elastin gene expression. J Biol Chem 1990; 265: 15544-15549
66. Tobias JW, Bern MM, Netland PA, et al. Monocyte adhesion to subendothelial components. Blood 1987; 69: 1265-1268
67. Bobryshev YV, Lord RS. Accumulation of co-localized unesterified cholesterol and neutral lipids within vacuolized elastin fibers in atheroprone areas of the human aorta. Atherosclerosis 1999; 142: 121-131
68. O'Blenes SB, Zaidi SH, Cheah AY, et al. Gene transfer of the serine elastase inhibitor elafin protects against vein graft degeneration. Circulation 2000; 102[suppl III]: III-289-III-295
69. Cowan B, Molossi C, Coulber C, et al. Interleukin (IL)-1B stimulated fibronectin synthesis in coronary smooth muscle cells requires endogenous vascular elastase activity. Mol Biol Cell 1994; 5: 429a
70. Baumgartner I, Pieczek A, Manor O, et al. Constitutive expression of phVEGF165 after intramuscular gene transfer promotes collateral vessel development in patients with critical limb ischemia. Circulation 1998; 97: 1114-1123
71. Rosengart TK, Lee LY, Patel SR, et al. Angiogenic gene therapy. Phase I assessment of direct intramyocardial administration of an adenovirus vector expressing VEGF121 cDNA to individuals with clinically significant severe coronary artery disease. Circulation 1999; 100: 468-74

72. Weig H-J, Laugwitz K-L, Moretti A, et al. Enhanced cardiac contractility after gene transfer of V2 vasopressin receptors in vivo by ultrasound-guided injection or transcoronary delivery. Circulation 2000; 101: 1578-1585
73. McNally PG, Watt PAC, Rimmer T, et al. Impaired contraction and endothelium-dependent relaxation in isolated resistance vessels from patients with insulin-dependent diabetes mellitus. Clin Sci 1994; 87: 31-36
74. McVeigh GE, Brennan GM, Johnston GD, et al. Impaired endothelium-dependent and independent vasodilatation in patients with type 2 (non-insulin-dependent) diabetes mellitus. Diabetologia 1992; 35: 771-776
75. Lund DD, Faraci FM, Ooboshi H, et al. Adenovirus-mediated gene transfer is augmented in basilar and carotid arteries of heritable hyperlipidemic rabbits. Stroke 1998; 29: 120-125
76. Ooboshi H, Rios CD, Chu Y, et al. Augmented adenovirus-mediated gene transfer in athero-sclerotic vessels. Arterioscler Thromb Vasc Biol 1997; 17: 1786-1792
77. Lund DD, Faraci FM, Miller FJ, et al. Gene transfer of endothelial nitric oxide synthase improves relaxation of carotid arteries from diabetic rabbits. Circulation 2000; 101: 1027-1033
78. Kamata K, Miyata N, Kasuya Y. Impairment of endothelium-dependent relaxation and changes in levels of cyclic GMP in aorta from streptozotocin-induced diabetic rats. Br J Pharmacol 1989; 97: 614-618
79. Meraji S, Joakody L, Senaratene MP, Thomson ABR, Kappagoda T. Endothelium-dependent relaxation in aorta of BB rat. Diabetes 1987; 36: 978-981
80. Pieper GM, Mei DA, Langenstroer P, et al. Bioassay of endothelium- derived relaxing factor in diabetic rat aorta. Am J Physiol 1988; 263: H676-H680
81. Hattori Y, Kawasaki H, Abe K, et al. Superoxide dismutase recovers altered endothelium-dependent relaxation in diabetic rat aorta. Am J Physiol 1991; 261: H1086-H1094
82. Pieper GM, Siebeneich W, Rosa AM, et al. Chronic treatment in vivo with dimethylthiourea, a hydroxyl radical scavenger, prevents diabetes-induced endothelial dysfunction. J Cardiovasc Pharmacol 1996; 28: 741-745
83. Pagano PJ, Griswold MC, Ravel D, et al. Vascular action of the hypoglycaemic agent gliclazide in diabetic rabbits. Diabetologia 1998; 41: 9-15
84. Lindquist S. The heat-shock response. Annu Rev Biochem 1986; 55: 1151-1191
85. Lindquist S, Craig EA. The heat-shock proteins. Annu Rev Genet 1988; 22: 631-677
86. Vayssier M, Polla BS. Heat shock proteins: chaperoning life and death. Cell Stress Chaperones 1998; 3: 221-227
87. Currie RW, Karmazyn M, Kloc M, et al. Heat-shock response is associated with enhanced postischemic ventricular recovery. Circ Res 1988; 63: 543-549
88. Amrani M, Corbett J, Allen NJ, et al. Induction of heat-shock proteins enhances myocardial and endothelial functional recovery after prolonged cardioplegic arrest. Ann Thorac Surg 1994; 57: 157-160
89. Jayakumar J, Suzuki K, Khan M, et al. Gene therapy for myocardial protection transfection of donor hearts with heat shock protein 70 gene protects cardiac function against ischemia-reperfusion injury. Circulation 2000; 102[suppl III]: III-302-III-306
90. Allen MD. Myocardial protection: is there a role for gene therapy? Ann Thorac Surg 1999; 68: 1924-1928. 25
91. Isner JM, Pieczek A, Schainfeld R, et al. Clinical evidence of angiogenesis after arterial gene transfer of phVEGF165 in patient with ischemic limb. Lancet 1996; 348: 370-4
92. Tsurumi Y, Takeshita S, Chen D, et al. Direct intramuscular gene transfer of naked DNA encoding vascular endothelial growth factor augments collateral development and tissue perfusion. Circulation 1996; 94: 3281-3290
93. Losordo DW, Vale PR, Symes JF, et al. Gene therapy for myocardial angiogenesis: initial clinical results with direct myocardial injection of phVEGF165 as sole therapy for myocardial ischemia. Circulation 1998; 98: 2800-2804
94. Vale PR, Losordo DW, Milliken CE, et al. Left ventricular electromechanical mapping to assess efficacy of phVEGF165 gene transfer for therapeutic angiogenesis in chronic myocardial ischemia. Circulation 2000; 102: 965-974
95. Baumgartner I, Rauh G, Pieczek A. et al. Lower-extremity edema associated with gene transfer of naked DNA vascular endothelial growth factor. Ann Int Med 2000; 132: 880-884
96. Lopez JJ, Laham RJ, Stamler A, et al. VEGF administration in chronic myocardial ischemia in pigs. Cardiovasc Res 1998; 40: 272-281
97. Henry TD, Annex BH, Azrin MA, et al. Final results of the VIVA trial of rhVEGF for human therapeutic angiogenesis. Circulation 1999; 100: I-476. (Abstract)
98. Guzman RJ, Lemarchand P, Crystal RG, et al. Efficient gene transfer into myocardium by direct injection of adenovirus vectors. Circ Res 1993; 73:1202-1207
99. Svensson EC, Marshall DJ, Woodard K, et al. Effi-

cient and stable transduction of cardiomyocytes after intramyocardial injection or intracoronary perfusion with recombinant adeno-associated virus vectors. Circulation 1999; 99: 201-205
100. Schumacher B, Pecher P, von Specht BU, et al. Induction of neoangiogenesis in ischemic myocardium by human growth factors: first clinical results of a new treatment of coronary heart disease. Circulation 1998; 97: 645-650
101. Sanborn TA, Tarazona N, Deutsch E, et al. Percutaneous endocardial gene therapy: in vivo gene transfer and expression. J Am Coll Cardiol 1999; 33(suppl A): 262A. Abstract
102. Kornowski R, Fuchs S, Vodovotz Y, et al. Successful gene transfer in a porcine ischemia model using the Biosense guided transendocardial injection catheter. J Am Coll Cardiol 1999; 33(suppl A): 355A. Abstract
103. Vale PR, Losordo DW, Tkebuchava T, et al. Catheter-based myocardial gene transfer utilizing nonfluoroscopic electromechanical left ventricular mapping. J Am Coll Cardiol 1999; 34: 246-254
104. Losordo DW, Vale PR, Hendel RC et al. Phase 1/2 placebo-controlled, double-blind, dose-escalating trial of myocardial vascular endothelial growth factor 2 gene transfer by catheter delivery in patients with chronic myocardial ischemia. Circulation 2002; 105: 2012-2018
104a. Schwarz ER, Speakman MT, Patterson M, Hale SS, Isner JM, Kedes LH, Kloner RA. Evaluation of the effects of intramyocardial injection of DNA expressing vascular endothelial growth factor (VEGF) in a myocardial infarction model in the rat–angiogenesis and angioma formation. J Am Coll Cardiol 2000; 35: 1323-30
105. Landau C, Jacobs AK, Haudenschild CC. Intrapericardial basic fibroblast growth factor induces myocardial angiogenesis in a rabbit model of chronic ischemia. Am Heart J 1995; 129: 924-931. 29
106. Uchida Y, Yanagisawa-Miwa A, Nakamura F, et al. Angiogenic therapy of acute myocardial infarction by intrapericardial injection of basic fibroblast growth factor and heparin sulfate: an experimental study. Am Heart J 1995; 130: 1182-1188
107. Lopez JJ, Edelman ER, Stamler A, et al. Angiogenic potential of perivascularly delivered aFGF in a porcine model of chronic myocardial ischemia. Am J Physiol 1998; 274: H930-H936
108. Laham RJ, Hung D, Simons M. Therapeutic myocardial angiogenesis using percutaneous intrapericardial drug delivery. Clin Cardiol 1999; 22(suppl 1): I-6-I-9
109. Lazarous DF, Shou M, Stiber JA, et al. Pharmacodynamics of basic fibroblast growth factor: route of administration determines myocardial and systemic distribution. Cardiovasc Res 1997; 36: 78-85
110. Laham RJ, Sellke FW, Ware JA, et al. Results of a randomized, double-blind, placebo-controlled study of local perivascular basic fibroblasts growth factor (bFGF) treatment in patients undergoing coronary artery bypass surgery. J Am Coll Cardiol 1999; 33(suppl A): 383A. Abstract
111. Harada K, Grossman W, Friedman M, et al. Basic fibroblast growth factor improves myocardial function in chronically ischemic porcine hearts. J Clin Invest 1994; 94: 623-30
112. Lopez JJ, Edelman ER, Stamler A, et al. Basic fibroblast growth factor in a porcine model of chronic myocardial ischemia: a comparison of angiographic, echocardiographic and coronary flow parameters. J Pharmacol Exp Ther 1997; 282: 385-90
113. March KL, Woody M, Mehdi K, et al. Efficient in vivo catheter-based pericardial gene transfer mediated by adenoviral vectors. Clin Cardiol 1999; 22: I23-I29
114. Giordano FJ, Ping P, Mckirnan D, et al. Intracoronary gene transfer of fibroblast growth factor-5 increases blood flow and contractile function in an ischemic region of the heart. Nat Med 1996; 2: 534-539
115. Weintraub WS, Culler SD, Kosinski A, et al. Economics, health-related quality of life, and cost-effectiveness methods for the TACTICS (Treat Angina With Aggrastat [tirofiban] and Determine Cost of Therapy with Invasive or Conservative Strategy)-TIMI 18 trial. Am J Cardiol 1999; 83: 317-22
116. Dougherty CM, Dewhurst T, Nichol WP, et al. Comparison of three quality of life instruments in stable angina pectoris: Seattle Angina Questionnaire, Short Form Health Survey (SF-36), and Quality of Life Index-Cardiac Version III. J Clin Epidemiol 1998; 51: 569-75
117. Thirumurti V, Shou M, Hodge E, et al. Lack of efficacy of intravenous basic fibroblast growth factor in promoting myocardial angiogenesis. J Am Coll Cardiol 1998; 31: 54A. Abstract
118. Unger EF, Banai S, Shou M, et al. Basic fibroblast growth factor enhances myocardial collateral flow in a canine model. Am J Physiol 1994; 266: H1588-H1595
119. Lazarous DF, Scheinowitz M, Shou M, et al. Effect of chronic systemic administration of basic fibroblast growth factor on collateral development in the canine heart. Circulation 1995; 91: 145-153
120. Yang R, Thomas GR, Bunting S, et al. Effects of vascular endothelial growth factor on hemodynamics and cardiac performance. J Cardiovasc Pharmacol 1996; 27: 838-844
121. Lopez J, Laham RJ, Carrozza JC, et al. Hemodynamic

effects of intracoronary VEGF delivery: evidence of tachyphylaxis and NO dependence of response. Am J Physiol 1997; 273: H1317-H1323
122. Sato K, Wu T, Laham RJ et al. Efficacy of intracoronary or intravenous VGEF-165 in a pig model of chronic myocardial ischemia. J Am Coll Cardiol 2001; 37: 616-23
123. Ziche M, Morbidelli L, Choudhuri R, et al. Nitric oxide synthase lies downstream from vascular endothelial growth factor-induced but not basic fibroblast growth factor-induced angiogenesis. J Clin Invest 1997; 99: 2625-34
124. Montrucchio G, Lupia E, de Martino A, et al. Nitric oxide mediates angiogenesis induced in vivo by platelet-activating factor and tumor necrosis factor-alpha. Am J Pathol 1997; 151: 557-63
125. Papapetropoulos A, Desai KM, Rudic RD, et al. Nitric oxide synthase inhibitors attenuate transforming-growth-factor-beta 1-stimulated capillary organization in vitro. Am J Pathol 1997; 150: 1835-44
126. Nabel EG, Yang ZY, Plautz G, et al. Recombinant fibroblast growth factor-1 promotes intimal hyperplasia and angiogenesis in arteries in vivo. Nature. 1993; 362: 844-846
127. Flugelman MY, Virmani R, Correa R, et al. Smooth muscle cell abundance and fibroblast growth factors in coronary lesions of patients with nonfatal unstable angina: a clue to the mechanism of transformation from the stable to the unstable clinical state. Circulation 1993; 88: 2493-2500
128. Inoue M, Itoh H, Ueda M, et al. Vascular endothelial growth factor (VEGF) expression in human coronary atherosclerotic lesions: possible pathophysiological significance of VEGF in progression of atherosclerosis. Circulation 1998; 98: 2108-2116
129. Siegel et al. Circulation 2000; 101: 2026-2029
130. Baffour R, Berman J, Garb JL, et al. Enhanced angiogenesis and growth of collaterals by in vivo administration of recombinant basic fibroblast growth factor in a rabbit model of acute lower limb ischemia: dose-dependent effect of basic fibroblast growth factor. J Vasc Surg 1992; 16: 181-191
131. Unger EC, McCreery TP, Sweitzer RH. Ultrasound enhances gene expression of liposomal transfection. Invest Radiol 1997; 32: 723-727
132. Feichheimer M, Boylan JF, Parker S, et al. Transfection loading of mammalian cells with plasmid DNA by scrape loading and sonication loading. Proc Natl Acad Sci USA 1987; 84: 8463-8467
133. Takeshita S, Isshiki T, Sato T. Increased expression of direct gene transfer into skeletal muscle observed after acute ischemic injury in rats. Lab Invest. 1996; 74: 1061-1065
134. Tata DB, Dunn F, Tindall DJ. Selective clinical ultrasound signals mediate differential gene transfer and expression in two human prostate cancer cell lines: LnCap and PC-3. Biochem Biophys Res Commun 1997; 23: 64-7
135. Kim HJ, Greenleaf JF, Kinnick RR, et al. Ultrasound mediated transfection of mammalian cells. Hum Gene Ther 1996; 7: 1339-46
136. Bao S, Thrall BD, Miller DL. Transfection of a reporter plasmid into cultured cells by sonoporation in vitro. Ultrasound Med Biol 1997; 23: 953-9
137. Lawrie A, Brisken AF, Francis SE, et al. Ultrasound enhances reporter gene expression after transfection of vascular cells in vitro. Circulation 1999; 99: 2617-20
138. Gao X, Huang L. Cationic liposome-mediated gene transfer. Gene Ther 1995; 2: 710-722
139. Tata DB, Dunn F. Interaction of ultrasound and model membrane systems: analyses and predictions. J Phys Chem 1992; 96: 3548-3555
140. Tata DB, Dunn F, Tindall DJ. Selective clinical ultrasound signals mediate differential gene transfer and expression in two human prostate cancer cell lines: LnCap and PC-3. Biochem Biophys Res Commun 1997; 234: 64-67
141. Greenleaf WJ, Bolander ME, Sarkar G, et al. Artificial cavitation nuclei significantly enhance acoustically induced cell transfection. Ultrasound Med Biol 1998; 24: 587-595
142. Kim HJ, Greenleaf JF, Kinnick RR, et al. Ultrasound-mediated transfection of mammalian cells. Hum Gene Ther 1996; 7: 1339-1346
143. Tata DB, Dunn F, Tindall DJ. Selective clinical ultrasound signals mediate differential gene transfer and expression in two human prostate cancer cell lines: LnCap and PC-3. Biochem Biophys Res Commun 1997; 234: 64-67
144. Ramirez A, Schwane JA, McFarland C, et al. The effect of ultrasound on collagen synthesis and fibroblast proliferation in vitro. Med Sci Sports Exerc. 1997; 29: 326-332
145. Koster R, Hamm CW, Terres W, et al. Effects of sonication with catheter-delivered low frequency ultrasound on proliferation, migration and drug uptake of vascular smooth muscle cells. J Am Coll Cardiol 1997; 29: 97554. Abstract
146. Amabile PG, Waugh JM, Lewis TN, et al. High-efficiency endovascular gene delivery via therapeutic ultrasound. J Am Coll Cardiol 2001; 37: 1975-1980
147. Campbell AIM, Monge JC, Latter DA, et al. Direct DNA injection of vascular endothelial growth factor induces angiogenesis in nonischemic myocardium. J Am Coll Cardiol 1998; 31: 25A
148. Skyba DM, Price RJ, Linka AZ, et al. Direct in vivo visualization of intravascular destruction of

microbubbles by ultrasound and its local effects on tissue. Circulation 1998; 98: 290-293
149. Price RJ, Skyba DM, Kaul S, et al. Delivery of colloidal particles and red blood cells to tissue through microvessel ruptures created by targeted microbubble destruction with ultrasound. Circulation 1998; 98: 1264-1267
150. Porter TR, Iversen PL, Li S, et al. Interaction of diagnostic ultrasound with synthetic oligonucleotide-labeled perfluorocarbon-exposed sonicated dextrose albumin microbubbles. J Ultrasound Med 1996; 15: 577-584
151. Main ML, Grayburn PA. Clinical applications of transpulmonary contrast echocardiography. Am Heart J 1999; 137 :144-153
152. Shohet RV, Chen S, Zhou VT, et al. Echocardiographic destruction of albumin microbubbles directs gene delivery to myocardium. Circulation 2000; 101: 2554-2556
153. Porter TR, Xie F, Kricsfeld D, Armbruster RW. Improved myocardial contrast with second harmonic transient ultrasound response imaging in humans using intravenous perfluorocarbon exposed sonicated dextrose albumin. J Am Coll Cardiol 1996; 27: 1497-501
154. Porter TR, Iversen PL, Shouping L, et al. Interaction of diagnostic ultrasound with synthetic oligonucleotide-labeled perfluorocarbon exposed sonicated dextrose albumin microbubbles. J Ultrasound Med 1996; 15: 577-84
155. Mukherjee D, Wong J, Griffin B, et al. Ten-fold augmentation of endothelial uptake of vascular endothelial growth factor with ultrasound after systemic administration. J Am Coll Cardiol. 2000; 35: 1678-1686
156. Wong J, Mukherjee D, Porter T, et al. Ultrasound enhances PESDA linked oligonucleotide deposition into myocardial tissue. J Am Soc Echo 1998; 11: RC
157. Henderson J, Willson K, Jago JR, Whittingham. A survey of the acoustic outputs of diagnostic ultrasound equipment in current clinical use. Ultrasound Med Biol 1995; 21: 699-705
158. Miller DL, Thomas RM, Frazier ME. Ultrasonic cavitation indirectly induces strand breaks in DNA of viable cells in vitro by the action of residual hydrogen peroxide. Ultrasound Med Biol 1991; 17: 729-35
159. Ashush H, Rozenszajin LA, Blass M, et al. Apoptosis induction of human myeloid leukemic cells by ultrasound exposure. Cancer Res 2000; 60: 1014-20
160. Miller MW, Miller DL, Brayman AA. A review of in vitro bioeffects of inertial ultrasonic cavitation from a mechanistic perspective. Ultrasound Med Biol 1996; 22: 1131-54
161. Kondo T, Kano E. Effect of free radicals induced by ultrasonic cavitation on cell killing. Int J Radiat Biol 1988; 54: 475-86
162. Huxley VH, Curry FE. Albumin modulation of capillary permeability: test of an adsorption mechanism. Am J Physiol 1985; 248(2 pt 2): H264-73
163. Ausprunk DH, Folkman J. Migration and proliferation of endothelial cells in preformed and newly formed blood vessels during tumor angiogenesis. Microvasc Res 1977; 14: 53-65
164. Sholley MM, Ferguson GP, Seibel HR. Mechanisms of revascularization: vascular sprouting can occur without proliferation of endothelial cells. Lab Invest 1984;54:624-34
165. Takeshita S, Pu L-Q, Zheng LP. Vascular endothelial growth factor induces dose-dependent revascularization in a rabbit model of persistent limb ischemia. Circulation 1994; 90: II-228-34
166. Zhou Z, Mukherjee D, Wang K, et al. Induction of angiogenesis in a canine model of chronic myocardial ischemia with intravenous infusion of vascular endothelial growth factor (VGEF) combined with ultrasound energy and echo contrast agent. Circulation, 2001 (Abstract)

MIX
Papier aus verantwortungsvollen Quellen
Paper from responsible sources
FSC® C105338

If you have any concerns about our products,
you can contact us on
ProductSafety@springernature.com

In case Publisher is established outside the EU,
the EU authorized representative is:
Springer Nature Customer Service Center GmbH
Europaplatz 3, 69115 Heidelberg, Germany

Printed by Libri Plureos GmbH
in Hamburg, Germany